REVIEWS ON SELECTED TOPICS OF TELOMERE BIOLOGY

Edited by **Bibo Li**

Reviews on Selected Topics of Telomere Biology
http://dx.doi.org/10.5772/2329
Edited by Bibo Li

Contributors

Radhika Muzumdar, Gil Atzmon, Sergey Shpiz, Alla Kalmykova, Jiří Nehyba, Radmila Hrdličková, Henry R. Bose, Jr., Güvem Gümüş-Akay, Ajlan Tükün, Didem Turgut Cosan, Ahu Soyocak, Sena Aydos, Cigir Biray Avci, Bibo Li, Arkasubhra Ghosh, Vinay Tergaonkar, Konrad Ocalewicz

Published by InTech

Janeza Trdine 9, 51000 Rijeka, Croatia

Publishing Process Manager Oliver Kurelic
Technical Editor InTech DTP team
Cover InTech Design team

Additional hard copies can be obtained from orders@intechopen.com

Hydrogen Storage, Edited by Lianjun Liu
p. cm.
ISBN 978-953-51-0731-6

For EU product safety concerns:
IN TECH d.o.o., Prolaz Marije Krucifikse Kozulić 3, 51000 Rijeka, Croatia,
info@intechopen.com or visit our website at intechopen.com.

Meet the editor

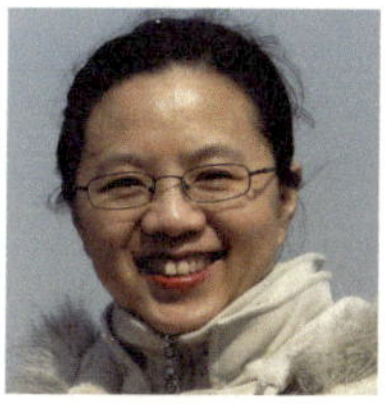

Dr. Bibo Li obtained her Ph.D. in Molecular Biology from Weill Cornell Medical College in 1997 and did her postdoctoral training working on telomere functions in humans. In 2002, Dr. Li started to study the telomere structure and functions in a protozoan parasite, Trypanosoma brucei, which causes human African trypanosomiasis. Dr. Li joined Cleveland State University in 2006 and became a tenured associate professor in 2011. Her work has led to the identification of T. brucei telomere proteins TRF and RAP1. She has shown that T. brucei RAP1 plays an essential role in silencing virulence genes located adjacent to telomeres, demonstrating for the first time that the telomere complex plays an important role in T. brucei pathogenesis and virulence regulation (Yang et al. 2009. Cell, as a cover story).

Contents

Preface

The sequence of Tetrahymena telomere DNA was the first to be determined among all eukaryotes by Elizabeth (Liz) Blackburn and Joseph Gall in 1978, and the yeast telomere was first cloned by Jack Szostak and Liz Blackburn in 1982. A few years later, the telomerase activity was first identified in Tetrahymena by Carol Greider and Liz Blackburn in 1985. These discoveries are miles stones marking the beginning of molecular era of telomere biology. Since then a tremendous amount of studies have demonstrated that telomeres are essential for genome stability and integrity, and maintaining telomere length homeostasis is the prerequisite for normal chromosome end protection. The significance of telomere study is highlighted by the 2009 Nobel prize in Physiology or Medicine awarded to Liz Blackburn, Carol Greider, and Jack Szostak for their discovery of how chromosomes are protected by telomeres and the enzyme telomerase. Although the award is no doubt one of the most exciting events in the history of telomere biology, by no means it signals that we have reached the peak of telomere research. The golden era of telomere studies continues, and the telomere field is still moving at a strong and fast pace. New findings about telomere functions and the underlying mechanisms are revealed every day. Particularly, there are more and more studies linking telomere dysfunction to a number of human diseases. Not only are telomere functions implicated in aging and age-related diseases, they are also important for microbial pathogen virulence. In addition, as our knowledge about telomere components expands, new non-telomeric roles of telomere proteins are revealed.

This book includes several current reviews on a few selected topics of telomere biology, including telomere length maintenance and its regulation, telomere and human diseases, novel extra-telomeric functions of telomere proteins, and finally a touch on telomere sequence evolution. We hope reviewing available data would help us to focus better on future research directions and make faster progresses in understanding various aspects of telomere functions.

Bibo Li
Center for Gene Regulation in Health & Disease Dept. of Biological,
Geo. & Env. Sciences, Cleveland State University,
USA

Section 1

Telomere Length and Its Regulation

1

Telomere Length and Aging

Radhika Muzumdar[1] and Gil Atzmon[2]
[1]*Department of Pediatrics, Children's Hospital at Montefiore, Diabetes Research and Training Center, Albert Einstein College of Medicine, Bronx, NY*
[2]*Diabetes Research and Training Center, Departments of Medicine and Genetic, Albert Einstein College of Medicine, Bronx, NY*
[1,2]*USA*

1. Introduction

Telomeres, the TTAGGG tandem repeats at the ends of chromosomes, become progressively shortened with each replication of cultured human somatic cells (reviewed in Wong and Collins (Wong & Collins 2003)) until a critical length is achieved, at which point the cell enters replicative senescence. This situation can be reversed by the enzyme named telomerase that is responsible for Telomere Length maintenance. Activation of the telomerase will result in telomere elongation and regulation of its activity can save the cell from senescence (Zvereva et al., 2010). Though increased activity of telomerase has been noted in cancer cell lines, telomere length could be in steady state suggesting alternative pathways for telomere length maintenance (Ouellette et al. 1999). The length of the telomere is longest at birth and decreases with increasing age. It has been demonstrated in cross-sectional analyses that age affects attrition of Telomere Length in white blood cells (Slagboom et al., 1994; Benetos et al., 2001; Nawrot et al., 2004). The rate of attrition is different between individuals and tissues and is influenced by multiple factors including oxidative stress and activity of telomerase enzyme. Telomere Length reflects the cumulative burden of oxidative stress and repeated cell replication (Serra et al., 2003), and such oxidative stress may represent the link between telomeres and aging-related disease in humans. Telomere shortening has been implicated as a mechanism explaining variations in life expectancy and aging-related diseases.

In this chapter we will review the alterations in Telomere Length with aging and its association with multiple age-related diseases. We will discuss the mechanism of telomere shortening and how it is affected by the aging process. Finally we will review the various genetic components that play a part in either telomere attrition or maintenance with aging.

2. Telomere Length and aging

It is well established that telomere shortens with age (figure 1). Cross-sectional studies have demonstrated that adult telomeres become shorter with age at a relatively constant rate. As demonstrated in figure 1, there is an individual variation of Telomere Length change with age but the cumulative trend is that telomeres shorten with age. It should be pointed out that many of the studies evaluating the association of Telomere Length with age contain relatively few subjects with exceptional longevity (Frenck et al., 1998; Rufer et al., 1999;

Cawthon et al., 2003). Age associated attrition in telomere is linked to many age related diseases and their complications. This raises an important question if the link between Telomere Length and age related diseases are associative or causative. In the subsequent sections, we will review the changes associated with Telomere Length in various age related diseases and their progression.

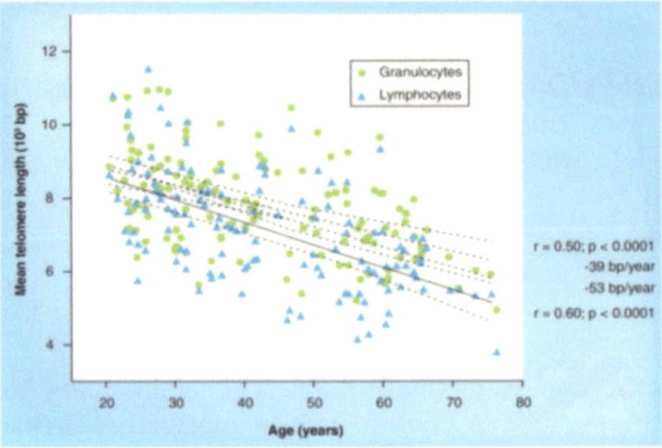

Fig. 1. Age-related telomere shortening in granulocytes and lymphocytes. (Hoffmann & Spyridopoulos 2011)

2.1 Telomere and age associated disease

"Chronological Aging" is a risk factor for multiple age-associated diseases (figure 2). However, the long and vivacious debate whether aging is a cause or effect is not settled. The supporters for chronological aging as a "cause" for age-related diseases put force the notion that age associated physiological deterioration, systems decline and immunological weakening resulting from the lost of natural shields, allows "chronological aging" to be an optimal situation for disease penetration. The opponents claim that the "physiological aging phenomenon" is a result of age-associated diseases. This hypothesis can be backed by the early onset of most of the claimed age associated diseases (i.e. Hypertension (HT), Diabetes, Cancer etc.) in the current western world. Can telomere pattern solve this debate?

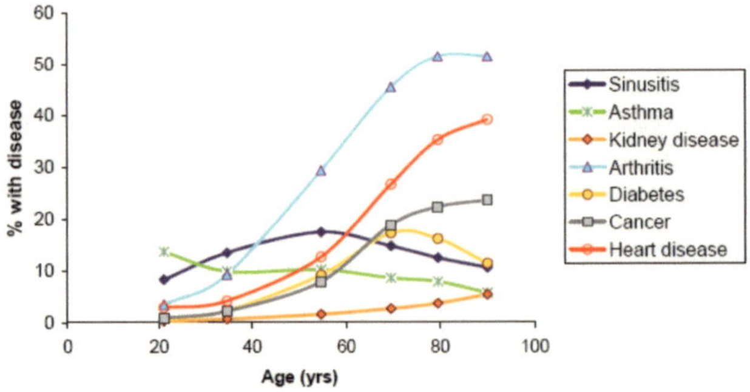

Fig. 2. Prevalence of selected chronic conditions, expressed in percentages, as a function of age for the US population (2002-2003 dataset). All forms of cancer and heart disease are featured. Source: National Center for Health Statistics, Data Warehouse on Trends in Health and Aging.

Telomere attrition with aging has been demonstrated in numerous studies, independent of the presence of any age related diseases. This supports the notion that shortened Telomere Length, seen in chronologic aging may serve as a biomarker of age independent of age-related diseases. In addition, occurrence of age-related diseases can accelerate the rate of telomere attrition. In fact older adults with one or more age associated diseases demonstrated higher attrition rate compare to healthy cohorts. Thus, aging and concurrent age-related diseases may play independent roles on Telomere Length; presence of both is synergistic in their effects on Telomere Length.

2.1.1 Telomere and hypertension

Hypertension is one of the most prevalent medical conditions among elderly. Almost 50% of the western world's 50 years old subjects suffer from high blood pressure. The prevalence increases with age to about 70% in the 80 years old. Multiple factors including environmental and genetic background and Telomere Length have been tied to this increased incidence. Though HT is more prevalent among elderly, a relationship between HT and Telomere Length has also been reported in the young; Jeanclos and colleagues (Jeanclos et al., 2000) had show that Telomere Length is shorter among younger patients with hypertension compared to healthy subjects at the same age. No studies have demonstrated a direct effect or established the mechanism by which Telomere Length affects blood pressure.

2.1.2 Telomere and Cardiovascular diseases

In addition to hypertension, age-associated Cardio Vascular Diseases (CVDs) include atherosclerosis, coronary artery disease, Myocardial infarction_(MI), and heart failure. Telomere Length has been proposed as a marker for biological aging of the cardiovascular system.

Telomere attrition and vascular aging

Studies (Benetos et al., 2004; Brouilette et al., 2007; Fitzpatrick et al., 2007) have shown that high rate of telomere attrition is associated with elevated CVD risk. Welleit et al. (Willeit et al., 2010) demonstrated higher rate of telomere shortening among people with CVD compared to people without CVD. In addition, Telomere Length has been established as independent risk predictor for myocardial infarction and stroke (figure 3). As presented in figure 3, while subjects among the higher tertile of Telomere Length have significantly lower hazard risk to develop MI, CVD, stroke and vascular death over 10 years of follow up, subjects in the middle or lower tertile are substantially at greater risk. Furthermore, in a 5 years longitudinal study, those individuals with shorter telomeres were at a higher risk of developing coronary artery disease (CAD). Risk factors for CVD such as smoking were associated with telomere shortening as well (Parks et al., 2011).

Mainous et al. (Mainous & Diaz 2010) studied the relationship between Telomere Length and atherosclerosis on the background of aging. He concluded that Telomere Length is inversely associated with arterial calcification and is highly correlated to arterial age rather than chronological age, supporting the notion of telomere being a yardstick for biological aging. Endothelial cells at the atherosclerotic plaque have been shown to have shorter telomeres compared to endothelial cells from subjects without CAD (Ogami et al., 2004).

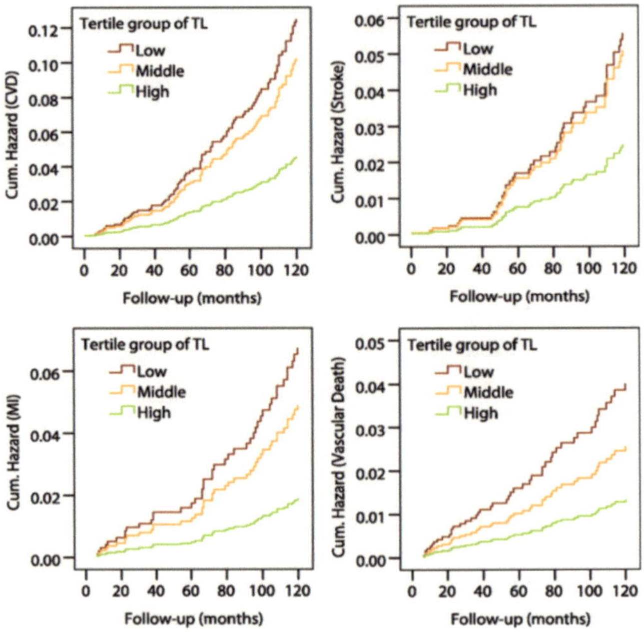

Fig. 3. Cumulative hazard curves for CVD, vascular death, myocardinal infraction, and stroke manifesting between 1995 and 2005. (Willeit et al. 2010)

In the first clinical observation, Samani et al. showed that severe coronary heart disease (CHD) is associated with shorter Telomere Length (Samani et al., 2001). Since then, many studies have shown that shortened Telomere Length is linked to severity of CVD (Table 1), (Hoffmann & Spyridopoulos 2011); however no causal role for shortened telomere in etiology of CVD or its progression has been established.

Accumulated evidence places oxidative stress as an accelerator of telomere attrition during cell replication (von Zglinicki 2002). Studies (Libby 2002; Stocker & Keaney 2004) denote inflammation and oxidative stress as the major contributors to pathophysiology of aging and age-related cardiovascular disease. In the Cardiovascular Health Study (CHS), in the face of subclinical and clinical cardiovascular disease and Telomere Length, the authors demonstrated negative correlation of IL-6 and C-reactive proteins with Telomere Length, highlighting the role of inflammation in Telomere Length regulation (Fitzpatrick et al., 2007). O'Donovan et al. reported of increased systemic inflammation with shorter Leukocyte Telomere Length in the Health, Aging and Body Composition Study (Health ABC) cohort (O'Donovan et al., 2011). Multiple studies have shown a relationship between oxidative stress and short telomeres. In the West of Scotland Coronary Prevention Study (WOSCOP) trial by Brouilette et al. (Brouilette et al., 2007), pravastatin treatment attenuated the risk of coronary heart disease even though the shorter telomeres persisted, illustrating that the short telomere is not causatively linked to coronary artery disease.

The review of literature unequivocally highlights the fact that the short Telomere Length is associated with CVD, risk factors for CVD such as hypertension and smoking and may be a prognostic indicator; however, no causative link between Telomere Length and CVD has been established.

Author (year)	Association with shorter Telomere Length
Leukocyte TL	
(Cawthon et al., 2003)	Cardiovascular mortality (+)
(Brouilette et al., 2003)	Premature myocardial infarction (+)
(Benetos et al., 2004)	Carotid atherosclerosis in hypertension (+)
(Valdes et al., 2005)	Smoking (+), obesity (+) in women
(Fitzpatrick et al., 2007)	Risk of myocardial infarction (+), diabetes (+)
(Kurz et al., 2006)	Degenerative aortic valve stenosis (+)
(Brouilette et al., 2007)	Occurrence of coronary heart disease (+)
(Collerton et al., 2007)	Left ventricular function in healthy 85 year olds (-)
(van der Harst et al., 2007)	Congestive heart failure (+)
(Farzaneh-Far et al., 2008)	Mortality in patients with stable coronary heart disease (+)
(Cherkas et al., 2008)	Physical activity (-)
(De Meyer et al., 2009)	Carotid plaque/intima media ratio (#)
(Vasan et al., 2009)	LV mass (-)
(Kuznetsova et al., 2010)	LV mass (-)
(Panayiotou et al., 2010)	Carotid intima-media thickness (+)
(Atturu et al., 2010)	Aortic abdominal aneurysm (+)
(Huzen et al., 2011)	CHD (-), carotid plaques (#)
Telomere Length in other cells	
(Wilson et al., 2008)	Patients with aortic abdominal aneurysm: aortic tissue (+)
(Spyridopoulos et al., 2008)	Patients with CHD: bone marrow cells (+)
(Spyridopoulos et al., 2009)	Patients with CHD: CD34+ progenitor cells (+), granulocytes (+), monocytes (+), T-cells (+), B-cells (+)

Table 1. **Selected cardiovascular studies measuring Telomere Length.** (adopted from Hoffmann & Spyridopoulos 2011), positive (+) or negative (-) association with shorter Telomere Length

2.1.3 Telomere and diabetes

Type 2 diabetes mellitus (T2DM) is estimated to affect 438 million people globally by 2030, and is recognized as an epidemic in most developed countries. T2DM is a chronic metabolic disease resulting from a combination of genetic susceptibility, environment, behavior, and as yet unexplained risk factors (Saxena et al., 2007). Considerable increased prevalence and earlier age of onset (Ness et al., 1999; Robbins et al., 2000) have been observed in older people (Dewan & Wilding 2003; Selvin et al., 2006), suggesting that genetic factors may influence both timing and prevalence with advance age. Earlier onset of diabetes could also be related to the global epidemic of obesity, leading to the coining of the relatively new term "Diabesity" (diabetes due to obesity). Today obesity is considered a pandemic as it affects 1.5 billion people across the world. This is a major economic and health care burden. However, obesity is just the beginning of cascade of physiologic events that results in a variety of age-associated diseases including diabetes. The relevant issues are how Leukocyte Telomere Length is associated with diabesity, how Telomere Length is regulated, and if Leukocyte Telomere Length is a coincidence, a biomarker or part of the mechanism.

Gardner et al. (Gardner et al., 2005) reported of shorter telomeres among diabesity patients. In addition, they show that earlier obesity increases the risk to develop diabesity, and these subjects had shorter telomeres. Thus, they put force the idea that telomere is a biomarker and showed negative correlation of Leukocyte Telomere Length with development of diabesity. Shorter Telomere Length has been observed in patients with insulin resistance, type 1 and type 2 diabetes mellitus. Al-Attas et al. determined the associations of Leukocyte Telomere Length to insulin resistance in middle-aged adult male and female Arabs with and without T2DM and show that Telomere Length is inversely associated with fasting insulin and homeostasis model assessment of insulin resistance (HOMA-IR). In this study, analysis revealed that HOMA-IR was the most significant predictor for Telomere Length in males. (Al-Attas et al., 2010).

Multiple variables related to glycemic control including glucose, HbA1C reveal negative correlation with Leukocyte Telomere Length (Olivieri et al., 2009). In subjects with diabetes, Telomere Length is linked to the duration of diabetes; patients with more than 10 years of diabetes had a shorter Telomere Length compared to patients with shorter duration of diabetes. Moreover, Telomere Length has been established as a marker for patients' overall condition; shorter leukocyte Telomere Length has been demonstrated in patients with diabetes complications compared to healthy control subjects. There is a positive correlation between telomere attrition and increased number of diabetes complications. (Fuller et al., 1990). Using multivariate analysis including diabetes, van der Harst et al. demonstrate that shorter Telomere Length is associated with a higher risk for death and thus can serve as a predictor for death or hospitalization in patients with heart problems. (van der Harst et al., 2010). In addition, short telomeres have been suggested by Fyhrquist et al. to be an independent predictor of progression of diabetic nephropathy in type 1 diabetes patients (Fyhrquist et al., 2010). Olivieri et al. showed that Leukocyte Telomere Length were shorter in elderly patients with both T2DM and MI compared to elders with just one of them. Similarly, Tentolouris showed that patients with both T2DM and microalbuminuria (MA) have shorter telomere compared to patients with MA only, this could partly be due to the observation that T2DM patients have increased arterial stiffness (Tentolouris et al., 2007). Indeed, significant telomere shortening among T2DM patients with atherosclerotic plaques has been reported compared to those without plaques (Adaikalakoteswari et al., 2007). Such trend between multiple risks and shorter telomere was reported in the central part of Italy (figure 4) (Testa et al., 2011). However, while in the study conducted by Fyhrquist et al., Telomere Length could serve as predictor of diabetic type 1 nephropathy progression (Fyhrquist et al., 2010), in a study reported by Astrup et al., Telomere Length did not differ between type 1 diabetic patients with or without nephropathy (Astrup et al., 2010).

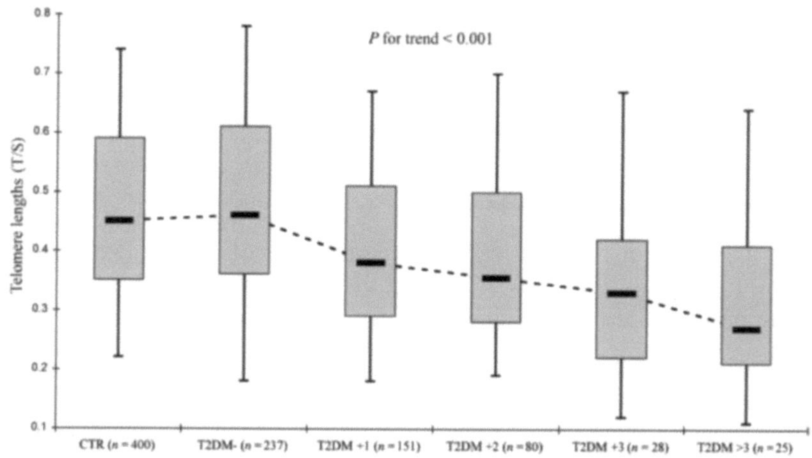

Fig. 4. Box plot of leukocyte Telomere Length (T/S) according to the number of diabetic complications. CTR -control, T2DM(–)- Diabetes only ,TSDM+N- for diabetes with complication. (Testa et al., 2011)

From a mechanistic standpoint, Verzola et al. demonstrated that telomere gets shorter when cultivated cells were introduced to high glucose level, leading them to propose that telomere shortening is due to replicative senescence. Indeed, investigation of kidney with T2DM nephropathy displays similar effects (accelerated senescence in various renal cell types under high glucose levels), suggesting diabetes may boost common pathways involving kidney cell senescence (Verzola et al., 2008). As indicated in the section on CVD, shorter Leukocyte Telomere Length could also be attributed to the high oxidative stress observed in patients with T2D (Salpea et al., 2010).

2.1.3.1 *Telomere and diabetes: genetic perspective*

Telomere Length, like most of the quantitative traits follows a polygenic mode of inheritance (Falconer & Mackay 1996). The most pronounced enzyme associated with telomere is Telomerase (which will be discussed further on sub chapter 3) including both a protein and an RNA subunit encoded by TERT and TERC. Telomerase activity contributes to telomere elongation, while other factors including exonucleases and end replication problem contribute to telomere shortening. The net Telomere Length depends on both telomere elongation and shortening factors. However, the attempt to explore the entire cascade of genetic elements that affecting Telomere Length are far from completion. Here we review this search on the background of diabetes. In the Women's Genome Health Study, genetic variation within the telomere-pathway gene loci has been associated with T2DM risk (Zee et al., 2011). Salpea et al. reported association of Leukocyte Telomere Length with functional variant in the promoter area of uncoupling proteins 2 (UCP2) among T2DM patients suggesting a link between mitochondrial production of reactive oxygen species and Leukocyte Telomere Length (Salpea et al., 2010). Whole-genome screening with a copy number variation by Kudo et al. in T2DM patients revealed that loss of copy number within the 1.3-Mb of chromosome 4p16.3 sub-telomeric region (contains 34 putative genes)was associated with early-onset T2DM. (Kudo et al., 2011).

In summary, there is mixed evidence for an association between short Telomere Length and diabetes, risk factors for diabetes, and complications of diabetes. Presence of more than one risk factor for diabetes does have a correlation with Telomere Length suggesting that it (Telomere Length) could be a cause rather than an effect; however, more studies are necessary before definitively drawing this conclusion.

2.1.4 Telomere and Alzheimer's disease

Alzheimer's is a neurodegenerative disease associated with aging (Rolyan et al., 2011). Currently, more than 35 million people around the world are effected, and this number is predicted to dramaticaly increase as life expectency is prolonged.

Memory deterioration and other cognitive domains decline are the main features of Alzheimer Disease (AD) which may lead to death in 3–9 years after diagnosis. Early signs of dementia, family history and potentially modifiable risk factors as well as biological factors such as Telomere Length and telomerase dysfunction can serve as early disease markers. (Lukens et al., 2009; Saeed et al., 2011).

Paul presented a different view of the role of Telomere Length in age-related diseases and suggested that the telomere dysfunction can be linked to certain diseases including Alzheimer's. In addition, he proposed that nutrients as well as epigenetic changes accompanied the disease progression, and can affect the telomerase activity and thus Telomere Length. (Paul 2011). Thomas et al. demonstrated significant differences of Telomere Length between Alzheimer patients and control subjects not only in the leukocytes but also in buccal and hippocampus cells. Interestingly enough, while the leukocyte and buccal cells telomere were shorter among the Alzheimer patients, in the hippocampus cells telomeres were longer, suggesting deferential telomere maintenance to protect the brain of Alzheimer's patients. (Thomas et al., 2008). Panossian et al. reported the immune system involvement in telomere maintenance among Alzheimer patients. However only T cell and B cell Telomere Length were correlated with Alzheimer's disease progression (Panossian et al., 2003).

A support for the notion that Telomere Length modulates disease progression came from a study done by Rolyan et al. Using aged telomerase knockout mice (G3Terc-/-), they show loss of neuron and impaired short-term memory in carriers of short telomere. Conversely, opposite effects were demonstrated in mouse model for Alzheimer's disease, both for memory decline as well as restoration of amyloid plaque, suggesting beneficial effects of telomere shortening with Alzheimer (Rolyan et al., 2011).

In contrast, Lukens et al. did not find any association between Alzheimer progression and cerebellum Telomere Length (figure 5) (Lukens et al., 2009). Similar results have been reported by Zekry at al. in a longitudinal study among large oldest old cohorts. After two years of follow-up, Alzheimer patients did not present significant shorter telomere compared to either demented or normal cognition groups (Zekry et al., 2010). Lof-Ohlin et al. compared Vascular demented patients versus Alzheimer patients and did not find any Telomere Length differences between the groups in such a way that it can serve as a predictor for either form of dementia (Lof-Ohlin et al., 2008). Though the exact association between Telomere Length and neurodegenerative diseases is inconclusive, there is evidence to suggest that "local" Telomere Length could be more relevant and a better index than Leukocyte Telomere Length.

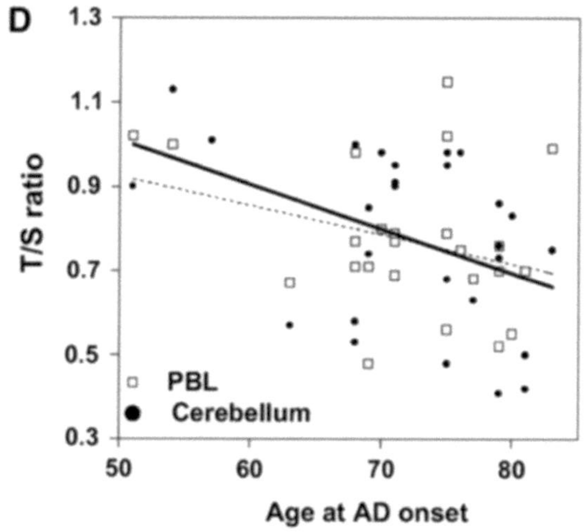

Fig. 5. Relationships between age of AD onset and cerebellar T/S ratio (n = 30, solid circles and solid line; $P = 0.027$) and peripheral blood leukocyte (PBL) T/S ratio (n = 29, open squares and dotted line; $P = 0.108$). (Lukens et al., 2009)

2.1.5 Telomere Length and cognition

Advances in technology and medical treatment increase the life expectancy substantially across the world, thus more people are living to their old age. One consequence of such trend is that number of people with dementia that are not much prevalent at young age is increasing (Matthews et al., 2009).

Cellular aging (senescence) is associated with telomere shortening but little is known about how it can affect dementia among the elderly. Harris et al. tested the hypothesis that telomere attrition with age can affect cognition changes, among the Lothian Birth Cohort 1921. Follow adjustment for multiple covariates including childhood IQ, they reported of an insignificance association (Harris et al., 2006). Harris et al. also checked whether Telomere Length can serve as a biomarker for cognitive function in 1000 elderly Scots from the Lothian Birth Cohort of 1936 and found significant evidence only with higher general cognitive ability scores (Harris et al., 2010). In the Leiden 85 plus study, Martin-Ruiz et al. reported the lack for association between Leukocyte Telomere Length and mini-mental state examination (MMSE) , and they demoted this observation to telomere instability in this highly frail population (Martin-Ruiz et al., 2005). Similar results have been obtained in the

Nurses' Health Study (NHS) of 2000 elderly subjects (Devore et al., 2011) as well as study preformed in two narrow age-range cohort of the Canberra-Queanbeyan region of Australia (Mather et al., 2010), suggesting that Telomere Length could not serve as predictor for memory decline.

In contrast, Valdes et al. reported association between sub sets of cognitive measurements and Leukocyte Telomere Length in the UK twin cohort study, suggesting Leukocyte Telomere Length as a potential biomarker of cognitive dysfunction with age (Valdes et al., 2010). Supporting such observation, Yaffe et al. have demonstrated that subject with better baseline Digit Symbol Substitution Test (DSST) scored have longer telomere in the Health ABC study (Yaffe et al., 2011). Canela et al. have used FISH to assess Telomere Length and found a significant correlation between telomere attrition and cognitive decline but only in subjects 60–69 years of age (Canela et al., 2007). Although brain aging research has progressed in the last decade, it is still poorly understood. The majority of the cognitive deficits are still attributable to either age associated senescence or AD (Gress 2001) and not Telomere Length.

2.2 Telomere and frailty

The prevalence of severe disability among older Americans is estimated to be as much as 37 percent (http://www.aoa.gov/PROF/Statistics/profile/2007/16.aspx.). This number is predicted to grow given the increased life expectancy and rise in conditions such as obesity (Manton 2008). Seniors with mobility disability experience worse quality of life than those without activity limitations with more falls, and more days of pain (CDC 1998; Ganz et al., 2005). They are more likely to be isolated from the community, suffer more morbidity and have higher incidence of mortality (Hirvensalo et al., 2000; Simonsick et al., 2001; Newman et al., 2003; Newman et al., 2006).

Frailty at a clinical level encompasses various chronic diseases associated with aging and therefore has been suggested to serve as a measure for biological ageing. Accumulated reports propose Telomere Length as an ageing biomarker. To test the theory that Telomere Length can serve as a biological marker for frailty, Woo et al. longitudinally studied healthy population using "frailty index" (figure 6) (Woo et al., 2008), and found no significant association between frailty index and telomere attrition either in whole group or after dichotomization for sex (Woo et al., 2008).

Various explanations have been proposed for the relationship between frailty and Telomere Length, Waltson suggested in his review that underlying molecular changes such as telomere shortening and reduced telomerase activity make the older humans more susceptible to frailty (Walston 2004). Sharpless and DePinho associated the lack of rejuvenate stem cells due to telomere shortening an unwanted consequence which may induce aging phenotype such as frailty (Sharpless & DePinho 2007). Kirkwood suggested "Evolutionary theory" supported by empirical evidence that accumulation of cell and tissue damage with age will result in frailty. Cell damage could be part of processes such as DNA damage or oxidative stress and the cures lie in system maintenance or natural biological processes that either fix the damage or substantially slow it down. Such examples to support this theory for better maintenance can be seen in some of the observed differences between long and short live species (Kirkwood 2002).

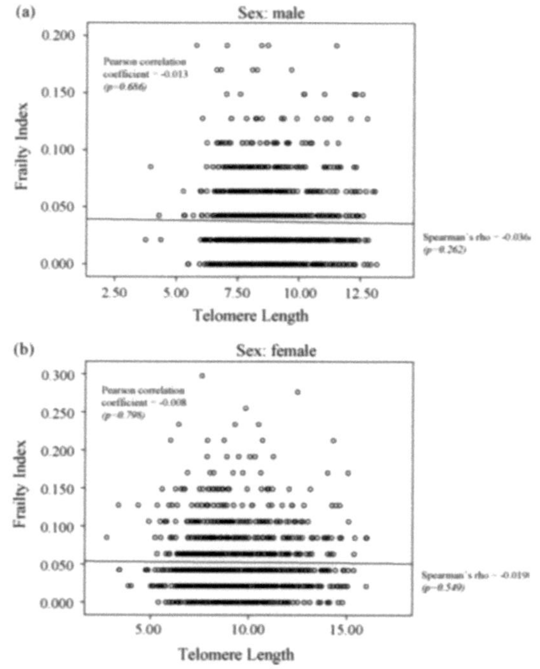

Fig. 6. Frailty index and Telomere Length (a) male and (b) female (Woo et al., 2008).

2.3 Telomere and bone structure

Aging accelerates osteoporosis and other bone diseases. More so, since the bone loses its flexibility with age, they become less sensitive to any treatment (Kepler et al., 2011). However, there are conflicting reports in the literature regarding the exact association of telomere shortening and age-related bone loss, pobably due to the different phenotypes that have been assessed. Sanders and collgue reported a lack of association between Telomere Length and Bone Mineral Density (BMD), osteoporosis, or fracture in older cohort in the Health ABC study (Sanders et al., 2009). In elder Chinese, similar observation has been seen with baseline BMD or bone loss over a 4-year period and Telomere Length (Table 2) (Tang et al., 2010).

Age (M/F)	TL1 vs. TL3 (OR (95% CI))	TL2 vs. TL3 (OR (95% CI))	p-Value	
			(TL1 vs. TL3)	(TL2 vs. TL3)
65-69 (963/904)	0.3 (0.06–1.52)/0.8 (0.36–1.81)	0.1 (0.01–1.29)/0.6 (0.26–1.44)	0.15/0.60	0.08/0.26
70-74 (963/904)	2.6 (0.47–14.21)/1.1 (0.51–2.58)	1.1 (0.17–7.32)/1.3 (0.54–2.92)	0.27/0.74	0.91/0.59
≥75 (963/904)	0.9 (0.33–2.33)/0.9 (0.42–1.89)	0.9 (0.33–2.30)/0.9 (0.43–1.99)	0.79/0.75	0.77/0.84

Table 2. Logistic regressions for association between (Bone Mineral Density)BMD and tertiled Telomere Length (TL) (Tang et al., 2010)

In contrast Valdes et al. (Valdes et al., 2007) reported that follow adjustments for multiple variants, BMD was correlated with Telomere Length. In addition, women with osteoporosis have shorter Telomere Lengths. Following their observation of negative correlation between Telomere Length and age and the association with bone loss, Bekaert et al. concluded that Telomere Length can serve as a predictor for bone loss (Bekaert et al., 2005). Kveiborg et al. took this comparison a step further and showed increased telomere attrition with age in cultured aging osteoblasts cells. However, this pattern was not observed in a groups of osteoporotic women and age matched elderly cohort, dismissing the notion that cell senescense occur much earlier in osteoporotic patients (Kveiborg et al., 1999).

Terc(-/-) mice (abolished telomerase activity) have been used to explore the mechanism behind telomere shortening in vivo and its association with bone loss. One of the phenotypes of this strain of mice is that they demonstrate accelerated rate of bone loss with age (Saeed et al., 2011). In cultured bone cells isolated from these mice, impaired osteogenic differentiation and reduced proliferation as well as accelerate senescence and DNA damage have been observed (Saeed et al., 2011). In addition, overexpression of proinflammatory genes involved in osteoclast differentiation was demonstrated by microarray screening. Thus, two mechanisms associate with bone deterioration with age have been demonstrated in telomerase deficient mice, suggesting presence of such a mechanism with aging: A) Bone cells damage and, B) Over expression of proinflammatory genes (Saeed et al., 2011). Similar observation of low bone mass phenotype and age-related osteoporosis has been reported in double knockout mice (the telomerase deficient and Wrn helicase which caused premature aging). In addition, mesenchymal stem cells (MSCs) from the double knockout mice have a short lifespan and impaired osteogenic *in vitro* (Pignolo et al., 2008).

2.4 Telomere and epigenetic

Chronological aging is a risk for numerous chronic diseases such as cardiovascular disease and type 2 diabetes mellitus (Resnick et al., 2000; Najjar et al., 2005) that affect the quality of life and lifespan. Epigenetics (acquired or heritable changes in gene function or phenotypes without changes in DNA sequence), has emerged as an important factor in gene expression and disease risk. Epigenetics refer to several mechanisms by which gene expression, DNA replication, DNA damage repair, and DNA recombination are modulated. In this section, we will review the advances in the research of epigenetics of aging and its relevance to Telomere Length.

Response of fetus to environmental stressors such as poor nutrition resulted in the early occurrence of age-associated diseases later in life (Barker Hypothesis). Such hypothesis was supported by animal models of IUGR (intra uterine growth restriction): these animals develop age-associated diseases significantly earlier than their normal birth cohorts. This observation was supported by growing evidence for the involvement of DNA methylation and histone modifications in gene expression during gestation, an effect leading to permanent cell damage and shorter Telomere Length (Barnes & Ozanne 2011).

A relationship between folate (precursors for nucleotide synthesis modulated by DNA methylation) and Telomere Length was proposed by Paul et al. Among a middle age and elderly cohort, subjects with higher folate plasma concentration had longer telomeres (Paul et al., 2009). Kim et al. proposed that artificial increase of folate in the diet can increase Telomere Length and telomerase activity, thus promoting healthy aging (Kim et al., 2009).

From a more mechanistic view, Gonzalez-Suarez & Gonzalo suggested that since aging is associated with increased chromatin defects as a result of alteration in processes associated with nuclear organization, an involvement of epigenetics in telomeric and subtelomeric region is crucial to decelerating cell senescence and therefore healthy aging. (Gonzalez-Suarez & Gonzalo 2008). Blasco report subtelomeric regions that are affected by histone modification of methyltransferases and DNA methyltransferases providing evidence for epigenetic regulation of telomere-length (Blasco 2007).

Another interestingly popular view was presented by Zeng, who hypothesized that the differentiation of undifferentiated Human Embryonic Stem Cells (hESCs) into somatic cell transforms them from immortal to mortal cells. Since the Telomere Length was maintained by active telomerase in the hESCs, transition to mortal cells results in loss of this maintenance and over time, will lead to cell death. Such a transition, the author argues, is modulated by epigenetic changes as the aging environment is changed. Controlling this environment by understanding the genomic and epigenetic of the immortal hESC can lead to successful control of somatic cell senescence and thus could offer a better treatment for age associated diseases (Zeng 2007). Tam et al. elaborated on this strategy and suggested reprogramming those cells by various techniques such as cell fusion, somatic cell nuclear transfer and more. Employing gene expression alteration or changing chromatin epigenetic state reverses the cellular ageing by controlling both Telomere Length and telomerase activity (Tam et al., 2007). Fraga et al. indicated a global perspective on hypomethylation and CpG island hypermethylation changes during aging to have their impact on cell senescence through the effect on telomere attrition and telomerase activity (Fraga et al., 2007). Thus, epigenetic regulation of Telomere Length is an extremely complex but potentially interesting avenue that could lead to modifications of disease risk and healthy aging.

2.5 Telomere and longevity

Extremely long life span or in its more common term "Longevity" is a result of multiple variables including genetic, epigenetic and environmental factors. Longevity, the right tail of life expectancy (increases steadily by quarter of a year every year (Oeppen & Vaupel 2002)) is more prevalent now due to improvements in not only medical treatment and knowledge, but also access to better nutrition, food availability, healthy environment, and overall self secure. Human longevity can be reached in many ways such as having a favourable genetic background (Schumacher et al., 2009), a low degree of disability (Terry et al., 2008), robust maintenance of physiological functions (Barzilai et al., 2010), diet (Hausman et al., 2011), front of the line healthcare (Michaud et al., 2011), environment (de Magalhaes et al., 2012), and cellular and DNA maintenance (Schumacher et al., 2009; Barzilai 2010). Can long Telomere Length be considered as one?

Telomere Length may play a role in the genetics of human longevity (Guan et al., 2007). The question is how and where? Guan et al. investigate this question among a wide range of aged people. They report decreased mean Telomere Length with age; a trend that was less steep among women (Guan et al., 2007). Friedrich et al. expanded their study to more advanced ages with three different sources of telomeres from the same donor. Interestingly, leukocytes demonstrated significantly shorter telomere compared to skin and synovial tissues within donors. In addition, the leucocyte and skin sources exhibit significant attrition with age, suggesting leukocytes as a surrogate indicator for Telomere Length for other tissues (Friedrich et al., 2000). Stindl reported similar results for both negative correlation between mean Telomere Length and longevity and shorter telomeres among men. Stindl attributes these sex differences to different body size and propose that increased height differences are the main reason why women outlive men in the western countries (Stindl 2004). Manestar-Blazic took a step backwards and suggests that Telomere Length and longevity depend on the telomere state in the germ line of the parents at conception. Telomere Length in the gametes of the parents is a yin-yang situation; the longer they are, the faster they attrite, the best composition between the two opposing mechanism will define the starting point for the offspring Telomere Length and thus their longevity (Manestar-Blazic 2004). This is supported by Njajou et al., who studied a large cohort of the Amish. Telomere Length was negatively associated with aging, was not different between genders and positively correlated with paternal lifespan when offspring and their parents were tested, suggesting a positive influence of Telomere Length and cross generation lifespan (Njajou et al., 2007). In a different view, Bakaysa et al. established Telomere Length as a biomarker for survival on Swedish twins excluding environmental and familial effects. In their study, subjects with shorter telomeres have shorter survival compared to his/her twin sibling with longer telomeres (Bakaysa et al., 2007). Kimura et al. demonstrated the same in the oldest old; a decline of overall mean Telomere Length with age and difference between genders with females having longer mean Telomere Length compared to men. Interestingly enough, the average shorter telomere observed in the oldest old could be due to a higher percentage of short telomere fragments compared to young age subjects (Kimura et al., 2007). Further support for this phenomenon has been observed in gray and white matter autopsy samples from 72 subjects aged 0-100 YO. The authors reported of a decline in mean Telomere Length until the age of 79 followed by an increase in Telomere Length with age in the higher age group (Nakamura et al., 2007).

On the other hand multiple studies have reported a lack of association between Telomere Length and longevity. Njajou et al., using leukocyte from peripheral blood from a large cohort of mixed ethnicity, found no association for either survival or early death from major age associated disease. However, Telomere Length was linked to healthy aging suggesting that Telomere Length may be an indirect biomarker for longevity (Njajou et al., 2009). Graakjaer et al. used different technology to measure Telomere Length by fluorescent in situ hybridization (FISH) and report unique length distribution within individuals (on the cell level) and between individuals. Interestingly enough, this unique Telomere Length distribution doesn't change much through life and is partially inherited, suggesting a lesser involvement of Telomere Length with longevity and more as an accompanied trait (Graakjaer et al., 2006).

Searching for the secret of long-lived life of extremely old individuals, Terry et al. studied centenarians. Telomere Length was significantly longer in the healthy group compared to the unwell centenarians, suggesting health as a major component of telomere maintenance and not necessarily longevity mechanism. Terry et al. concluded that survival to old age is not a factor of Telomere Length rather than a signature for healthy performance (Terry et al., 2008). Taking extended centenarian cohort, we found that centenarian and their offspring exhibit longer telomeres compared to controls. Since this phenomenon was across the board including healthy and non healthy centenarians, we suggested Telomere Length as a longevity associated trait especially since the offspring of centenarians (inherited at least half of the genetic background of their extremely performed parents) demonstrate the same trend. We attributed this observation to slow attrition rate, suggesting higher telomere maintenance among families with longevity (figure 7) (Atzmon et al., 2010). Same observation was reported by Ishikawa et al.. Cross sectional (0 and 100 years) measurement of Telomere Length in normal pituitary glands revealed decline in Telomere Length with age until certain point where the trend of Telomere Length attrition reversed and show longer telomere among the oldest old (Ishikawa et al., 2011). Such observation points to the fact that different mechanism of telomere maintenance exists in the extremely old people. This also suggests that observation of longer Telomere Length compared to age-matched controls in a cross-sectional assessment early in life could be a surrogate indicator for longevity.

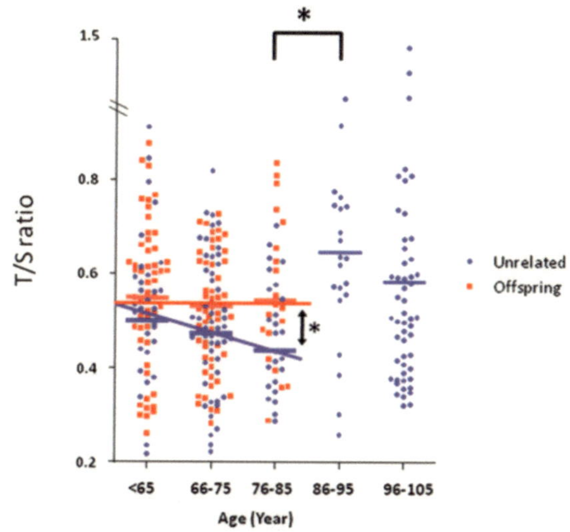

Fig. 7. Comparison of Telomere Length among Ashkenazi Jewish centenarians (n = 86), their offspring (n = 175), and controls (n = 93). Values are adjusted for age at recruitment and gender in the offspring and control groups and for gender alone in the centenarian group *P < 0.05. (Atzmon et al., 2010)

3. Telomere maintenance mechanisms

One of the critical mechanisms by which telomere is maintained, is through the enzyme telomerase reverse transcriptase (TERT) activity. Telomerase is the enzyme that is responsible for the elongation of the telomere, an action that reverses the telomere attrition. Higher telomerase activity would increase Telomere Length and extend cell proliferation potential, while lower activity would result in shorter telomere (Nicholls et al., 2011).

Using telomerase-deficient mice, Jaskelioff et al. demonstrated the crucial role of Telomere Length in cell senescence. Under conditional mutation, the mice that lack telomerase activity developed age associated phenotypes including shorter telomeres and increased DNA damage. Reactivation of the telomerase activity reversed the aging phenotypes and restored Telomere Length that in turn led to less DNA damage. This elegant study reemphasized the importance of Telomere Length and its maintenance by the telomerase activity for cell proliferation and longevity, supporting the notion of telomerase as longevity precursor (Jaskelioff et al., 2011)

The importance of telomerase activity in telomere maintenance and cell senescence was demonstrated by introducing an alternative strategy for telomere maintenance (ALT) (Wu et al.). This strategy is executed in telomerase deficient cells in order to preserve cell growth and maintain the balance between cell senescence and tumorigenesis. However, this introduced substantial Telomere Length variability, and therefore more complexity (Wu et al., 2009). Royle et al. expanded the ALT mechanism by including processes that are activated in the absence of telomerase activity such as telomere chromatid exchange elevation, blocking t-loops and activation of recombination-based processes that restore replication capability (Royle et al., 2009). Cell proliferation has been crafted through evolution to the point that each system is in harmony with its environment; hence any changes in this balance (although there are alternatives) will have deleterious impact. Pessos et al. suggested telomere attrition as the cause for cellular senescence, a mechanism that is similar to tumor suppressing. However, evidence exists for involvement of multiple processes in cell senescence such as mitochondrial function, ROS, chromatin, and functional and biochemical complexes (Passos et al., 2009). An alternative view of the impact of stress on Telomere Length was reviewed by Epel et al. They proposed a model of two opposing systems to demonstrate the effect of psychological function on Telomere Length; a. stress condition which increases cortisol, insulin and oxidative stress, all of which shorten telomere and lower telomerase activity; and b. positive cognition which increases androgen, GH axis activity and vagal tone and therefore telomere maintenance (figure 8) (Epel et al., 2009). Involvement of sex hormones in telomere maintenance and telomerase activity were further elucidated by Li et al.. Reviewing the role of estrogen in cell proliferation, Li et al. suggested mechanisms by which estrogen regulates the telomerase activity and therefore Telomere Length (Li et al., 2010). Since estrogen declines with age, its role as telomere homeostasis regulator are limited, thus other mechanisms are introduced to compensate for its absence (Li et al., 2010). On the protein level, The RecQ helicases (mainly WRN and BLM) were introduced by Bohr, as a protein family that is responsible for telomere maintenance, and defects in these proteins are associated with poor telomere maintenance and early aging. Interaction of the main proteins (i.e. WRN and BLM) with the telomere region exposes DNA damage and activates damage responses. The various mechanisms by which

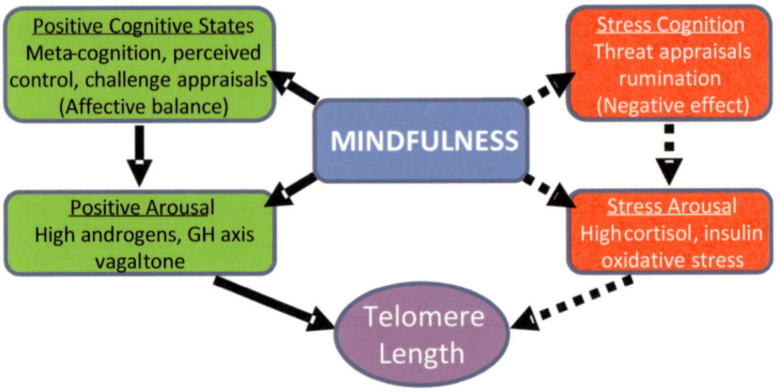

Fig. 8. Effects of Mindfulness Meditation on Telomere Length through Positive and Stressful Cognitive States. The dotted arrows represent inverse relationships specifically, we propose that positive arousal promotes and stress arousal prevents telomere maintenance (Epel et al., 2009)

RecQ helicases offer genome and specifically telomere maintenance can provide us with a clue towards successful aging (Bohr 2008). Stem cell research offers another interesting point of view. This source for cell renewal functionality declines with age; the same process was observed in telomerase deficient mice (Song et al., 2009). This connection has been further strengthened by demonstration of over expression of 4 genome maintenance proteins in plasma during aging in humans. Furthermore, this has been demonstrated in older people with age associated diseases suggesting that provocation of the DNA damage machinery interacts closely with telomere dysfunction status (Jiang et al., 2008).

4. Telomere Length in the genomic era

Candidate gene approach has been a major source in the revelation of the underline genetic mechanisms involved in telomerase activity and telomere maintenance. However, these discoveries were loci dependent, providing explanation very specifically on the immediate genetic components affecting telomerase activity and Telomere Length. Recent advances in genomic tools provide us with a more global view as well as network interaction on the genetic basis of telomerase activity and Telomere Length. From this perspective, Codd et al. conducted GWAS with mean leukocyte Telomere Length and demonstrate an area near the TERC locus that is significantly associated with mean Leukocyte Telomere Length (Codd et al., 2010). Similar analysis has been performed in a consortium of four Caucasian cohorts. In this study, the strength of the unbiased screening revealed new genes associated with Leukocyte Telomere Length such as OBFC1 and the cytokine CXCR4 as well as the TERC, demonstrating multi-component genetic effects on Telomere Length that could only have been discovered through unbiased genomic screening (Levy et al., 2010). Gu et al. conducted a multistage GWAS and found a locus next to a gene that involves in cytokine production PELI2 that is significantly associated with Leukocyte Telomere Length, thus increasing the palette of possible genes associated with Leukocyte Telomere Length (Gu et al., 2011). Prescott et al. replicated previously identified GWAS loci TERC in the Nurses' Health Study but failed to replicate other locus or identify any new loci significant associated with Telomere Length (Prescott et al., 2011). Shen et al., not surprisingly detected the TERC locus to have significant effect on Leukocyte Telomere Length in Chinese population through unbiased genome screening (Shen et al., 2011); the same two SNPs were found to be associated with Telomere Length as well as longevity in the oldest-old Danes (Soerensen et al., 2011).

Although there is evidence for association with Telomere Length in multiple facets of aging and age-related diseases, neither a conclusive causative link nor a predictable association has been established. Thus, the main question whether Telomere Length drives the aging process or is influenced by aging or age-associated diseases remains unresolved. Advance in technologies in genomics, more studies using animal models and human cells as well as improved understanding of telomere maintenance will help us answer this question unequivocally leading to the use of Telomere Length as a biomarker and ultimately personalized medicine.

5. References

Centers for Disease Control and Prevention (CDC) 1998). Health-related quality of life and activity limitation--eight states, 1995. *MMWR Morb Mortal Wkly Rep* Vol. 47, No. 7, (Feb 27 1998), pp. 134-140,

Adaikalakoteswari, A., M. Balasubramanyam, R. Ravikumar, et al. (2007). Association of telomere shortening with impaired glucose tolerance and diabetic macroangiopathy. *Atherosclerosis* Vol. 195, No. 1, (Nov 2007), pp. 83-89, 1879-1484 (Electronic) 0021-9150 (Linking).

Al-Attas, O. S., N. M. Al-Daghri, M. S. Alokail, et al. (2010). Adiposity and insulin resistance correlate with Telomere Length in middle-aged Arabs: the influence of circulating adiponectin. *Eur J Endocrinol* Vol. 163, No. 4, (Oct 2010), pp. 601-607, 1479-683X (Electronic) 0804-4643 (Linking).

Astrup, A. S., L. Tarnow, A. Jorsal, et al. (2010). Telomere Length predicts all-cause mortality in patients with type 1 diabetes. *Diabetologia* Vol. 53, No. 1, (Jan 2010), pp. 45-48, 1432-0428 (Electronic) 0012-186X (Linking).

Atturu, G., S. Brouilette, N. J. Samani, et al. (2010). Short leukocyte Telomere Length is associated with abdominal aortic aneurysm (AAA). *Eur J Vasc Endovasc Surg* Vol. 39, No. 5, (May 2010), pp. 559-564, 1532-2165 (Electronic) 1078-5884 (Linking).

Atzmon, G., M. Cho, R. M. Cawthon, et al. (2010). Evolution in health and medicine Sackler colloquium: Genetic variation in human telomerase is associated with Telomere Length in Ashkenazi centenarians. *Proc Natl Acad Sci U S A* Vol. 107 Suppl 1, No. (Jan 26 2010), pp. 1710-1717, 1091-6490 (Electronic) 0027-8424 (Linking).

Bakaysa, S. L., L. A. Mucci, P. E. Slagboom, et al. (2007). Telomere Length predicts survival independent of genetic influences. *Aging Cell* Vol. 6, No. 6, (Dec 2007), pp. 769-774, 1474-9726 (Electronic) 1474-9718 (Linking).

Barnes, S. K. & S. E. Ozanne (2011). Pathways linking the early environment to long-term health and lifespan. *Prog Biophys Mol Biol* Vol. 106, No. 1, (Jul 2011), pp. 323-336, 1873-1732 (Electronic) 0079-6107 (Linking).

Barzilai, A. (2010). DNA damage, neuronal and glial cell death and neurodegeneration. *Apoptosis* Vol. 15, No. 11, (Nov 2010), pp. 1371-1381, 1573-675X (Electronic) 1360-8185 (Linking).

Barzilai, N., I. Gabriely, G. Atzmon, et al. (2010). Genetic studies reveal the role of the endocrine and metabolic systems in aging. *J Clin Endocrinol Metab* Vol. 95, No. 10, (Oct 2010), pp. 4493-4500, 1945-7197 (Electronic) 0021-972X (Linking).

Bekaert, S., I. Van Pottelbergh, T. De Meyer, et al. (2005). Telomere Length versus hormonal and bone mineral status in healthy elderly men. *Mech Ageing Dev* Vol. 126, No. 10, (Oct 2005), pp. 1115-1122, 0047-6374 (Print) 0047-6374 (Linking).

Benetos, A., J. P. Gardner, M. Zureik, et al. (2004). Short telomeres are associated with increased carotid atherosclerosis in hypertensive subjects. *Hypertension* Vol. 43, No. 2, (Feb 2004), pp. 182-185, 1524-4563 (Electronic) 0194-911X (Linking).

Benetos, A., K. Okuda, M. Lajemi, et al. (2001). Telomere Length as an indicator of biological aging: the gender effect and relation with pulse pressure and pulse wave velocity. *Hypertension* Vol. 37, No. 2 Part 2, (Feb 2001), pp. 381-385, Blasco, M. A. (2007). The epigenetic regulation of mammalian telomeres. *Nat Rev Genet* Vol. 8, No. 4, (Apr 2007), pp. 299-309, 1471-0056 (Print) 1471-0056 (Linking).

Bohr, V. A. (2008). Rising from the RecQ-age: the role of human RecQ helicases in genome maintenance. *Trends Biochem Sci* Vol. 33, No. 12, (Dec 2008), pp. 609-620, 0968-0004 (Print) 0968-0004 (Linking).

Brouilette, S., R. K. Singh, J. R. Thompson, et al. (2003). White cell Telomere Length and risk of premature myocardial infarction. *Arterioscler Thromb Vasc Biol* Vol. 23, No. 5, (May 1 2003), pp. 842-846, 1524-4636 (Electronic) 1079-5642 (Linking).

Brouilette, S. W., J. S. Moore, A. D. McMahon, et al. (2007). Telomere Length, risk of coronary heart disease, and statin treatment in the West of Scotland Primary Prevention Study: a nested case-control study. *Lancet* Vol. 369, No. 9556, (Jan 13 2007), pp. 107-114, 1474-547X (Electronic) 0140-6736 (Linking).

Canela, A., E. Vera, P. Klatt, et al. (2007). High-throughput Telomere Length quantification by FISH and its application to human population studies. *Proc Natl Acad Sci U S A* Vol. 104, No. 13, (Mar 27 2007), pp. 5300-5305, 0027-8424 (Print) 0027-8424 (Linking).

Cawthon, R. M., K. R. Smith, E. O'Brien, et al. (2003). Association between Telomere Length in blood and mortality in people aged 60 years or older. *Lancet* Vol. 361, No. 9355, (Feb 1 2003), pp. 393-395, 0140-6736 (Print) 0140-6736 (Linking).

Cawthon, R. M., K. R. Smith, E. O'Brien, et al. (2003). Association between Telomere Length in blood and mortality in people aged 60 years or older. *The Lancet* Vol. 361, No. 9355, (2003/2/1 2003), pp. 393-395,

Cherkas, L. F., J. L. Hunkin, B. S. Kato, et al. (2008). The association between physical activity in leisure time and leukocyte Telomere Length. *Arch Intern Med* Vol. 168, No. 2, (Jan 28 2008), pp. 154-158, 0003-9926 (Print) 0003-9926 (Linking).

Codd, V., M. Mangino, P. van der Harst, et al. (2010). Common variants near TERC are associated with mean Telomere Length. *Nat Genet* Vol. 42, No. 3, (Mar 2010), pp. 197-199, 1546-1718 (Electronic) 1061-4036 (Linking).

Collerton, J., C. Martin-Ruiz, A. Kenny, et al. (2007). Telomere Length is associated with left ventricular function in the oldest old: the Newcastle 85+ study. *Eur Heart J* Vol. 28, No. 2, (Jan 2007), pp. 172-176, 0195-668X (Print) 0195-668X (Linking).

de Magalhaes, J. P., D. Wuttke, S. H. Wood, et al. (2012). Genome-environment interactions that modulate aging: powerful targets for drug discovery. *Pharmacol Rev* Vol. 64, No. 1, (Jan 2012), pp. 88-101, 1521-0081 (Electronic) 0031-6997 (Linking).

De Meyer, T., E. R. Rietzschel, M. L. De Buyzere, et al. (2009). Systemic Telomere Length and preclinical atherosclerosis: the Asklepios Study. *Eur Heart J* Vol. 30, No. 24, (Dec 2009), pp. 3074-3081, 1522-9645 (Electronic) 0195-668X (Linking).

Devore, E. E., J. Prescott, I. De Vivo, et al. (2011). Relative Telomere Length and cognitive decline in the Nurses' Health Study. *Neurosci Lett* Vol. 492, No. 1, (Mar 29 2011), pp. 15-18, 1872-7972 (Electronic) 0304-3940 (Linking).

Dewan, S. & J. P. Wilding (2003). Obesity and type-2 diabetes in the elderly. *Gerontology* Vol. 49, No. 3, (May-Jun 2003), pp. 137-145,

Epel, E., J. Daubenmier, J. T. Moskowitz, et al. (2009). Can meditation slow rate of cellular aging? Cognitive stress, mindfulness, and telomeres. *Ann N Y Acad Sci* Vol. 1172, No. (Aug 2009), pp. 34-53, 1749-6632 (Electronic) 0077-8923 (Linking).

Falconer, D. S. & T. F. C. Mackay (1996). Introduction to Quantitative Genetics. Essex, UK, Addison Wesley Longman.

Farzaneh-Far, R., R. M. Cawthon, B. Na, et al. (2008). Prognostic value of leukocyte Telomere Length in patients with stable coronary artery disease: data from the Heart and

Soul Study. *Arterioscler Thromb Vasc Biol* Vol. 28, No. 7, (Jul 2008), pp. 1379-1384, 1524-4636 (Electronic) 1079-5642 (Linking).

Fitzpatrick, A. L., R. A. Kronmal, J. P. Gardner, et al. (2007). Leukocyte Telomere Length and cardiovascular disease in the cardiovascular health study. *Am J Epidemiol* Vol. 165, No. 1, (Jan 1 2007), pp. 14-21, 0002-9262 (Print) 0002-9262 (Linking).

Fraga, M. F., R. Agrelo & M. Esteller (2007). Cross-talk between aging and cancer: the epigenetic language. *Ann N Y Acad Sci* Vol. 1100, No. (Apr 2007), pp. 60-74, 0077-8923 (Print) 0077-8923 (Linking).

Frenck, R. W., Jr., E. H. Blackburn & K. M. Shannon (1998). The rate of telomere sequence loss in human leukocytes varies with age. *Proc Natl Acad Sci U S A* Vol. 95, No. 10, (May 12 1998), pp. 5607-5610,

Friedrich, U., E. Griese, M. Schwab, et al. (2000). Telomere Length in different tissues of elderly patients. *Mech Ageing Dev* Vol. 119, No. 3, (Nov 15 2000), pp. 89-99, 0047-6374 (Print) 0047-6374 (Linking).

Fuller, K. A., D. Pearl & C. C. Whitacre (1990). Oral tolerance in experimental autoimmune encephalomyelitis: serum and salivary antibody responses. *J Neuroimmunol* Vol. 28, No. 1, (Jun 1990), pp. 15-26, 0165-5728 (Print) 0165-5728 (Linking).

Fyhrquist, F., A. Tiitu, O. Saijonmaa, et al. (2010). Telomere Length and progression of diabetic nephropathy in patients with type 1 diabetes. *J Intern Med* Vol. 267, No. 3, (Mar 2010), pp. 278-286, 1365-2796 (Electronic) 0954-6820 (Linking).

Fyhrquist, F., A. Tiitu, O. Saijonmaa, et al. (2010). Telomere Length and progression of diabetic nephropathy in patients with type 1 diabetes. *J Intern Med* Vol. 267, No. 3, (Mar 2010), pp. 278-286, 1365-2796 (Electronic) 0954-6820 (Linking).

Ganz, D. A., T. Higashi & L. Z. Rubenstein (2005). Monitoring falls in cohort studies of community-dwelling older people: effect of the recall interval. *J Am Geriatr Soc* Vol. 53, No. 12, (Dec 2005), pp. 2190-2194,

Gardner, J. P., S. Li, S. R. Srinivasan, et al. (2005). Rise in insulin resistance is associated with escalated telomere attrition. *Circulation* Vol. 111, No. 17, (May 3 2005), pp. 2171-2177, 1524-4539 (Electronic) 0009-7322 (Linking).

Gonzalez-Suarez, I. & S. Gonzalo (2008). Crosstalk between chromatin structure, nuclear compartmentalization, and telomere biology. *Cytogenet Genome Res* Vol. 122, No. 3-4, 2008), pp. 202-210, 1424-859X (Electronic) 1424-8581 (Linking).

Graakjaer, J., J. A. Londono-Vallejo, K. Christensen, et al. (2006). The pattern of chromosome-specific variations in Telomere Length in humans shows signs of heritability and is maintained through life. *Ann N Y Acad Sci* Vol. 1067, No. (May 2006), pp. 311-316, 0077-8923 (Print) 0077-8923 (Linking).

Gress, D. R. (2001). Aging and dementia: more gray hair and less gray matter. *AJNR Am J Neuroradiol* Vol. 22, No. 9, (Oct 2001), pp. 1641-1642, 0195-6108 (Print) 0195-6108 (Linking).

Gu, J., M. Chen, S. Shete, et al. (2011). A genome-wide association study identifies a locus on chromosome 14q21 as a predictor of leukocyte Telomere Length and as a marker of susceptibility for bladder cancer. *Cancer Prev Res (Phila)* Vol. 4, No. 4, (Apr 2011), pp. 514-521, 1940-6215 (Electronic) 1940-6215 (Linking).

Guan, J. Z., T. Maeda, M. Sugano, et al. (2007). Change in the Telomere Length distribution with age in the Japanese population. *Mol Cell Biochem* Vol. 304, No. 1-2, (Oct 2007), pp. 353-360, 0300-8177 (Print) 0300-8177 (Linking).

Harris, S. E., I. J. Deary, A. MacIntyre, et al. (2006). The association between Telomere Length, physical health, cognitive ageing, and mortality in non-demented older people. *Neurosci Lett* Vol. 406, No. 3, (Oct 9 2006), pp. 260-264, 0304-3940 (Print) 0304-3940 (Linking).

Harris, S. E., C. Martin-Ruiz, T. von Zglinicki, et al. (2010). Telomere Length and aging biomarkers in 70-year-olds: the Lothian Birth Cohort 1936. *Neurobiol Aging* Vol. 1558-1497 (Electronic) 0197-4580 (Linking), No. (Dec 29 2010), pp. 1558-1497 (Electronic) 0197-4580 (Linking).

Hausman, D. B., J. G. Fischer & M. A. Johnson (2011). Nutrition in centenarians. *Maturitas* Vol. 68, No. 3, (Mar 2011), pp. 203-209, 1873-4111 (Electronic) 0378-5122 (Linking).

Hirvensalo, M., T. Rantanen & E. Heikkinen (2000). Mobility difficulties and physical activity as predictors of mortality and loss of independence in the community-living older population. *J Am Geriatr Soc* Vol. 48, No. 5, (May 2000), pp. 493-498,

Hoffmann, J. & I. Spyridopoulos (2011). Telomere Length in cardiovascular disease: new challenges in measuring this marker of cardiovascular aging. *Future Cardiol* Vol. 7, No. 6, (Nov 2011), pp. 789-803, 1744-8298 (Electronic) 1479-6678 (Linking). http://www.aoa.gov/PROF/Statistics/profile/2007/16.aspx.

Huzen, J., W. Peeters, R. A. de Boer, et al. (2011). Circulating leukocyte and carotid atherosclerotic plaque Telomere Length: interrelation, association with plaque characteristics, and restenosis after endarterectomy. *Arterioscler Thromb Vasc Biol* Vol. 31, No. 5, (May 2011), pp. 1219-1225, 1524-4636 (Electronic) 1079-5642 (Linking).

Ishikawa, N., K. I. Nakamura, N. Izumiyama, et al. (2011). Telomere Length dynamics in the human pituitary gland: robust preservation throughout adult life to centenarian age. *Age (Dordr)* Vol. 1574-4647 (Electronic), No. (Jul 7 2011), pp. 1574-4647 (Electronic).

Jaskelioff, M., F. L. Muller, J. H. Paik, et al. (2011). Telomerase reactivation reverses tissue degeneration in aged telomerase-deficient mice. *Nature* Vol. 469, No. 7328, (Jan 6 2011), pp. 102-106, 1476-4687 (Electronic) 0028-0836 (Linking).

Jeanclos, E., N. J. Schork, K. O. Kyvik, et al. (2000). Telomere Length inversely correlates with pulse pressure and is highly familial. *Hypertension* Vol. 36, No. 2, (Aug 2000), pp. 195-200, 0194-911X (Print) 0194-911X (Linking).

Jiang, H., E. Schiffer, Z. Song, et al. (2008). Proteins induced by telomere dysfunction and DNA damage represent biomarkers of human aging and disease. *Proc Natl Acad Sci U S A* Vol. 105, No. 32, (Aug 12 2008), pp. 11299-11304, 1091-6490 (Electronic) 0027-8424 (Linking).

Kepler, C. K., D. G. Anderson, C. Tannoury, et al. (2011). Intervertebral disk degeneration and emerging biologic treatments. *J Am Acad Orthop Surg* Vol. 19, No. 9, (Sep 2011), pp. 543-553, 1067-151X (Print) 1067-151X (Linking).

Kim, K. C., S. Friso & S. W. Choi (2009). DNA methylation, an epigenetic mechanism connecting folate to healthy embryonic development and aging. *J Nutr Biochem* Vol. 20, No. 12, (Dec 2009), pp. 917-926, 1873-4847 (Electronic) 0955-2863 (Linking).

Kimura, M., M. Barbieri, J. P. Gardner, et al. (2007). Leukocytes of exceptionally old persons display ultra-short telomeres. *Am J Physiol Regul Integr Comp Physiol* Vol. 293, No. 6, (Dec 2007), pp. R2210-2217, 0363-6119 (Print) 0363-6119 (Linking).

Kirkwood, T. B. (2002). Molecular gerontology. *J Inherit Metab Dis* Vol. 25, No. 3, (May 2002), pp. 189-196, 0141-8955 (Print) 0141-8955 (Linking).

Kudo, H., M. Emi, Y. Ishigaki, et al. (2011). Frequent loss of genome gap region in 4p16.3 subtelomere in early-onset type 2 diabetes mellitus. *Exp Diabetes Res* Vol. 2011, No. 2011), pp. 498460, 1687-5303 (Electronic) 1687-5214 (Linking).

Kurz, D. J., B. Kloeckener-Gruissem, A. Akhmedov, et al. (2006). Degenerative aortic valve stenosis, but not coronary disease, is associated with shorter Telomere Length in the elderly. *Arterioscler Thromb Vasc Biol* Vol. 26, No. 6, (Jun 2006), pp. e114-117, 1524-4636 (Electronic) 1079-5642 (Linking).

Kuznetsova, T., V. Codd, S. Brouilette, et al. (2010). Association between left ventricular mass and Telomere Length in a population study. *Am J Epidemiol* Vol. 172, No. 4, (Aug 15 2010), pp. 440-450, 1476-6256 (Electronic) 0002-9262 (Linking).

Kveiborg, M., M. Kassem, B. Langdahl, et al. (1999). Telomere shortening during aging of human osteoblasts in vitro and leukocytes in vivo: lack of excessive telomere loss in osteoporotic patients. *Mech Ageing Dev* Vol. 106, No. 3, (Jan 15 1999), pp. 261-271, 0047-6374 (Print) 0047-6374 (Linking).

Levy, D., S. L. Neuhausen, S. C. Hunt, et al. (2010). Genome-wide association identifies OBFC1 as a locus involved in human leukocyte telomere biology. *Proc Natl Acad Sci U S A* Vol. 107, No. 20, (May 18 2010), pp. 9293-9298, 1091-6490 (Electronic) 0027-8424 (Linking).

Li, H., E. R. Simpson & J. P. Liu (2010). Oestrogen, telomerase, ovarian ageing and cancer. *Clin Exp Pharmacol Physiol* Vol. 37, No. 1, (Jan 2010), pp. 78-82, 1440-1681 (Electronic) 0305-1870 (Linking).

Libby, P. (2002). Inflammation in atherosclerosis. *Nature* Vol. 420, No. 6917, (Dec 19-26 2002), pp. 868-874, 0028-0836 (Print) 0028-0836 (Linking).

Lof-Ohlin, Z. M., N. O. Hagnelius & T. K. Nilsson (2008). Relative Telomere Length in patients with late-onset Alzheimer's dementia or vascular dementia. *Neuroreport* Vol. 19, No. 12, (Aug 6 2008), pp. 1199-1202, 1473-558X (Electronic) 0959-4965 (Linking).

Lukens, J. N., V. Van Deerlin, C. M. Clark, et al. (2009). Comparisons of Telomere Lengths in peripheral blood and cerebellum in Alzheimer's disease. *Alzheimers Dement* Vol. 5, No. 6, (Nov 2009), pp. 463-469, 1552-5279 (Electronic) 1552-5260 (Linking).

Mainous, A. G. & V. A. Diaz (2010). Telomere Length as a risk marker for cardiovascular disease: the next big thing? *Expert Rev Mol Diagn* Vol. 10, No. 8, (Nov 2010), pp. 969-971, 1744-8352 (Electronic) 1473-7159 (Linking).

Manestar-Blazic, T. (2004). Hypothesis on transmission of longevity based on Telomere Length and state of integrity. *Med Hypotheses* Vol. 62, No. 5, 2004), pp. 770-772, 0306-9877 (Print) 0306-9877 (Linking).

Manton, K. G. (2008). Recent declines in chronic disability in the elderly U.S. population: risk factors and future dynamics. *Annu Rev Public Health* Vol. 29, No. 2008), pp. 91-113,

Martin-Ruiz, C. M., J. Gussekloo, D. van Heemst, et al. (2005). Telomere Length in white blood cells is not associated with morbidity or mortality in the oldest old: a population-based study. *Aging Cell* Vol. 4, No. 6, (Dec 2005), pp. 287-290, 1474-9718 (Print) 1474-9718 (Linking).

Mather, K. A., A. F. Jorm, K. J. Anstey, et al. (2010). Cognitive performance and leukocyte Telomere Length in two narrow age-range cohorts: a population study. *BMC Geriatr* Vol. 10, No. 2010), pp. 62, 1471-2318 (Electronic) 1471-2318 (Linking).

Matthews, F. E., C. Brayne, J. Lowe, et al. (2009). Epidemiological pathology of dementia: attributable-risks at death in the Medical Research Council Cognitive Function and Ageing Study. *PLoS Med* Vol. 6, No. 11, (Nov 2009), pp. e1000180, 1549-1676 (Electronic) 1549-1277 (Linking).

Michaud, P. C., D. Goldman, D. Lakdawalla, et al. (2011). Differences in health between Americans and Western Europeans: Effects on longevity and public finance. *Soc Sci Med* Vol. 73, No. 2, (Jul 2011), pp. 254-263, 1873-5347 (Electronic) 0277-9536 (Linking).

Najjar, S. S., A. Scuteri & E. G. Lakatta (2005). Arterial aging: is it an immutable cardiovascular risk factor? *Hypertension* Vol. 46, No. 3, (Sep 2005), pp. 454-462, 1524-4563 (Electronic) 0194-911X (Linking).

Nakamura, K., K. Takubo, N. Izumiyama-Shimomura, et al. (2007). Telomeric DNA length in cerebral gray and white matter is associated with longevity in individuals aged 70 years or older. *Exp Gerontol* Vol. 42, No. 10, (Oct 2007), pp. 944-950, 0531-5565 (Print) 0531-5565 (Linking).

Nawrot, T. S., J. A. Staessen, J. P. Gardner, et al. (2004). Telomere Length and possible link to X chromosome. *The Lancet* Vol. 363, No. 9408, (2004/2/14 2004), pp. 507-510,

Ness, J., D. Nassimiha, M. I. Feria, et al. (1999). Diabetes mellitus in older African-Americans, Hispanics, and whites in an academic hospital-based geriatrics practice. *Coron Artery Dis* Vol. 10, No. 5, (Jul 1999), pp. 343-346, 0954-6928 (Print).

Newman, A. B., C. L. Haggerty, S. B. Kritchevsky, et al. (2003). Walking performance and cardiovascular response: associations with age and morbidity--the Health, Aging and Body Composition Study. *J Gerontol A Biol Sci Med Sci* Vol. 58, No. 8, (Aug 2003), pp. 715-720,

Newman, A. B., E. M. Simonsick, B. L. Naydeck, et al. (2006). Association of long-distance corridor walk performance with mortality, cardiovascular disease, mobility limitation, and disability. *Jama* Vol. 295, No. 17, (May 3 2006), pp. 2018-2026,

Nicholls, C., H. Li, J. Q. Wang, et al. (2011). Molecular regulation of telomerase activity in aging. *Protein Cell* Vol. 2, No. 9, (Sep 2011), pp. 726-738, 1674-8018 (Electronic).

Njajou, O. T., R. M. Cawthon, C. M. Damcott, et al. (2007). Telomere Length is paternally inherited and is associated with parental lifespan. *Proc Natl Acad Sci U S A* Vol. 104, No. 29, (Jul 17 2007), pp. 12135-12139, 0027-8424 (Print) 0027-8424 (Linking).

Njajou, O. T., W. C. Hsueh, E. H. Blackburn, et al. (2009). Association between Telomere Length, specific causes of death, and years of healthy life in health, aging, and body composition, a population-based cohort study. *J Gerontol A Biol Sci Med Sci* Vol. 64, No. 8, (Aug 2009), pp. 860-864, 1758-535X (Electronic) 1079-5006 (Linking).

O'Donovan, A., M. S. Pantell, E. Puterman, et al. (2011). Cumulative inflammatory load is associated with short leukocyte Telomere Length in the Health, Aging and Body

Composition Study. *PLoS One* Vol. 6, No. 5, 2011), pp. e19687, 1932-6203 (Electronic) 1932-6203 (Linking).

Oeppen, J. & J. W. Vaupel (2002). Demography. Broken limits to life expectancy. *Science* Vol. 296, No. 5570, (May 10 2002), pp. 1029-1031,

Ogami, M., Y. Ikura, M. Ohsawa, et al. (2004). Telomere shortening in human coronary artery diseases. *Arterioscler Thromb Vasc Biol* Vol. 24, No. 3, (Mar 2004), pp. 546-550, 1524-4636 (Electronic) 1079-5642 (Linking).

Olivieri, F., M. Lorenzi, R. Antonicelli, et al. (2009). Leukocyte telomere shortening in elderly Type2DM patients with previous myocardial infarction. *Atherosclerosis* Vol. 206, No. 2, (Oct 2009), pp. 588-593, 1879-1484 (Electronic) 0021-9150 (Linking).

Ouellette, M. M., Aisner, D.L., Savre-Train, I., Wright, W. E., . Shay J. W. (1999). Telomerase Activity Does Not Always Imply Telomere Maintenance. *Biochemical and Biophysical Research Communications* Vol. **254**, (Jan 1999), pp.795–803, 0006-291X (Print) 0006-291X (Linking)

Panayiotou, A. G., A. N. Nicolaides, M. Griffin, et al. (2010). Leukocyte Telomere Length is associated with measures of subclinical atherosclerosis. *Atherosclerosis* Vol. 211, No. 1, (Jul 2010), pp. 176-181, 1879-1484 (Electronic) 0021-9150 (Linking).

Panossian, L. A., V. R. Porter, H. F. Valenzuela, et al. (2003). Telomere shortening in T cells correlates with Alzheimer's disease status. *Neurobiol Aging* Vol. 24, No. 1, (Jan-Feb 2003), pp. 77-84, 0197-4580 (Print) 0197-4580 (Linking).

Parks, C. G., L. A. DeRoo, D. B. Miller, et al. (2011). Employment and work schedule are related to Telomere Length in women. *Occup Environ Med* Vol. 68, No. 8, (Aug 2011), pp. 582-589, 1470-7926 (Electronic) 1351-0711 (Linking).

Passos, J. F., C. Simillion, J. Hallinan, et al. (2009). Cellular senescence: unravelling complexity. *Age (Dordr)* Vol. 31, No. 4, (Dec 2009), pp. 353-363, 1574-4647 (Electronic).

Paul, L. (2011). Diet, nutrition and Telomere Length. *J Nutr Biochem* Vol. 22, No. 10, (Oct 2011), pp. 895-901, 1873-4847 (Electronic) 0955-2863 (Linking).

Paul, L., M. Cattaneo, A. D'Angelo, et al. (2009). Telomere Length in peripheral blood mononuclear cells is associated with folate status in men. *J Nutr* Vol. 139, No. 7, (Jul 2009), pp. 1273-1278, 1541-6100 (Electronic) 0022-3166 (Linking).

Pignolo, R. J., R. K. Suda, E. A. McMillan, et al. (2008). Defects in telomere maintenance molecules impair osteoblast differentiation and promote osteoporosis. *Aging Cell* Vol. 7, No. 1, (Jan 2008), pp. 23-31, 1474-9726 (Electronic) 1474-9718 (Linking).

Prescott, J., P. Kraft, D. I. Chasman, et al. (2011). Genome-wide association study of relative Telomere Length. *PLoS One* Vol. 6, No. 5, 2011), pp. e19635, 1932-6203 (Electronic) 1932-6203 (Linking).

Resnick, H. E., M. I. Harris, D. B. Brock, et al. (2000). American Diabetes Association diabetes diagnostic criteria, advancing age, and cardiovascular disease risk profiles: results from the Third National Health and Nutrition Examination Survey. *Diabetes Care* Vol. 23, No. 2, (Feb 2000), pp. 176-180, 0149-5992 (Print) 0149-5992 (Linking).

Robbins, J. M., V. Vaccarino, H. Zhang, et al. (2000). Excess type 2 diabetes in African-American women and men aged 40-74 and socioeconomic status: evidence from the Third National Health and Nutrition Examination Survey. *J Epidemiol Community Health* Vol. 54, No. 11, (Nov 2000), pp. 839-845,

Rolyan, H., A. Scheffold, A. Heinrich, et al. (2011). Telomere shortening reduces Alzheimer's disease amyloid pathology in mice. *Brain* Vol. 134, No. Pt 7, (Jul 2011), pp. 2044-2056, 1460-2156 (Electronic) 0006-8950 (Linking).

Royle, N. J., A. Mendez-Bermudez, A. Gravani, et al. (2009). The role of recombination in Telomere Length maintenance. *Biochem Soc Trans* Vol. 37, No. Pt 3, (Jun 2009), pp. 589-595, 1470-8752 (Electronic) 0300-5127 (Linking).

Rufer, N., T. H. Brummendorf, S. Kolvraa, et al. (1999). Telomere fluorescence measurements in granulocytes and T lymphocyte subsets point to a high turnover of hematopoietic stem cells and memory T cells in early childhood. *J Exp Med* Vol. 190, No. 2, (Jul 19 1999), pp. 157-167,

Saeed, H., B. M. Abdallah, N. Ditzel, et al. (2011). Telomerase-deficient mice exhibit bone loss owing to defects in osteoblasts and increased osteoclastogenesis by inflammatory microenvironment. *J Bone Miner Res* Vol. 26, No. 7, (Jul 2011), pp. 1494-1505, 1523-4681 (Electronic) 0884-0431 (Linking).

Salpea, K. D., P. J. Talmud, J. A. Cooper, et al. (2010). Association of Telomere Length with type 2 diabetes, oxidative stress and UCP2 gene variation. *Atherosclerosis* Vol. 209, No. 1, (Mar 2010), pp. 42-50, 1879-1484 (Electronic) 0021-9150 (Linking).

Samani, N. J., R.Boultby, R. Butler, J. R. Thompson, A. H. Goodall, (2001). Telomere shortening in atherosclerosis. *Lancet* Vol. 358, (Aug 2001), pp. 472-3, 0140-6736 (Print) 0140-6736 (Linking).

Sanders, J. L., J. A. Cauley, R. M. Boudreau, et al. (2009). Leukocyte Telomere Length Is Not Associated With BMD, Osteoporosis, or Fracture in Older Adults: Results From the Health, Aging and Body Composition Study. *J Bone Miner Res* Vol. 24, No. 9, (Sep 2009), pp. 1531-1536, 1523-4681 (Electronic) 0884-0431 (Linking).

Saxena, R., B. F. Voight, V. Lyssenko, et al. (2007). Genome-wide association analysis identifies loci for type 2 diabetes and triglyceride levels. *Science* Vol. 316, No. 5829, (Jun 1 2007), pp. 1331-1336,

Schumacher, B., J. H. Hoeijmakers & G. A. Garinis (2009). Sealing the gap between nuclear DNA damage and longevity. *Mol Cell Endocrinol* Vol. 299, No. 1, (Feb 5 2009), pp. 112-117, 0303-7207 (Print) 0303-7207 (Linking).

Selvin, E., J. Coresh & F. L. Brancati (2006). The burden and treatment of diabetes in elderly individuals in the u.s. *Diabetes Care* Vol. 29, No. 11, (Nov 2006), pp. 2415-2419,

Serra, V., T. von Zglinicki, M. Lorenz, et al. (2003). Extracellular Superoxide Dismutase Is a Major Antioxidant in Human Fibroblasts and Slows Telomere Shortening. *J. Biol. Chem.* Vol. 278, No. 9, (February 21, 2003 2003), pp. 6824-6830,

Sharpless, N. E. & R. A. DePinho (2007). How stem cells age and why this makes us grow old. *Nat Rev Mol Cell Biol* Vol. 8, No. 9, (Sep 2007), pp. 703-713, 1471-0080 (Electronic) 1471-0072 (Linking).

Shen, Q., Z. Zhang, L. Yu, et al. (2011). Common variants near TERC are associated with leukocyte Telomere Length in the Chinese Han population. *Eur J Hum Genet* Vol. 19, No. 6, (Jun 2011), pp. 721-723, 1476-5438 (Electronic) 1018-4813 (Linking).

Simonsick, E. M., P. S. Montgomery, A. B. Newman, et al. (2001). Measuring fitness in healthy older adults: the Health ABC Long Distance Corridor Walk. *J Am Geriatr Soc* Vol. 49, No. 11, (Nov 2001), pp. 1544-1548,

Slagboom, P. E., S. Droog & D. I. Boomsma (1994). Genetic determination of telomere size in humans: a twin study of three age groups. *Am J Hum Genet* Vol. 55, No. 5, (Nov 1994), pp. 876-882,

Soerensen, M., M. Thinggaard, M. Nygaard, et al. (2011). Genetic variation in TERT and TERC and human leukocyte Telomere Length and longevity: a cross sectional and longitudinal analysis. *Aging Cell* Vol. 1474-9726 (Electronic) 1474-9718 (Linking), No. (Dec 2 2011), pp. 1474-9726 (Electronic) 1474-9718 (Linking).

Song, Z., Z. Ju & K. L. Rudolph (2009). Cell intrinsic and extrinsic mechanisms of stem cell aging depend on telomere status. *Exp Gerontol* Vol. 44, No. 1-2, (Jan-Feb 2009), pp. 75-82, 1873-6815 (Electronic) 0531-5565 (Linking).

Spyridopoulos, I., Y. Erben, T. H. Brummendorf, et al. (2008). Telomere gap between granulocytes and lymphocytes is a determinant for hematopoetic progenitor cell impairment in patients with previous myocardial infarction. *Arterioscler Thromb Vasc Biol* Vol. 28, No. 5, (May 2008), pp. 968-974, 1524-4636 (Electronic) 1079-5642 (Linking).

Spyridopoulos, I., J. Hoffmann, A. Aicher, et al. (2009). Accelerated telomere shortening in leukocyte subpopulations of patients with coronary heart disease: role of cytomegalovirus seropositivity. *Circulation* Vol. 120, No. 14, (Oct 6 2009), pp. 1364-1372, 1524-4539 (Electronic) 0009-7322 (Linking).

Stindl, R. (2004). Tying it all together: telomeres, sexual size dimorphism and the gender gap in life expectancy. *Med Hypotheses* Vol. 62, No. 1, 2004), pp. 151-154, 0306-9877 (Print) 0306-9877 (Linking).

Stocker, R. & J. F. Keaney, Jr. (2004). Role of oxidative modifications in atherosclerosis. *Physiol Rev* Vol. 84, No. 4, (Oct 2004), pp. 1381-1478, 0031-9333 (Print) 0031-9333 (Linking).

Tam, W. L., Y. S. Ang & B. Lim (2007). The molecular basis of ageing in stem cells. *Mech Ageing Dev* Vol. 128, No. 1, (Jan 2007), pp. 137-148, 0047-6374 (Print) 0047-6374 (Linking).

Tang, N. L., J. Woo, E. W. Suen, et al. (2010). The effect of Telomere Length, a marker of biological aging, on bone mineral density in elderly population. *Osteoporos Int* Vol. 21, No. 1, (Jan 2010), pp. 89-97, 1433-2965 (Electronic) 0937-941X (Linking).

Tentolouris, N., R. Nzietchueng, V. Cattan, et al. (2007). White blood cells Telomere Length is shorter in males with type 2 diabetes and microalbuminuria. *Diabetes Care* Vol. 30, No. 11, (Nov 2007), pp. 2909-2915, 1935-5548 (Electronic) 0149-5992 (Linking).

Terry, D. F., V. G. Nolan, S. L. Andersen, et al. (2008). Association of longer telomeres with better health in centenarians. *J Gerontol A Biol Sci Med Sci* Vol. 63, No. 8, (Aug 2008), pp. 809-812, 1079-5006 (Print) 1079-5006 (Linking).

Terry, D. F., P. Sebastiani, S. L. Andersen, et al. (2008). Disentangling the roles of disability and morbidity in survival to exceptional old age. *Arch Intern Med* Vol. 168, No. 3, (Feb 11 2008), pp. 277-283, 0003-9926 (Print) 0003-9926 (Linking).

Testa, R., F. Olivieri, C. Sirolla, et al. (2011). Leukocyte Telomere Length is associated with complications of type 2 diabetes mellitus. *Diabet Med* Vol. 28, No. 11, (Nov 2011), pp. 1388-1394, 1464-5491 (Electronic) 0742-3071 (Linking).

Thomas, P., O. C. NJ & M. Fenech (2008). Telomere Length in white blood cells, buccal cells and brain tissue and its variation with ageing and Alzheimer's disease. *Mech Ageing Dev* Vol. 129, No. 4, (Apr 2008), pp. 183-190, 0047-6374 (Print) 0047-6374 (Linking).

Valdes, A. M., T. Andrew, J. P. Gardner, et al. (2005). Obesity, cigarette smoking, and Telomere Length in women. *Lancet* Vol. 366, No. 9486, (Aug 20-26 2005), pp. 662-664, 1474-547X (Electronic) 0140-6736 (Linking).

Valdes, A. M., I. J. Deary, J. Gardner, et al. (2010). Leukocyte Telomere Length is associated with cognitive performance in healthy women. *Neurobiol Aging* Vol. 31, No. 6, (Jun 2010), pp. 986-992, 1558-1497 (Electronic)0197-4580 (Linking).

Valdes, A. M., J. B. Richards, J. P. Gardner, et al. (2007). Telomere Length in leukocytes correlates with bone mineral density and is shorter in women with osteoporosis. *Osteoporos Int* Vol. 18, No. 9, (Sep 2007), pp. 1203-1210, 0937-941X (Print) 0937-941X (Linking).

van der Harst, P., R. A. de Boer, N. J. Samani, et al. (2010). Telomere Length and outcome in heart failure. *Ann Med* Vol. 42, No. 1, 2010), pp. 36-44, 1365-2060 (Electronic) 0785-3890 (Linking).

van der Harst, P., G. van der Steege, R. A. de Boer, et al. (2007). Telomere Length of circulating leukocytes is decreased in patients with chronic heart failure. *J Am Coll Cardiol* Vol. 49, No. 13, (Apr 3 2007), pp. 1459-1464, 1558-3597 (Electronic) 0735-1097 (Linking).

Vasan, R. S., S. Demissie, M. Kimura, et al. (2009). Association of leukocyte Telomere Length with echocardiographic left ventricular mass: the Framingham heart study. *Circulation* Vol. 120, No. 13, (Sep 29 2009), pp. 1195-1202, 1524-4539 (Electronic) 0009-7322 (Linking).

Verzola, D., M. T. Gandolfo, G. Gaetani, et al. (2008). Accelerated senescence in the kidneys of patients with type 2 diabetic nephropathy. *Am J Physiol Renal Physiol* Vol. 295, No. 5, (Nov 2008), pp. F1563-1573, 1931-857X (Print) 1522-1466 (Linking).

von Zglinicki, T. (2002). Oxidative stress shortens telomeres. *Trends Biochem Sci* Vol. 27, No. 7, (Jul 2002), pp. 339-344, 0968-0004 (Print) 0968-0004 (Linking).

Walston, J. (2004). Frailty--the search for underlying causes. *Sci Aging Knowledge Environ* Vol. 2004, No. 4, (Jan 28 2004), pp. pe4, 1539-6150 (Electronic) 1539-6150 (Linking).

Willeit, P., J. Willeit, A. Brandstatter, et al. (2010). Cellular aging reflected by leukocyte Telomere Length predicts advanced atherosclerosis and cardiovascular disease risk. *Arterioscler Thromb Vasc Biol* Vol. 30, No. 8, (Aug 2010), pp. 1649-1656, 1524-4636 (Electronic) 1079-5642 (Linking).

Wilson, W. R., K. E. Herbert, Y. Mistry, et al. (2008). Blood leucocyte telomere DNA content predicts vascular telomere DNA content in humans with and without vascular disease. *Eur Heart J* Vol. 29, No. 21, (Nov 2008), pp. 2689-2694, 1522-9645 (Electronic) 0195-668X (Linking).

Wong, J. M. & K. Collins (2003). Telomere maintenance and disease. *The Lancet* Vol. 362, No. 9388, (2003/9/20 2003), pp. 983-988,

Woo, J., N. L. Tang, E. Suen, et al. (2008). Telomeres and frailty. *Mech Ageing Dev* Vol. 129, No. 11, (Nov 2008), pp. 642-648, 0047-6374 (Print)0047-6374 (Linking).

Wu, X. M., W. R. Tang & Y. Luo (2009). [ALT--alternative lengthening of telomere]. *Yi Chuan* Vol. 31, No. 12, (Dec 2009), pp. 1185-1191, 0253-9772 (Print) 0253-9772 (Linking).

Yaffe, K., K. Lindquist, M. Kluse, et al. (2011). Telomere Length and cognitive function in community-dwelling elders: findings from the Health ABC Study. *Neurobiol Aging* Vol. 32, No. 11, (Nov 2011), pp. 2055-2060, 1558-1497 (Electronic) 0197-4580 (Linking).

Zee, R. Y., P. M. Ridker & D. I. Chasman (2011). Genetic variants of 11 telomere-pathway gene loci and the risk of incident type 2 diabetes mellitus: the Women's Genome Health Study. *Atherosclerosis* Vol. 218, No. 1, (Sep 2011), pp. 144-146, 1879-1484 (Electronic) 0021-9150 (Linking).

Zekry, D., F. R. Herrmann, I. Irminger-Finger, et al. (2010). Telomere Length is not predictive of dementia or MCI conversion in the oldest old. *Neurobiol Aging* Vol. 31, No. 4, (Apr 2010), pp. 719-720, 1558-1497 (Electronic) 0197-4580 (Linking).

Zeng, X. (2007). Human embryonic stem cells: mechanisms to escape replicative senescence? *Stem Cell Rev* Vol. 3, No. 4, (Dec 2007), pp. 270-279, 1550-8943 (Print)1550-8943 (Linking).

Zvereva, M. I., D. M. Shcherbakova & O. A. Dontsova (2010). Telomerase: structure, functions, and activity regulation. *Biochemistry (Mosc)* Vol. 75, No. 13, (Dec 2010), pp. 1563-1583, 1608-3040 (Electronic) 0006-2979 (Linking).

2

Control of Telomere Length in *Drosophila*

Sergey Shpiz and Alla Kalmykova
Institute of Molecular Genetics, Russian Academy of Sciences, Moscow
Russia

1. Introduction

The problem of incomplete end replication of DNA was originally raised by the Russian scientist Aleksey Olovnikov (Olovnikov, 1971, 1973). The main function of telomeric DNA is the compensation of end degradation. In most eukaryotes, telomeric DNA is maintained by the action of telomerase, which is responsible for the synthesis of short 6-9 nucleotide repeats using an RNA component as a template (Greider and Blackburn, 1985). In contrast, telomeres of *Drosophila* are maintained as a result of retrotransposition of specialized telomeric non-long terminal repeat retrotransposons (Biessmann et al., 1990a; Biessmann et al., 1992a; Levis et al., 1993; Abad et al., 2004b).

Retrotransposons are also found in telomeric regions of such organisms as the silkworm *Bombix mori* (Okazaki et al., 1995; Takahashi et al., 1997), the green alga *Chlorella vulgaris* (Higashiyama et al., 1997) and a flagellated protozoan parasite *Giardia lamblia* (Arkhipova and Morrison, 2001). In *Bombyx mori* and *Chlorella,* there is a mixed type of telomere elongation: telomeric retrotransposons are inserted into telomerase-generated sequences (Fig.1). In *Drosophila* genomes, no telomerase orthologs have been found (Osanai et al., 2006). Elongation of *Drosophila* telomeres is mediated by specialized telomeric retroelement transpositions onto chromosome ends (Biessmann et al. 1992a; Levis et al. 1993). Recombination represents a bypass mechanism for chromosome length maintenance (Mikhailovsky et al. 1999; Kahn et al. 2000).

This review is focused on the mechanism of telomeric transposition control, which is a crucial step in *Drosophila* telomere elongation. Telomeric retroelements are arranged in *Drosophila* telomeres in mixed tandem head-to-tail arrays, with their 3′ ends orientated toward the centromere. Telomeric element transcripts serve as a template for transposition according to target-primed reverse transcription. In this case, as well as in telomerase encoding organisms, telomere elongation utilizes reverse transcription, i.e., synthesis of DNA from an RNA template. *Drosophila* represents a unique model system with an alternative mechanism of telomere maintenance. A characteristic feature of *Drosophila* telomeres is that the RNA template for telomere elongation is encoded by the telomeric sequences themselves, in contrast to a telomerase RNA component encoded by a separate cellular gene. Regulation of the activity of genes encoding telomerase and the RNA template as well as changes in concentration of the telomere repeat binding proteins play a crucial role in telomere length control in organisms that use telomerase. To understand the mechanism of length control of *Drosophila* telomeres, it is important to know how the addition of retrotransposon elements onto chromosome ends is regulated. This process is directly associated with the transcriptional regulation of telomeric retrotransposons and chromatin structure in the telomeric region. Components of the telomere capping protein complex are involved in *Drosophila* telomere length control. Recent studies of *Drosophila* telomeres have demonstrated the importance of the RNA interference (RNAi) pathway in *Drosophila* telomere homeostasis. In the *Drosophila* germline, retrotransposons are silenced by the PIWI-interacting RNA (piRNA) pathway (Aravin et al. 2007). The telomeric retroelements *HeT-A, TART* and *TAHRE,* which are involved in telomere maintenance in *Drosophila,* are also the targets of the piRNA-mediated silencing. The abundance of telomeric retroelement transcripts, both sense and antisense, as well as the frequency of their transpositions onto chromosome ends, are controlled by a piRNA-mediated mechanism (Savitsky et al., 2006; Shpiz et al., 2007). piRNAs induce transcriptional silencing of the telomeric retrotransposons (Shpiz et al., 2011), suggesting a putative role for the piRNA pathway in the formation of the telomeric chromatin that protects chromosome ends from fusion and is involved in meiotic and mitotic telomere behavior.

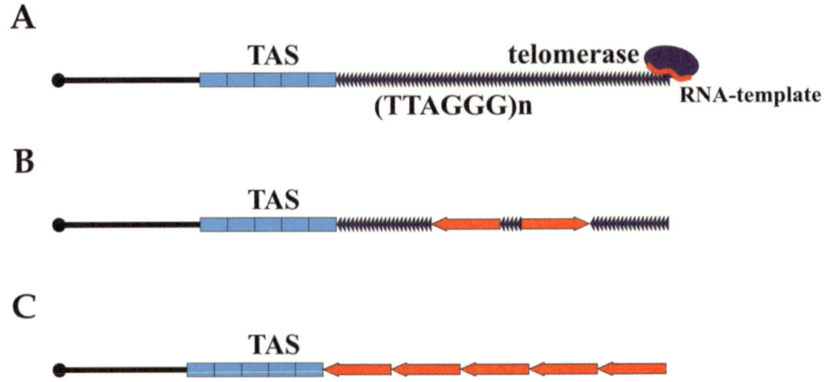

Fig. 1. Different modes of telomere elongation. (A) Telomeric DNA is maintained by telomerase, which synthesizes short 6-9 nucleotide arrays using an RNA component as a template. The human-specific telomeric repeat is shown. (B) A mixed type of telomere elongation: the telomeric retrotransposons are inserted into the short repeats formed by telomerase (*Bombyx mori, Chlorella*). (C) *Drosophila* telomeres are formed as a result of retrotransposition of specialized telomeric retrotransposons. Telomere-associated sequences (TASs) are indicated.

2. Structure of *Drosophila* telomeres

Telomeres are nucleoprotein complexes localized at the ends of linear chromosomes. Based on this, *Drosophila* telomeres can be subdivided into three domains (Andreyeva et al., 2005; Biessmann et al., 2005; Frydrychova et al., 2008) (Fig.2). The very end of the chromosome is protected by a special protein complex, the so-called telomeric cap. This structure prevents chromosome ends from end-to-end fusions and degradation by DNA repair mechanisms. The second domain accommodates the telomeric retrotransposon arrays that replace telomerase-generated repeats and supports chromosome end elongation. Lastly, proximally located repetitive complex sequences form subtelomeric or telomere associated sequences (TASs). These domains are characterized by specific chromatin structures that ensure proper telomere functioning.

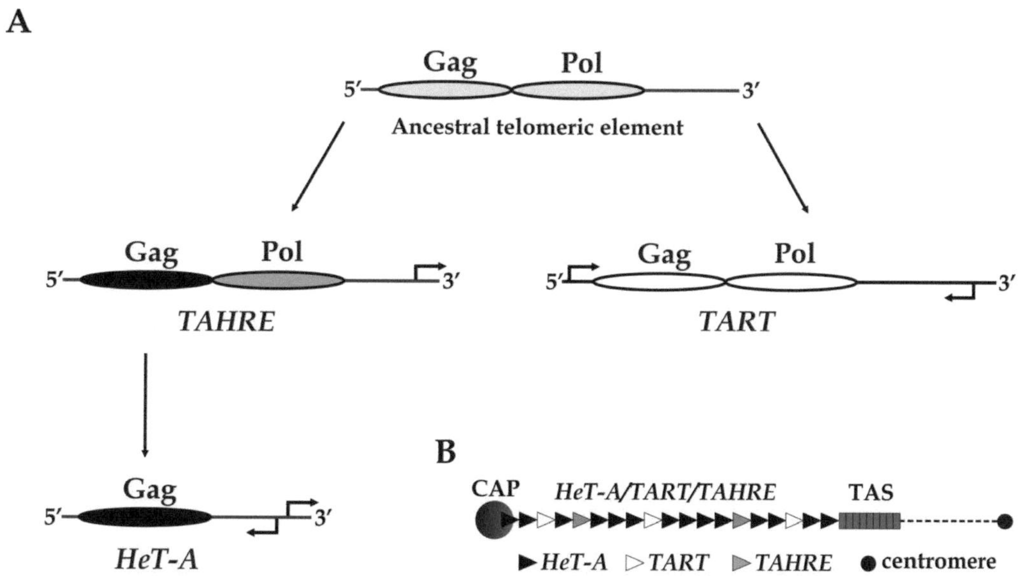

Fig. 2. *Drosophila* telomeres. (A) Putative evolutionary relationship between *D. melanogaster* telomeric retrotransposons. Transcription start sites are indicated by arrows. Ovals correspond to ORFs for Gag and Pol proteins. (B) *Drosophila* telomere region. The head-to-tail array of *HeT-A, TART,* and *TAHRE* retrotransposons is shown. The satellite-like TASs are located proximally. The protective protein cap complex is formed at the chromosome end.

2.1 *Drosophila* telomeric retrotransposons

The telomeres of *Drosophila melanogaster* consist of the specialized telomeric retrotransposons *HeT-A, TART* and *TAHRE* (Biessmann et al., 1992a; Levis et al., 1993; Abad et al., 2004b). They are LINE (long interspersed nucleic elements) or non-LTR (long terminal repeat)-type retroelements. Spontaneous transpositions of *HeT-A, TART* and *TAHRE* to telomeres have been observed, indicating that all three retrotransposon families participate in *Drosophila* telomere maintenance (Biessmann et al., 1992b; Sheen and Levis, 1994; Kahn et al., 2000; Golubovsky et al., 2001; Shpiz et al., 2007). *HeT-A, TART* and *TAHRE* are present at *Drosophila* telomeres in mixed tandem head-to-tail arrays; their oligo(A) tails always face proximally, towards the centromere. LINE elements use a target-primed reverse transcription mechanism for their transposition (Luan et al., 1993). It has been suggested that *Drosophila* telomeric retrotransposons can use the 3′ protruding end of the chromosome as a primer, but the mechanism of site-specific transpositions of telomeric retroelements to the chromosome end remains unclear. Telomere targeting of retrotransposon mRNA is the most crucial stage in telomere elongation. It has been proposed that Gag proteins target the telomeric retroelement mRNA to chromosome termini in cultured *Drosophila* cells (Rashkova et al., 2002; Rashkova et al., 2003; Fuller et al., 2010).

HeT-A, the most abundant *Drosophila* telomeric element, contains a single open reading frame (ORF) encoding a Gag-like RNA-binding protein but lacks reverse transcriptase (RT). *TART* has two ORFs, encoding the Gag and Pol proteins. The ORF2 has both endonuclease and RT domains. Both elements have unusually long 3′ and 5′ untranslated regions (UTR).

TAHRE as well as *TART* has two ORFs ; ORF2 of *TAHRE* is similar to that of *TART*. The 5′ UTR, ORF1 and 3′ UTR of *TAHRE* are similar to the corresponding regions of *HeT-A*, which prompted the designation of a newly discovered telomeric element *TAHRE* (Telomere-Associated and *HeT-A*-Related Element) (Abad et al., 2004b). It was proposed that a putative ancestral element evolved to provide telomere maintenance in *Drosophila* (Fig.2A). *TART* and *TAHRE* diverged from a common ancestor. *HeT-A* lacks ORF2 and may have derived from a processed copy of *TAHRE* (Abad et al., 2004b). All of the analyzed *D. melanogaster* stocks have both *HeT-A* and *TART* elements, and the copy numbers are approximately 30 *HeT-A* and 10 *TART* per genome (Abad et al., 2004a; George et al., 2006). A single complete and three truncated *TAHRE* were identified in the genome of the *Drosophila* stock sequenced by the Genome Project (Abad et al., 2004b). Obviously, the structural role is not a primary function for *TART* and *TAHRE*, as some telomeres contain neither *TART* nor *TAHRE* elements (Levis et al., 1993; Abad et al., 2004a; Shpiz et al., 2007). It has been proposed that the RT activity necessary for *HeT-A* transposition might be provided by *TART* or *TAHRE* (Levis et al., 1993; Rashkova et al., 2002; Abad et al., 2004b). It is noteworthy that autonomous and nonautonomous telomere-specific retrotransposons were described in the genomes of evolutionary distant *Drosophila* species (Villasante et al., 2007). One of the reasons for the cooperation of several telomeric elements throughout evolution may be the distribution of different roles among elements.

Most of the non-LTR retrotransposons utilize an internal 5′UTR promoter to transcribe a full-length RNA that serves as a template for transposition. An unusual feature of the telomeric retroelements is that the promoters of *HeT-A* and *TAHRE* are localized in the 3′ UTR and drive transcription of a downstream element (Danilevskaya et al., 1997; Shpiz et al., 2007). An antisense promoter was detected in close proximity to the *HeT-A* promoter, which drives sense expression (Shpiz et al., 2009). It appears as if the common promoter drives bidirectional expression of *HeT-A*. The *TART* element was shown to also be transcribed bidirectionally from internal sense and antisense promoters that are localized within non-terminal direct repeats in the *TART* 5′ and 3′ regions (Danilevskaya et al., 1999; Maxwell et al., 2006). An unusual feature of non-coding *HeT-A* and *TART* antisense transcripts is that they are spliced (Maxwell et al., 2006; Shpiz et al., 2009). The role of antisense transcripts in the RNA silencing of the telomeric retrotransposons will be discussed below.

According to cytological and genetic data, chromatin in the region of telomeric retrotransposon arrays exhibits euchromatic characteristics. There are several examples of *white* transgene integration into coding and promoter regions of *HeT-A*, *TART* and *TAHRE*. In most cases, when the insertion is far from a TAS, the normal activity of a reporter gene is observed (Biessmann et al., 2005). The longer the *HeT-A* array is upstream of the telomeric *white* transgene located between the TAS and telomeric retroelements, the higher the expression of the reporter gene (Golubovsky et al., 2001). This indicates that telomeric retrotransposon arrays may activate the expression of nearby genes; however, the mechanism of this *trans*-activation remains unknown. Cytological studies have also characterized the region of telomeric retroelements as a zone of decondensed chromatin similar to euchromatin (Andreyeva et al., 2005; Biessmann et al., 2005). It is noteworthy that in organisms encoding telomerase, proteins binding to the telomerase-generated repeats form a heterochromatic silencing complex (Schoeftner and Blasco, 2009).

2.2 Structure of the *Drosophila* capping complex

The protein complex at the chromosome end forms a cap that protects DNA ends against the repair system and prevents telomere fusions. The formation of the *Drosophila* cap does not require specific telomeric sequences at the chromosome ends. Terminally deleted chromosomes in the absence of telomeric and subtelomeric sequences may form a cap as well as natural telomeres (Fanti et al., 1998; Perrini et al., 2004). Several proteins that protect *Drosophila* telomeres from end-to-end fusion events have been identified (Cenci et al., 2005). Among them are HOAP (Heterochromatin Protein 1/origin recognition complex-associated protein), HipHop, Moi (Modigliani) and Ver (Verrocchio), which are the founding components of a *Drosophila* capping complex (Cenci et al., 2003; Raffa et al., 2009; Gao et al., 2010; Raffa et al., 2010). These proteins are highly enriched at telomeres. The HOAP/Ver/Moi complex is a functional analog of shelterin, a protein complex that protects human chromosome ends (Palm and de Lange, 2008). This complex was named "terminin" (Raffa et al., 2009). Terminin accumulation at chromosome ends prevents telomere fusion and helps in recruiting nonterminin components of the *Drosophila* capping complex. It was proposed that *Drosophila* lost the shelterin that binds telomeric DNA in a sequence-specific fashion and evolved terminin to bind chromosome ends independent of the terminal DNA sequence. HP1 (heterochromatic protein 1) is another important structural component of the *Drosophila* chromosome cap (Fanti et al., 1998). In addition to the chromosome cap, this protein is also associated with centromeric regions and many euchromatic sites. Mutations in the HP1 coding gene cause aberrant chromosome associations and telomeric fusions in neuroblast cells, imaginal disks, early embryos and male meiotic cells, providing evidence that HP1 mediates normal telomere behavior in different *Drosophila* cells and tissues (Fanti et al., 1998). Mutations in genes encoding ATM and ATR kinases, which are the main enzymes of the cell response to DNA damage, and components of the MRN repair complex also cause telomere fusions (Bi et al., 2004; Ciapponi et al., 2004; Oikemus et al., 2004; Silva et al., 2004; Song et al., 2004; Bi et al., 2005). However, these proteins are not stable cap components and, most likely, they mediate HP1/HOAP/Moi recruitment at chromosome ends (Fig.3).

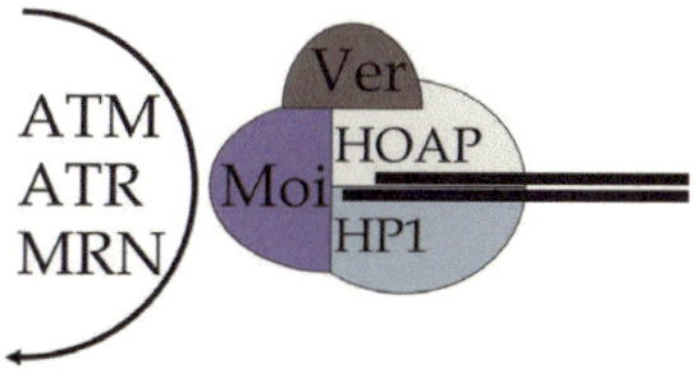

Fig. 3. *Drosophila* telomeric cap structure. The main structural cap components HOAP, Moi, Ver and HP1 are recruited to the chromosome ends by the assistance of the ATM, ATR and MRN components of the DNA damage response.

It has been suggested that transient interactions between DNA repair factors and terminal DNA sequences facilitate association of HOAP-HP1 with chromosome termini, which in turn would recruit Moi. A specific feature of the cap assembly is the redundancy of the pathways that affect capping protein recruitment to the telomere. For example, telomeric localization of both HP1 and HOAP requires functional Mre11/Rad50 components of the MRN complex. However, even in the absence of this complex, mitotic chromosomes retain the ability to recruit low levels of HOAP (Ciapponi et al., 2004). ATM and ATR kinases act redundantly in telomere protection (Bi et al., 2005). ATM may fully compensate ATR's absence in telomere capping while ATR may partially compensate for the loss of ATM (Bi et al., 2005). The mutations in the *effete* and *woc* genes, which encode an ubiquitin conjugating enzyme and a putative transcriptional factor, respectively, result in *Drosophila* telomere fusions; however, their role in telomere capping is still unclear (Cenci et al., 1997; Raffa et al., 2005). Heterochromatic proteins such as HP2 (a partner of HP1), Su(var)3-7 (a protein of pericentromere chromatin containing zinc fingers) and SUUR (a protein localized in late replicated regions, which is typical for heterochromatin) bind to polythene chromosome ends in the salivary glands (Andreyeva et al., 2005), suggesting that cap represents condensed chromatin structure. The repressive effect of the cap on the expression of terminally located genes extends as far as 4 kb (Mikhailovsky et al., 1999; Melnikova et al., 2004). Thus, in natural telomeres, only very distal telomeric retroelement may be affected by the capping complex.

Capping complexes might control telomere length by affecting the accessibility of the chromosome termini for telomeric element transposition. This process is of great importance in germinal cells. However, the majority of available data regarding cap structure was obtained by inspecting somatic cells, such as interphase salivary gland cells and mitotic larval brain cells. It should be noted that cap structure and the mechanisms of its assembly appear to differ in distinct cells and/or during the cell cycle. For example, a mutation in the gene *tefu* encoding ATM did not change the localization of HOAP at the telomeres of mitotic chromosomes, but it did decrease the amount of HOAP and HP1 at the telomeres of salivary gland polytene chromosomes (Bi et al., 2004; Oikemus et al., 2004). No detailed information about the cap structure of the germ cell chromosomes has been obtained. HP1 has been found at the ends of normal chromosomes as well as of terminally deleted chromosomes in the nuclei of nurse cells in *Drosophila* ovaries by immunohistochemistry (Shpiz et al., 2011) . Chromatin immunoprecipitation (ChIP) analysis revealed binding of both HP1 and HOAP with *HeT-A* in ovaries (Khurana et al., 2010). These data indicate that at least HP1 and HOAP provide chromosome capping in ovarian cells. Recent studies revealed a role of the piRNA pathway components in the assembly of the telomere capping complex in early embryogenesis (Khurana et al., 2010). piRNAs are essential for the retrotransposon silencing in the germline (Vagin et al., 2006; Brennecke et al., 2007; Aravin et al. 2007). *armi* and *aub* piRNA pathway components, which encode a putative RNA helicase and a piRNA binding Argonaute protein, respectively, are needed for telomere resolution during mitotic divisions in early embryos (Khurana et al., 2010). Maternally deposited piRNA pathway proteins likely function at this developmental stage (Brennecke et al., 2008). ChIP analysis on mutant *armi* and *aub* embryos revealed reduction (but not elimination) of the HOAP and HP1 binding to *HeT-A*, indicating the role of these components in telomere cap assembly. It is noteworthy that neither *ago3* nor *rhi* piRNA components affect HOAP or HP1 binding to *HeT-A*. A subpopulation of *HeT-A*-specific piRNAs was proposed to direct assembly of the telomere cap (Khurana et al., 2010). However, in *Drosophila*, chromosome capping is a sequence-independent process. *aub* and *armi* likely provide a redundant pathway for the recruitment of telomere capping proteins in early embryogenesis.

2.3 Subtelomeric region

The TAS is an extended heterochromatic chromosome region that is proximally adjacent to telomeric repeats in different organisms, the function of which remains unclear. In *Drosophila*, TASs consist of 15-25 kb of satellite-like repeats or fragments of mobile elements. TASs differ in length and sequence among chromosome arms, although some repeats share similarity. 2L TAS has homology with 3L TAS, while X TAS shares homology with 2R and 3R TAS. For example, TASs of the 2L and 3L chromosome arms are similar 460 bp repeats. X TASs are more complex repeats that are 0.9 and 1.8 kb in size (Karpen and Spradling, 1992; Wallrath and Elgin, 1995). The small fourth chromosome of *Drosophila* has a special TAS structure that is made of fragments of various mobile elements (Cryderman et al., 1999). *Drosophila* salivary gland polytene chromosome subtelomeric regions look cytologically more condensed when compared with a region resembling euchromatin and containing telomeric retrotransposons (Andreyeva et al., 2005; Biessmann et al., 2005). The eye color reporter gene *white* becomes silenced after insertion into a TAS (Karpen and Spradling, 1992; Cryderman et al., 1999; Golubovsky et al., 2001). Inactivation of a reporter gene inserted into a subtelomeric region is referred to as telomeric position effect (TPE). Transgenes in a TAS or close to a TAS demonstrate repressed and variegated expression. The silencing effect spreads to the limited distance from the TAS into the telomeric retrotransposon array (Frydrychova et al., 2007). As mentioned above, the reporter genes in the terminal *HeT-A, TAHRE,* or *TART* retroelements do not exhibit repressed expression (Biessmann et al., 2005).

In contrast to the classic position effect related to the suppression of a gene integrated into pericentric heterochromatin, *Drosophila* TPE does not depend on HP1 and known modifiers of the position effect. An exception is the fourth chromosome, where TPE depends on HP1 (Cryderman et al., 1999). This is not surprising because the fourth chromosome is cytologically located in the chromocenter, a region enriched with heterochromatic proteins. The TAS regions of most chromosome arms contain motifs recognized by the repressors of the Polycomb (PcG) protein family (Cryderman et al., 1999; Boivin et al., 2003; Andreyeva et al., 2005). The chromatin of the TAS region is enriched with methylated Lys27 of histone H3 (H3Me3K27) due to the activity of the histone methyltransferase E(z) (Czermin et al., 2002; Andreyeva et al., 2005). E(z) is a member of the Polycomb group proteins and exhibits chromomethylase activity toward Lys9 and 27 of histone H3 (Czermin et al., 2002). Methylation at these positions is a label that attracts PcG repressor proteins, which results in gene silencing. Interestingly, translocations of the second chromosome TAS to the fourth chromosome and vice versa retained the structure of the chromatin and TPE features in the translocated regions (Cryderman et al., 1999). The translocation of the fourth chromosome TAS to the second chromosome caused a sharp decrease in TPE-induced transgene silencing while dependence of TPE on HP1 within the translocated fragment was retained (Cryderman et al., 1999). This phenomenon may be attributed to changes in nuclear localization of the translocated fragment. Indeed, the fourth chromosome is usually positioned in the chromocenter that is enriched with heterochromatic proteins, whereas translocation transfers it to the periphery of the nucleus. These results suggest that TASs provide sequence-specific assembly of protein complexes involved in larger protein nuclear compartments. In addition, flies with a TAS deficiency on chromosome 2L show an increase in the expression level of telomeric *white* transgenes located both at homologous and non-homologous chromosomes, suggesting long-range telomere communication in the nucleus (Golubovsky et al., 2001; Mason et al., 2003; Frydrychova et al., 2007). Based on these data, it is tempting to propose that TASs and associated proteins play a key role in processes related to telomere positioning inside the nucleus.

3. Mechanisms of *Drosophila* telomere length control

Telomeres formed by telomerase consist of short repeats like TTAGGG in vertebrates. These repeats form a double-stranded DNA sequence of several thousand base pairs and a single strand 3′ overhang of several hundred nucleotides in length. Embedding of the single strand end into the telomeric DNA duplex forms a telomeric t-loop (de Lange, 2004). The telomeric repeats as well as the t-loop are recognized by specific DNA-binding telomeric proteins, representing a platform for assembly of the telomere–protein complex. This complex stabilizes the structure of the t-loop, protects the chromosome end against degradation and controls telomere length by regulating the accessibility of the chromosome end for telomerase (Smogorzewska and de Lange, 2004). In vertebrates, conservative DNA-binding telomeric proteins TRF1 and TRF2 directly bind the duplex of telomeric repeats and recruit other proteins to the telomere (such as the tankyrases and RAP1). TRF1 and TRF2 also associate with proteins of the DNA repair system including the heterodimer Ku70/Ku80, the MRN complex (MRE11, RAD50, NBS1) and ATM-kinase (Chan and Blackburn, 2002; Goytisolo and Blasco, 2002; Smogorzewska and de Lange, 2004). Several dozen proteins are involved in the formation of the telomere complex in mammals. The mode of the complex formation is similar for different organisms and includes sequence-specific recognition of telomeric repeats.

The heterogeneity of terminal sequences distinguishes *Drosophila* telomeres from the telomeres formed by short repeats. The transposition of three various retroelements to the chromosome end and the process of end degradation results in varied terminal nucleotide sequences, even between chromosomes of the same individual. It remains unclear whether *Drosophila* telomeres terminate with the long 3′ overhang and form the t-loop like structure. Indirect evidence for this possibility is that *Drosophila* telomeres can be elongated as a result of the recombination of tandem repeats located on the same chromosome (Kahn et al., 2000; Savitsky et al., 2002; Melnikova et al., 2005). It is possible that recombination is facilitated by integration of the chromosome end into the internal region of terminal DNA. Nevertheless, no evidence for the existence of a stable t-loop in *Drosophila* has been obtained by molecular or cytological methods. Thus, *Drosophila* telomeres contain neither specific terminal sequences nor t-loop configuration. Although regulation of telomere length in telomerase-expressing organisms is a complex process that depends on numerous factors, it may be described as protein titration on telomeric DNA: a decrease in telomeric proteins on a shortened telomere increases its susceptibility to telomerase in germinal cells or represents a signal for arrest of somatic cell division (Chan and Blackburn, 2002; Smogorzewska and de Lange, 2004).

The activity of genes encoding telomerase and the RNA template are also important factors regulating telomere length (Nugent and Lundblad, 1998). In *Drosophila,* no specific signaling pathway responsible for the retrotransposon addition to the shortened telomere has been discovered so far. Taking into account the peculiarities of *Drosophila* telomere structure, one may suggest that two steps are crucial for its telomere elongation: accessibility of the chromosome end for transpositions and control of the transposition frequency through the regulation of the telomeric retrotransposon expression. Table 1 represents a list of genes or genomic loci that affect *Drosophila* telomere length that confirm this hypothesis and demonstrate a striking crosstalk between the mechanisms of telomere protection and regulation of telomeric retrotransposon expression.

Protein/ Function	**Mutant allele**	**Mutant phenotype**				**Reference**
		Increased transpositions to TD	Increased length of natural chromosomes	Increased HeT-A/TART expression	Telomere fusions	
HP1/hetero chromatic protein	*Su(var)2-5*^{02} *Su(var)2-5*^{04} *Su(var)2-5*^{05}	+ + +	+ + +	+ (s) + (s) + (s)	- + +	Savitsky et al. 2002 Fanti et al. 1998 Perrini et al. 2004
Ku70/Ku80/ DNA repair system	deficiencies	+	+	-	-	Melnikova et al. 2005, Cenci et al. 2005
Tel/genomic locus controlling telomere length	*Tel* (from natural *Gaiano* stock)	ND	+	+ * (s)	-	Siriaco et al. 2002
SpnE/piRNA pathway, RNA helicase	*spnE*^{1}/ *spnE*^{hls3987}	+	-	+ (ov)	ND	Savitsky et al. 2006
Aub/ piRNA pathway, PIWI subfamily protein	*aub*^{QC42}/ *aub*^{HN}	+	-	+ (ov)	+	Savitsky et al. 2006, Khurana et al. 2010
Armi/ piRNA pathway, RNA helicase	*armi*^{1}/ *armi*$^{72.1}$	ND	+	+ (ov)	+	Khurana et al. 2010, Malone et al. 2009
Rhi/piRNA pathway, germline-specific homologue of HP1	*rhi*^{02086}/ *rhi*^{KG00910}	ND	+	+ (ov)	-	Khurana et al. 2010, Klattenhoff et al. 2009
Ago3/ piRNA pathway, PIWI subfamily protein	*ago3*^{4931}/ *ago3*^{3658}	ND	+	+ (ov)	-	Khurana et al. 2010, Li et al. 2009, Malone et al. 2009

TD terminally deleted chromosome; *ND* not determined; *s* somatic tissues; *ov* ovaries
* The increased level of *HeT-A* transcripts in the *Gaiano* stock is likely a consequence of high *HeT-A* copy number in the *Gaiano* telomeres (Savitsky et al. 2002).

Table 1. Negative regulators of *Drosophila* telomere length.

3.1 Role of the capping complex in *Drosophila* telomere length control

The frequency of spontaneous *HeT-A* transpositions to the chromosome end has been estimated to be in the range of 10^{-5} to 10^{-3} (Biessmann et al., 1992a; Kahn et al., 2000). Mutations in the *Su(var)2-5* gene encoding the major heterochromatic protein and cap component HP1 increase the addition of *HeT-A/TART* to the ends of terminally truncated chromosomes by more than a hundred times (Savitsky et al., 2002). HP1 mutations cause significant increases in *HeT-A* and *TART* expression. *Drosophila* lines harboring *Su(var)2-5* mutations maintain extremely long *HeT-A/TART* arrays at the natural chromosome termini (Savitsky et al., 2002; Perrini et al., 2004). Telomere elongation and *HeT-A/TART* derepression are observed in all studied *Su(var)2-5* mutants, but one of these mutations that disrupts the chromodomain does not influence HP1 capping capacity (Fanti et al., 1998; Perrini et al., 2004). It appears that the HP1 silencing effect on telomeric retrotransposon expression is more crucial for the negative control of telomere length than its role in the telomere capping. It should be noted here that the expression of *HeT-A/TART* and cap formation was studied in the somatic tissues of *Su(var)2-5* mutants, while terminal attachments causing telomere elongation that are detectable in the progeny take place in the germ cells. Thus, to elucidate the specific role of HP1 in the control of telomere length, its impact on the telomere biology in the germline should be investigated.

The Ku70/Ku80 heterodimer, a component of the DNA repair system, is an essential component of the human telomeric protein complex (Song et al., 2000; d'Adda di Fagagna et al., 2004; Jaco et al., 2004; Myung et al., 2004). A decrease in *Ku70* or *Ku80* gene dosage in *Drosophila* causes a sharp increase in the frequency of *HeT-A* and *TART* attachments to broken chromosome ends and in terminal DNA elongation by gene conversion (Melnikova et al., 2005). Ku70 mutant flies have elongated telomeres that contain an increased number of *HeT-A* and *TART* elements (Cenci et al., 2005). At the same time, a reduced concentration of Ku70 or Ku80 does not affect *HeT-A* transcript abundance in flies, and Ku70 null mutation does not cause telomeric fusions (Cenci et al., 2005; Melnikova et al., 2005). A role of the Ku complex in the accessibility of *Drosophila* chromosome termini for transpositions has been suggested (Melnikova et al., 2005).

In the HOAP mutants, as well as in the double ATM/ATR mutants, *HeT-A* expression is increased (Bi et al., 2005). However, it is currently unknown whether mutations of other than HP1 cap components lead to excessive telomere elongation.

The dominant factor *Telomere elongation (Tel)* was genetically identified in the natural *Drosophila Gaiano* stock that has unusually long telomeres (Siriaco et al., 2002). *E(tc)* locus, which affects terminal gene conversion, was also mapped to the same chromosome region (Melnikova and Georgiev, 2002). These factors might be different alleles of the same, but as yet unidentified, gene involved in *Drosophila* telomere length control.

3.2 Mechanisms of regulation of telomeric retrotransposon expression in somatic tissues

Telomeric retrotransposon transcripts serve as templates for the synthesis of proteins necessary for transposition as well as for reverse transcription primed by the 3′ end of the telomeric DNA. As a result of end underreplication, *Drosophila* telomeres shorten by 75 bp per generation (Biessmann and Mason, 1988; Levis, 1989; Biessmann et al., 1990b), whereas transposition of full-size retrotransposon results in chromosome elongation by 6-12 kb. Evidently, maintenance of normal length of telomeres requires strict control of transposition frequency and transcriptional activity of telomeric retroelements. In spite that the telomeric array exhibits euchromatic features telomeric retrotransposon expression is repressed in somatic tissues. Several negative regulators of telomeric element expression have been shown, such as HP1, ATM and ATR kinases, and PROD protein (Savitsky et al., 2002; Bi et al., 2005; Torok et al., 2007). It was proposed that a special chromatin structure forms along telomeric retrotransposon array providing retrotransposon silencing (Frydrychova et al., 2008). The mechanism of the telomeric element silencing in the somatic tissues is unknown. The role of RNA interference system in this process is still not clear. Twenty-one nucleotide long endogenous siRNAs (endo-siRNAs) have been identified in the somatic cells of *D. melanogaster* (Czech et al. 2008; Ghildiyal et al. 2008; Kawamura et al. 2008). This class of short RNAs is produced in a Dicer-2-dependent manner and can direct AGO2 to cleave target RNAs. A subset of endo-siRNAs that are homologous to retrotransposons including *HeT-A* was identified. However, *HeT-A* expression was not significantly affected by the RNAi pathway disruption in cell culture or imago tissues (Ghildiyal et al. 2008). It should be noted that the *HeT-A* promoter is active in replicating diploid larval tissues (George and Pardue, 2003). Evidently, endo-siRNAs control the steady-state abundance of *HeT-A* RNA only in those somatic tissues where the *HeT-A* promoter is active. Detailed histological analysis is needed to learn more about the contribution of the endo-siRNA pathway to telomeric retrotransposon silencing in the fly soma.

Importantly, we found that the expression of telomeric retrotransposons and the frequency of their transpositions onto chromosome ends are specifically regulated by an RNAi-based mechanism in the germline where heritable transpositions occur (Savitsky et al., 2006). These data are significant for the understanding of the control of *Drosophila* telomere length.

3.3 Role of the piRNA pathway in *Drosophila* telomeric retrotransposon expression in the germline

The piRNA pathway is directed by a distinct class of 24-30-nucleotide-long RNAs called PIWI-interacting RNAs (piRNAs), which are produced by a Dicer-independent mechanism and associated with Argonaute proteins from the PIWI subfamily (Brennecke et al., 2007; Aravin et al., 2008) (Fig.4). The piRNA pathway protects the genome in germ cells from transposable element activity. Piwi, Aubergine (Aub) and Argonaute 3 (AGO3) bind piRNAs and serve as core components of the piRNA machinery in *Drosophila* ovaries (Saito et al. 2006; Brennecke et al. 2007; Gunawardane et al. 2007; Li et al. 2009; Malone et al. 2009). These proteins are engaged in an amplification loop to mediate the generation of sense and antisense piRNAs from the transposon transcripts (Brennecke et al., 2007). Other proteins such as RNA helicases Spindle-E (Spn-E) and Armitage (Armi), nucleases Zucchini (Zuc) and Squash (Squ), the germline-specific homologue of HP1 Rhino and the product of the *vasa* locus are involved in transposon silencing in the germline and are required for piRNA production/stabilization (Cook et al. 2004; Vagin et al. 2004; Vagin et al. 2006; Pane et al. 2007; Klattenhoff and Theurkauf 2008; Klattenhoff et al. 2009; Malone et al. 2009). Transposon derepression and transpositions are observed in piRNA pathway mutants, pointing to the primary role of this system in the silencing of parasitic elements (Aravin et al. 2001; Sarot et al. 2004; Vagin et al. 2004; Kalmykova et al. 2005).

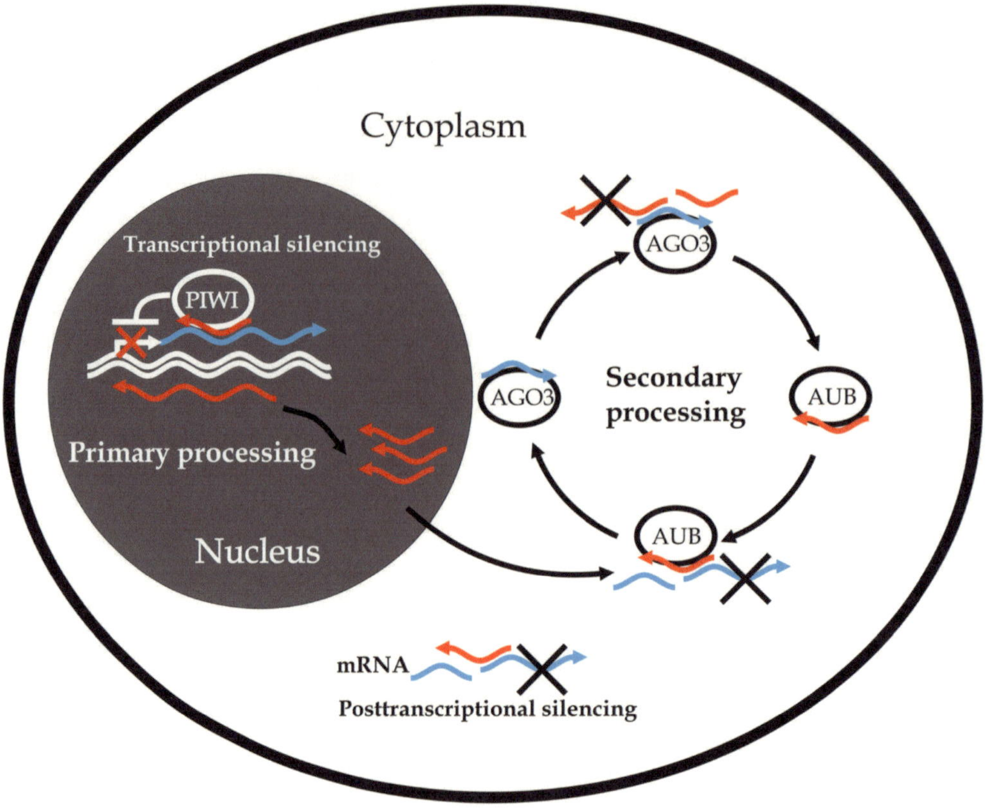

Fig. 4. piRNA pathway. The diagram shows the principal steps of the production and actions of piRNAs. piRNA-mediated protein complexes cleave complementary mRNAs in the cytoplasm or silence homologous loci in the nucleus.

In spite of their vital genomic function, *Drosophila* telomeric retroelements as well as other parasitic transposons were shown to be targets of the piRNA-mediated silencing pathway (Vagin et al., 2004; Savitsky et al., 2006; Shpiz et al., 2007; Shpiz et al., 2009). Mutations in the *spn-E, aub, piwi, squ* and *zuc* genes and *vasa* locus result in accumulation of telomeric element transcripts in ovaries (Vagin et al. 2004; Savitsky et al. 2006; Pane et al. 2007; Shpiz et al. 2007; Shpiz et al. 2009), but the same mutations do not affect telomeric element expression in *Drosophila* testes (A.K., unpublished data). *In situ* RNA hybridization analysis has revealed different patterns of accumulation of *HeT-A, TART* and *TAHRE* transcripts in the ovaries of piRNA mutants (Savitsky et al., 2006; Shpiz et al., 2007). *TART* transcripts accumulate in supporting nurse cells predominantly at the late stages of oogenesis, whereas *HeT-A* and *TAHRE* transcripts are detected in a growing oocyte from the earlier stages of oogenesis. This finding suggests that *TAHRE* rather than *TART* is a source of reverse transcriptase for the transpositions of non-autonomous *HeT-A* elements. Sense and antisense piRNAs specific to telomeric retrotransposons have been revealed in libraries of short RNAs and by Northern analysis (Saito et al. 2006; Savitsky et al. 2006; Brennecke et al. 2007; Shpiz et al. 2007; Malone et al. 2009; Shpiz et al. 2009). Their levels are dramatically lower in the ovaries of piRNA mutants, which correlate with increased expression.

Antisense transcripts of transposable elements are important intermediates in the piRNA pathway because they serve as templates for piRNA generation (Brennecke et al., 2007; Gunawardane et al., 2007). Interestingly, both *HeT-A* and *TART* produce long non-coding processed antisense transcripts from their internal promoters (Maxwell et al., 2006; Shpiz et al., 2009). The *HeT-A* antisense transcription start site was mapped to the 3′ UTR of this element 150 bp upstream of the sense transcription start site. *HeT-A* and *TART* antisense transcripts are targets of the piRNA pathway and accumulate in the germ cell nuclei of the piRNA pathway mutants. Thus, steady-state expression of *HeT-A* and *TART* retrotransposons could be a result of an intricate piRNA-mediated interplay of their sense and antisense transcripts (Shpiz et al., 2009). Thus, the piRNA system suppresses excessive retrotransposon activity and maintains transcripts at low levels because this system requires the presence of sense and antisense transcripts to act as triggers of this mechanism.

3.4 Role of the piRNA pathway in *Drosophila* telomere length control and telomeric chromatin assembly

We have shown that increased expression of *HeT-A/TART* in the piRNA pathway mutants results in an increased rate of their transpositions onto chromosome ends, i.e., telomere elongation (Savitsky et al., 2006). To screen for new transpositions on chromosome ends in the piRNA pathway mutants, we used truncated X chromosomes (designated y^{TD}) with a break in the *yellow* locus that controls body and bristle pigmentation. The break is located in the upstream regulatory region and results in the y^2-like fly phenotype with yellow aristae (a bristle-like part of the antenna). The addition of *HeT-A* or *TART* retroelements can be monitored by a yellow-to-black change in aristae pigmentation (Savitsky et al., 2002; Savitsky et al., 2006) (Fig.5).

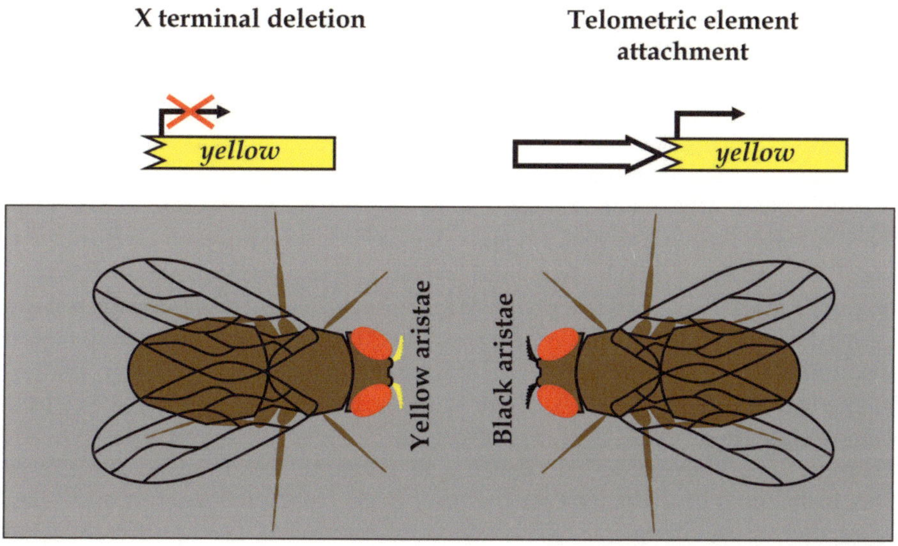

Fig. 5. Genetic assay to measure the frequency of telomeric element attachments to the broken chromosome end. Schematic representation of the telomeric retrotransposon attachments to the broken *yellow* gene located at the end of the terminally deleted X chromosome. As a result of terminal attachment, *yellow* is activated, causing yellow-to-black change in aristae pigmentation.

Both *spn-E* and *aub* mutations have a strong dominant effect on the frequency of attachments, resulting in a 20- to 100-fold increase in the appearance of flies with black-colored aristae. In flies carrying a single copy of the *spn-E* or *aub* mutant allele, the majority of the new transpositions were *TART*, whereas in the ovaries of sterile homozygous *spn-E* females, *HeT-A* transpositions were more frequent. This difference might be explained by peculiarities of the dosage effect of the piRNA mutations on *HeT-A/TART* expression. Clusters of flies with identical *TART* attachments were isolated in the progeny of *spn-E* and *aub* mutants, indicating that piRNA-mediated control of terminal transpositions occurs in premeiotic cells. It is noteworthy that despite the greatly increased frequency of *HeT-A* and *TART* attachments to the broken ends observed in this assay, *spn-E* or *aub* mutant lines do not have detectably longer telomeres on their native chromosomes (Savitsky et al., 2006; Khurana et al., 2010). This indicates that the truncated chromosome end is more sensitive to telomeric element attachments than the native telomere. Despite the fact that the protein cap can be formed on the broken chromosome ends, they lack both telomeric retrotransposons and subtelomeric repeats, which results in considerably different chromatin structure. The attachment of retrotransposons to native telomeres is likely impeded compared to the truncated chromosome. A recent study detected an increase in *HeT-A* copy number in *rhi*, *armi* and *ago3* piRNA pathway mutant stocks (Khurana et al., 2010). Among them, only the *armi* mutation affects HOAP and HP1 capping protein recruitment in early embryogenesis, whereas all of them cause telomeric element derepression in the germline. It seems that transcript accumulation is a main reason for telomere elongation in piRNA pathway mutants. However, piRNAs may affect not only transcript abundance but also chromatin structure.

Distinct short RNA-mediated silencing mechanisms have been described. Short RNAs have been shown to target the associated protein complex to degrade complementary mRNAs that mediate post-transcriptional silencing (Elbashir et al., 2001). Short-RNA-mediated heterochromatin assembly was described in fission yeast, plants and ciliates (Hamilton et al., 2002; Volpe et al., 2002; Liu et al., 2004). In this case, heterochromatinization diminishes the transcriptional capacity of the target locus, resulting in transcriptional silencing. In mice, transposon-specific piRNAs drive transposon promoter methylation in the male germline (Aravin et al., 2008; Kuramochi-Miyagawa et al., 2008). In the *Drosophila* model, the mechanism of the piRNA-mediated gene silencing has remained obscure. The three *Drosophila* PIWI proteins PIWI, Aub and Ago3 cleave complementary RNA *in vitro,* suggesting their involvement in the post-transcriptional degradation of mRNA (Saito et al., 2006; Brennecke et al., 2007; Gunawardane et al., 2007). piRNAs were shown to mediate post-transcriptional retrotransposon mRNA degradation into cytoplasmic bodies in the *Drosophila* germline (Lim et al., 2009). There is also evidence for the influence of piRNAs on the chromatin state (Josse et al., 2007; Klenov et al., 2007). In our recent study, we addressed the mechanism of piRNA-mediated silencing of telomeric retrotransposons (Shpiz et al., 2011). This problem is of great interest because, in the case of transcriptional silencing, it might be related to the formation of the telomeric chromatin. Using different approaches, we have shown that transcriptional activity of the telomeric retroelements substantially increased in the piRNA pathway mutants. Nuclear run-on assay (Jackson et al., 1998; Core et al., 2008) on ovarian tissues has been used to estimate the density of transcriptionally active RNA-polymerase complexes at telomeric loci. An increase in the nascent transcripts emerging from telomeric loci as well as from some other retrotransposons has been shown.

This observation was confirmed by the observation of enrichment of retrotransposon sequences in piRNA pathway mutants with two histone H3 modifications known to be linked to the RNA polymerase II activity (dimethylation of lysines 4 and 79). These data provided strong evidence for piRNA-mediated transcriptional silencing of the telomeric retrotransposon loci in the *Drosophila* germline. Most likely, transposon defense in the germline is a combination of the piRNA-mediated post-transcriptional and transcriptional silencing. This suggests that piRNAs are important participants in telomeric chromatin assembly.

Telomeric retrotransposon arrays as mentioned above display the features of open chromatin, however, no actively elongating RNA polymerase isoforms have been detected in this region (Andreyeva et al., 2005; Biessmann et al., 2005). We suggest that piRNAs mediate sequence-specific binding of the inhibition protein complex locally at the *HeT-A* promoter in the germ cells rather than heterochromatinization along telomeric arrays. Components of the transcription initiation complex of the telomeric retrotransposons may be considered as a putative link between piRNAs and inhibition of the transcription (Fig.6). However, little is known about the transcription factors that regulate telomeric element expression. The PROD protein, which is involved in heterochromatin formation, represses *HeT-A* expression (Torok et al., 2007). JIL-1 and Z4, which are associated with decompacted chromatin regions, are recruited to the telomeric retrotransposon array and colocalize with euchromatin-specific histone H3 trimethylated at lysine 4 in somatic tissues (Andreyeva et al., 2005).

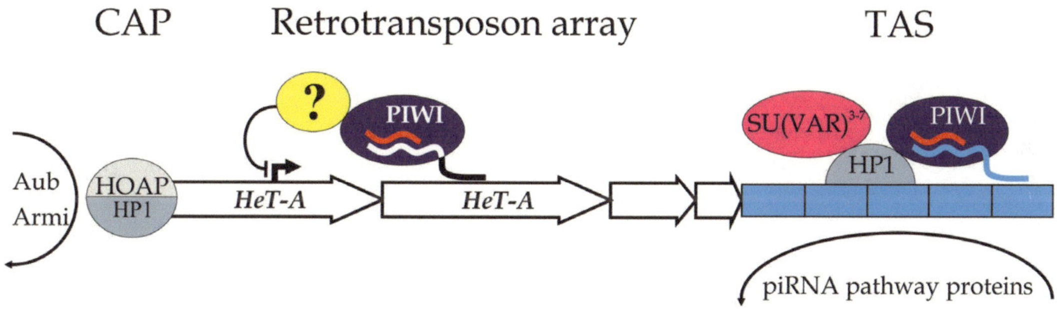

Fig. 6. Putative role of the piRNA pathway in *Drosophila* telomere functions in the germline. The piRNA/PIWI complex is proposed to mediate binding of the transcriptional inhibitors at the *HeT-A* promoter (yellow filled circle). The piRNA pathway components *aub* and *armi* are involved in telomere cap protein recruitment. TAS-specific piRNAs mediate chromatin assembly in this region.

HeT-A/TART derepression was recently reported to be a result of loss of histone H3 lysine 9 trimethylation by the methyltransferase dSETDB1 in the germline (Rangan et al., 2011). dSETDB1 was proposed to be required for piRNA production. This result underlined the importance of chromatin structure for piRNA-mediated expression of telomeric retrotransposons. Thus, piRNAs affect not only transcript abundance but changes in the chromatin state of telomeric retroelements as well. We believe that both factors cause the excessive telomere length detected in piRNA pathway mutants (Table 1). These data underscore the importance of the piRNA pathway in *Drosophila* telomere homeostasis.

However, there are still more open questions than clear answers in this field. Telomere fusions in early embryos are observed only in *aub* and *armi* piRNA mutants, which affect cap formation (Khurana et al., 2010), whereas an increase in the *HeT-A* copy number was detected in most investigated piRNA pathway mutants. Moreover, TAS regions also produce piRNAs (Brennecke et al., 2007; Yin and Lin, 2007; Todeschini et al., 2010). The study of transgenes inserted in TASs led to the discovery of a phenomenon called a telomeric trans-silencing effect (TSE) (Ronsseray et al., 2003). A transgene inserted in a TAS can *in trans* repress the expression of a homologous transgene in the germline. In recent studies, TSE was found to depend on the piRNA silencing pathway and heterochromatin components (Josse et al., 2007; Todeschini et al., 2010), suggesting that TAS may be considered as a platform for piRNA-mediated chromatin assembly.

As mentioned above, the telomeric region of *D. melanogaster* is subdivided into three distinct subdomains based on DNA composition and chromatin structure: the cap, the retrotransposon array and the TAS region. Interestingly, in spite of the distinct features of these domains, the chromatin structure of each is under the control of the piRNA silencing pathway. This may suggest that there are several levels of *Drosophila* telomere length regulation and that the piRNA pathway is one of the important participants in this complex process (Fig. 6).

4. Role of RNAi in the telomere function in different organisms

In the fission yeast *Schizosaccharomyces pombe*, RNAi is required for heterochromatin assembly (Hall et al., 2002; Volpe et al., 2002). Short RNAs guide histone methyltransferase to the target locus to methylate lysine 9 of histone H3 (H3K9) with subsequent binding of the heterochromatic protein Swi6. Specific repeated elements (dg and dh) that are present at all major heterochromatic regions, including pericentromeric regions, subtelomeres and the mating-type locus, have been shown to act as targets of RNAi-mediated silencing (Hall et al., 2002; Volpe et al., 2002). Disruption of the RNAi system leads to defects in telomere clustering during mitosis and meiosis, although the silencing of transgenes inserted within subtelomeric loci, telomere length and telomeric Swi6 localization are not affected (Hall et al., 2003; Sugiyama et al., 2005). It was shown that fission yeast employs two independent mechanisms to maintain gene silencing at telomeres (Fig. 7). A chromatin-remodeling complex is recruited to yeast telomeres via interaction with the telomeric repeat binding proteins Ccq1 and Taz1 or the RNAi machinery that acts through dg and dh repeats embedded within subtelomeric regions (Kanoh et al., 2005; Hansen et al., 2006; Sugiyama et al., 2007). Thus, the maintenance of telomeric chromatin depends on redundant RNAi-dependent and RNAi-independent mechanisms. The removal of genes encoding RNAi components has little impact on the maintenance of the silencing of reporters or on telomere length; however, it affects telomere dynamics during mitosis and meiosis. The RNAi machinery was proposed to be essential for higher-order chromatin organization at telomeres (Sugiyama et al., 2005).

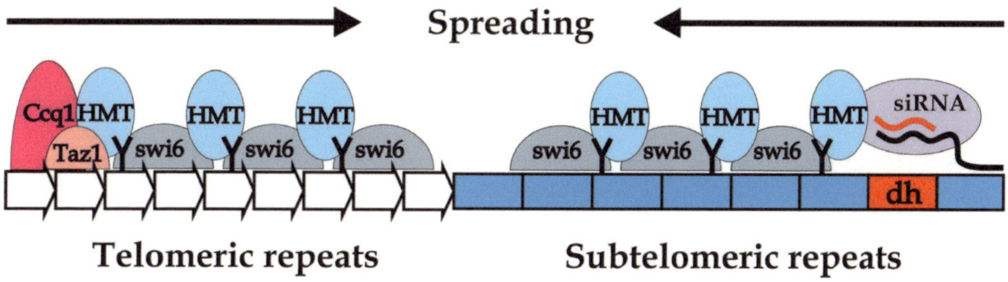

Fig. 7. Telomeric chromatin assembly in *S. pombe.* A chromatin-remodeling complex is recruited to yeast telomeres via redundant RNAi-dependent and RNAi-independent mechanisms. Subtelomeric repeats generate siRNAs that guide histone methyltransferase to methylate lysine 9 of histone H3 (H3K9me) with subsequent binding of the heterochromatic protein Swi6. Alternatively, telomere binding proteins Ccq1 and Taz1 induce the methylation of histone H3-K9 to recruit Swi6, which results in establishment of telomere heterochromatin.

In *Tetrahymena,* mutation of the *Dcl1p* gene that encodes the germline-specific ortholog of the RNase III enzyme Dicer causes serious impairments in meiotic chromosome behavior (Mochizuki and Gorovsky, 2005). The chromosome "bouquet" (i.e., telomere clustering in one region of the nuclear periphery) formation preceding homologous pairing did not occur in meiotic prophase, which resulted in impairments of chromosome segregation and higher lethality of progeny. This observation points to an important role of the RNAi component Dcl1 in chromosome segregation and telomere dynamics during conjugation in *Tetrahymena* (Mochizuki and Gorovsky, 2005). Taken together, these data suggest that a requirement for RNAi machinery in telomere function is probably conserved among eukaryotes. Telomere and/or subtelomeric arrays in different organisms irrespective of the mode of telomere elongation contain repetitive sequences, which are a potential source of short RNAs and the putative targets for RNAi.

5. Conclusion

Despite the different mode of chromosome end elongation (telomerase or transpositions), eukaryotic telomeres are functionally equal. They restore receding chromosome ends, protect them from the cell repair system, and are involved in the processes of chromosome positioning in the nucleus and chromosome condensation in meiosis and mitosis. The role of piRNAs in the expression of *Drosophila* telomeric retrotransposons, control of telomere length and assembly of the telomeric chromatin clearly indicates the importance of the piRNA pathway in *Drosophila* telomere homeostasis. Mutations in the RNAi machinery have been shown to disrupt telomere function in both *S. pombe* and *Tetrahymena.* RNAi likely mediates telomeric chromatin assembly, which plays a crucial role in telomere dynamics. It is tempting to speculate that RNA silencing plays a universal role in telomere function in various organisms irrespective of the mode of telomere elongation.

6. Acknowledgements

This work was supported by grants to A.K from the Russian Academy of Sciences program for Molecular and Cell Biology and the Russian Foundation for Basic Researches (09-04-00305).

7. References

Abad, J.P.; De Pablos, B.; Osoegawa, K.; De Jong, P.J.; Martin-Gallardo, A. & Villasante, A. (2004a). Genomic analysis of Drosophila melanogaster telomeres: full-length copies of HeT-A and TART elements at telomeres. *Mol Biol Evol*, Vol.21, No.9, Sep, pp. 1613-1619

Abad, J.P.; De Pablos, B.; Osoegawa, K.; De Jong, P.J.; Martin-Gallardo, A. & Villasante, A. (2004b). TAHRE, a novel telomeric retrotransposon from Drosophila melanogaster, reveals the origin of Drosophila telomeres. *Mol Biol Evol*, Vol.21, No.9, Sep, pp. 1620-1624

Andreyeva, E.N.; Belyaeva, E.S.; Semeshin, V.F.; Pokholkova, G.V. & Zhimulev, I.F. (2005). Three distinct chromatin domains in telomere ends of polytene chromosomes in Drosophila melanogaster Tel mutants. *J Cell Sci*, Vol.118, No.Pt 23, Dec 1, pp. 5465-5477

Aravin, A.A.; Naumova, N.M.; Tulin, A.V.; Vagin, V.V.; Rozovsky, Y.M. & Gvozdev, V.A. (2001). Double-stranded RNA-mediated silencing of genomic tandem repeats and transposable elements in the D. melanogaster germline. *Curr Biol*, Vol.11, No.13, Jul 10, pp. 1017-1027

Aravin, A.A.; Hannon G.J. & Brennecke J. 2007. The Piwi-piRNA pathway provides an adaptive defense in the transposon arms race. *Science*, Vol.318, No.5851, Nov 2, pp. 761-764

Aravin, A.A.; Sachidanandam, R.; Bourc'his, D.; Schaefer, C.; Pezic, D.; Toth, K.F.; Bestor, T. & Hannon, G.J. (2008). A piRNA pathway primed by individual transposons is linked to de novo DNA methylation in mice. *Mol Cell*, Vol.31, No.6, Sep 26, pp. 785-799

Arkhipova, I.R. & Morrison, H.G. (2001). Three retrotransposon families in the genome of Giardia lamblia: two telomeric, one dead. *Proc Natl Acad Sci U S A*, Vol.98, No.25, Dec 4, pp. 14497-14502

Bi, X.; Wei, S.C. & Rong, Y.S. (2004). Telomere protection without a telomerase; the role of ATM and Mre11 in Drosophila telomere maintenance. *Curr Biol*, Vol.14, No.15, Aug 10, pp. 1348-1353

Bi, X.; Srikanta, D.; Fanti, L.; Pimpinelli, S.; Badugu, R.; Kellum, R. & Rong, Y.S. (2005). Drosophila ATM and ATR checkpoint kinases control partially redundant pathways for telomere maintenance. *Proc Natl Acad Sci U S A*, Vol.102, No.42, Oct 18, pp. 15167-15172

Biessmann, H. & Mason, J.M. (1988). Progressive loss of DNA sequences from terminal chromosome deficiencies in Drosophila melanogaster. *Embo J*, Vol.7, No.4, Apr, pp. 1081-1086

Biessmann, H.; Mason, J.M.; Ferry, K.; d'Hulst, M.; Valgeirsdottir, K.; Traverse, K.L. & Pardue, M.L. (1990a). Addition of telomere-associated HeT DNA sequences "heals" broken chromosome ends in Drosophila. *Cell*, Vol.61, No.4, May 18, pp. 663-673

Biessmann, H.; Carter, S.B. & Mason, J.M. (1990b). Chromosome ends in Drosophila without telomeric DNA sequences. *Proc Natl Acad Sci U S A*, Vol.87, No.5, Mar, pp. 1758-1761

Biessmann, H.; Champion, L.E.; O'Hair, M.; Ikenaga, K.; Kasravi, B. & Mason, J.M. (1992a). Frequent transpositions of Drosophila melanogaster HeT-A transposable elements to receding chromosome ends. *Embo J*, Vol.11, No.12, Dec, pp. 4459-4469

Biessmann, H.; Valgeirsdottir, K.; Lofsky, A.; Chin, C.; Ginther, B.; Levis, R.W. & Pardue, M.L. (1992b). HeT-A, a transposable element specifically involved in "healing" broken chromosome ends in Drosophila melanogaster. *Mol Cell Biol*, Vol.12, No.9, Sep, pp. 3910-3918

Biessmann, H.; Prasad, S.; Semeshin, V.F.; Andreyeva, E.N.; Nguyen, Q.; Walter, M.F. & Mason, J.M. (2005). Two distinct domains in Drosophila melanogaster telomeres. *Genetics*, Vol.171, No.4, Dec, pp. 1767-1777

Boivin, A.; Gally, C.; Netter, S.; Anxolabehere, D. & Ronsseray, S. (2003). Telomeric associated sequences of Drosophila recruit polycomb-group proteins in vivo and can induce pairing-sensitive repression. *Genetics*, Vol.164, No.1, May, pp. 195-208

Brennecke, J.; Aravin, A.A.; Stark, A.; Dus, M.; Kellis, M.; Sachidanandam, R. & Hannon, G.J. (2007). Discrete small RNA-generating loci as master regulators of transposon activity in Drosophila. *Cell*, Vol.128, No.6, Mar 23, pp. 1089-1103

Brennecke, J.; Malone, C.D.; Aravin, A.A.; Sachidanandam, R.; Stark, A. & Hannon, G.J. (2008). An epigenetic role for maternally inherited piRNAs in transposon silencing. *Science*, Vol.322, No.5906, Nov 28, pp. 1387-1392

Cenci, G.; Rawson, R.B.; Belloni, G.; Castrillon, D.H.; Tudor, M.; Petrucci, R.; Goldberg, M.L.; Wasserman, S.A. & Gatti, M. (1997). UbcD1, a Drosophila ubiquitin-conjugating enzyme required for proper telomere behavior. *Genes Dev*, Vol.11, No.7, Apr 1, pp. 863-875

Cenci, G.; Siriaco, G.; Raffa, G.D.; Kellum, R. & Gatti, M. (2003). The Drosophila HOAP protein is required for telomere capping. *Nat Cell Biol*, Vol.5, No.1, Jan, pp. 82-84

Cenci, G.; Ciapponi, L. & Gatti, M. (2005). The mechanism of telomere protection: a comparison between Drosophila and humans. *Chromosoma*, Vol.114, No.3, Aug, pp. 135-145

Chan, S.W. & Blackburn, E.H. (2002). New ways not to make ends meet: telomerase, DNA damage proteins and heterochromatin. *Oncogene*, Vol.21, No.4, Jan 21, pp. 553-563

Ciapponi, L.; Cenci, G.; Ducau, J.; Flores, C.; Johnson-Schlitz, D.; Gorski, M.M.; Engels, W.R. & Gatti, M. (2004). The Drosophila Mre11/Rad50 complex is required to prevent both telomeric fusion and chromosome breakage. *Curr Biol*, Vol.14, No.15, Aug 10, pp. 1360-1366

Cook, H.A.; Koppetsch, B.S.; Wu, J. & Theurkauf, W.E. (2004). The Drosophila SDE3 homolog armitage is required for oskar mRNA silencing and embryonic axis specification. *Cell*, Vol.116, No.6, Mar 19, pp. 817-829

Core, L.J.; Waterfall, J.J. & Lis, J.T. (2008). Nascent RNA sequencing reveals widespread pausing and divergent initiation at human promoters. *Science*, Vol.322, No.5909, Dec 19, pp. 1845-1848

Cryderman, D.E.; Morris, E.J.; Biessmann, H.; Elgin, S.C. & Wallrath, L.L. (1999). Silencing at Drosophila telomeres: nuclear organization and chromatin structure play critical roles. *Embo J*, Vol.18, No.13, Jul 1, pp. 3724-3735

Czermin, B.; Melfi, R.; McCabe, D.; Seitz, V.; Imhof, A. & Pirrotta, V. (2002). Drosophila enhancer of Zeste/ESC complexes have a histone H3 methyltransferase activity that marks chromosomal Polycomb sites. *Cell*, Vol.111, No.2, Oct 18, pp. 185-196

Czech, B.; Malone C.D.; Zhou R.; Stark A.; Schlingeheyde C.; Dus M.; Perrimon N.; Kellis M.; Wohlschlegel J.A.; Sachidanandam R. et al. 2008. An endogenous small interfering RNA pathway in Drosophila. *Nature*, Vol.453, No.7196, Jun 5, pp. 798-802

d'Adda di Fagagna, F.; Teo, S.H. & Jackson, S.P. (2004). Functional links between telomeres and proteins of the DNA-damage response. *Genes Dev*, Vol.18, No.15, Aug 1, pp. 1781-1799

Danilevskaya, O.N.; Arkhipova, I.R.; Traverse, K.L. & Pardue, M.L. (1997). Promoting in tandem: the promoter for telomere transposon HeT-A and implications for the evolution of retroviral LTRs. *Cell*, Vol.88, No.5, Mar 7, pp. 647-655

Danilevskaya, O.N.; Traverse, K.L.; Hogan, N.C.; DeBaryshe, P.G. & Pardue, M.L. (1999). The two Drosophila telomeric transposable elements have very different patterns of transcription. *Mol Cell Biol*, Vol.19, No.1, Jan, pp. 873-881

de Lange, T. (2004). T-loops and the origin of telomeres. *Nat Rev Mol Cell Biol*, Vol.5, No.4, Apr, pp. 323-329

Elbashir, S.M.; Lendeckel, W. & Tuschl, T. (2001). RNA interference is mediated by 21- and 22-nucleotide RNAs. *Genes Dev*, Vol.15, No.2, Jan 15, pp. 188-200

Fanti, L.; Dorer, D.R.; Berloco, M.; Henikoff, S. & Pimpinelli, S. (1998). Heterochromatin protein 1 binds transgene arrays. *Chromosoma*, Vol.107, No.5, Nov, pp. 286-292

Frydrychova, R.C.; Biessmann, H.; Konev, A.Y.; Golubovsky, M.D.; Johnson, J.; Archer, T.K. & Mason, J.M. (2007). Transcriptional activity of the telomeric retrotransposon HeT-A in Drosophila melanogaster is stimulated as a consequence of subterminal deficiencies at homologous and nonhomologous telomeres. *Mol Cell Biol*, Vol.27, No.13, Jul, pp. 4991-5001

Frydrychova, R.C.; Mason, J.M. & Archer, T.K. (2008). HP1 is distributed within distinct chromatin domains at Drosophila telomeres. *Genetics*, Vol.180, No.1, Sep, pp. 121-131

Fuller, A.M.; Cook, E.G.; Kelley, K.J. & Pardue, M.L. (2010). Gag proteins of Drosophila telomeric retrotransposons: collaborative targeting to chromosome ends. *Genetics*, Vol.184, No.3, Mar, pp. 629-636

Gao, G.; Walser, J.C.; Beaucher, M.L.; Morciano, P.; Wesolowska, N.; Chen, J. & Rong, Y.S. (2010). HipHop interacts with HOAP and HP1 to protect Drosophila telomeres in a sequence-independent manner. *Embo J*, Vol.29, No.4, Feb 17, pp. 819-829

George, J.A. & Pardue, M.L. (2003). The promoter of the heterochromatic Drosophila telomeric retrotransposon, HeT-A, is active when moved into euchromatic locations. *Genetics*, Vol.163, No.2, Feb, pp. 625-635

George, J.A.; DeBaryshe, P.G.; Traverse, K.L.; Celniker, S.E. & Pardue, M.L. (2006). Genomic organization of the Drosophila telomere retrotransposable elements. *Genome Res*, Vol.16, No.10, Oct, pp. 1231-1240

Golubovsky, M.D.; Konev, A.Y.; Walter, M.F.; Biessmann, H. & Mason, J.M. (2001). Terminal retrotransposons activate a subtelomeric white transgene at the 2L telomere in Drosophila. *Genetics*, Vol.158, No.3, Jul, pp. 1111-1123

Ghildiyal, M.; Seitz H.; Horwich M.D.; Li C.; Du T.; Lee S.; Xu J.; Kittler E.L.; Zapp M.L.; Weng Z. et al. 2008. Endogenous siRNAs derived from transposons and mRNAs in Drosophila somatic cells. *Science*, Vol.320, No.5879, May 23, pp. 1077-1081

Goytisolo, F.A. & Blasco, M.A. (2002). Many ways to telomere dysfunction: in vivo studies using mouse models. *Oncogene*, Vol.21, No.4, Jan 21, pp. 584-591

Greider, C.W. & Blackburn, E.H. (1985). Identification of a specific telomere terminal transferase activity in Tetrahymena extracts. *Cell*, Vol.43, No.2 Pt 1, Dec, pp. 405-413

Gunawardane, L.S.; Saito, K.; Nishida, K.M.; Miyoshi, K.; Kawamura, Y.; Nagami, T.; Siomi, H. & Siomi, M.C. (2007). A slicer-mediated mechanism for repeat-associated siRNA 5' end formation in Drosophila. *Science*, Vol.315, No.5818, Mar 16, pp. 1587-1590

Hall, I.M.; Shankaranarayana, G.D.; Noma, K.; Ayoub, N.; Cohen, A. & Grewal, S.I. (2002). Establishment and maintenance of a heterochromatin domain. *Science*, Vol.297, No.5590, Sep 27, pp. 2232-2237

Hall, I.M.; Noma, K. & Grewal, S.I. (2003). RNA interference machinery regulates chromosome dynamics during mitosis and meiosis in fission yeast. *Proc Natl Acad Sci U S A*, Vol.100, No.1, Jan 7, pp. 193-198

Hamilton, A.; Voinnet, O.; Chappell, L. & Baulcombe, D. (2002). Two classes of short interfering RNA in RNA silencing. *Embo J*, Vol.21, No.17, Sep 2, pp. 4671-4679

Hansen, K.R.; Ibarra, P.T. & Thon, G. (2006). Evolutionary-conserved telomere-linked helicase genes of fission yeast are repressed by silencing factors, RNAi components and the telomere-binding protein Taz1. *Nucleic Acids Res*, Vol.34, No.1, pp. 78-88

Higashiyama, T.; Noutoshi, Y.; Fujie, M. & Yamada, T. (1997). Zepp, a LINE-like retrotransposon accumulated in the Chlorella telomeric region. *Embo J*, Vol.16, No.12, Jun 16, pp. 3715-3723

Jackson, D.A.; Iborra, F.J.; Manders, E.M. & Cook, P.R. (1998). Numbers and organization of RNA polymerases, nascent transcripts, and transcription units in HeLa nuclei. *Mol Biol Cell*, Vol.9, No.6, Jun, pp. 1523-1536

Jaco, I.; Munoz, P. & Blasco, M.A. (2004). Role of human Ku86 in telomere length maintenance and telomere capping. *Cancer Res*, Vol.64, No.20, Oct 15, pp. 7271-7278

Josse, T.; Teysset, L.; Todeschini, A.L.; Sidor, C.M.; Anxolabehere, D. & Ronsseray, S. (2007). Telomeric trans-silencing: an epigenetic repression combining RNA silencing and heterochromatin formation. *PLoS Genet*, Vol.3, No.9, Sep, pp. 1633-1643

Kahn, T.; Savitsky, M. & Georgiev, P. (2000). Attachment of HeT-A sequences to chromosomal termini in Drosophila melanogaster may occur by different mechanisms. *Mol Cell Biol*, Vol.20, No.20, Oct, pp. 7634-7642

Kalmykova, A.I.; Klenov, M.S. & Gvozdev, V.A. (2005). Argonaute protein PIWI controls mobilization of retrotransposons in the Drosophila male germline. *Nucleic Acids Res*, Vol.33, No.6, pp. 2052-2059

Kanoh, J.; Sadaie, M.; Urano, T. & Ishikawa, F. (2005). Telomere binding protein Taz1 establishes Swi6 heterochromatin independently of RNAi at telomeres. *Curr Biol*, Vol.15, No.20, Oct 25, pp. 1808-1819

Karpen, G.H. & Spradling, A.C. (1992). Analysis of subtelomeric heterochromatin in the Drosophila minichromosome Dp1187 by single P element insertional mutagenesis. *Genetics*, Vol.132, No.3, Nov, pp. 737-753

Kawamura, Y.; Saito, K.; Kin, T.; Ono, Y.; Asai, K.; Sunohara, T.; Okada, T.N.; Siomi, M.C. & Siomi, H. (2008). Drosophila endogenous small RNAs bind to Argonaute 2 in somatic cells. *Nature*, Vol.453, No.7196, Jun 5, pp. 793-797

Khurana, J.S.; Xu, J.; Weng, Z. & Theurkauf, W.E. (2010). Distinct functions for the Drosophila piRNA pathway in genome maintenance and telomere protection. *PLoS Genet*, Vol.6, No.12, pp. e1001246

Klattenhoff, C. & Theurkauf, W. (2008). Biogenesis and germline functions of piRNAs. *Development*, Vol.135, No.1, Jan, pp. 3-9

Klattenhoff, C.; Xi, H.; Li, C.; Lee, S.; Xu, J.; Khurana, J.S.; Zhang, F.; Schultz, N.; Koppetsch, B.S.; Nowosielska, A. et al. (2009). The Drosophila HP1 homolog Rhino is required for transposon silencing and piRNA production by dual-strand clusters. *Cell*, Vol.138, No.6, Sep 18, pp. 1137-1149

Klenov, M.S.; Lavrov, S.A.; Stolyarenko, A.D.; Ryazansky, S.S.; Aravin, A.A.; Tuschl, T. & Gvozdev, V.A. (2007). Repeat-associated siRNAs cause chromatin silencing of retrotransposons in the Drosophila melanogaster germline. *Nucleic Acids Res*, Vol.35, No.16, pp. 5430-5438

Kuramochi-Miyagawa, S.; Watanabe, T.; Gotoh, K.; Totoki, Y.; Toyoda, A.; Ikawa, M.; Asada, N.; Kojima, K.; Yamaguchi, Y.; Ijiri, T.W. et al. (2008). DNA methylation of retrotransposon genes is regulated by Piwi family members MILI and MIWI2 in murine fetal testes. *Genes Dev*, Vol.22, No.7, Apr 1, pp. 908-917

Levis, R.W. (1989). Viable deletions of a telomere from a Drosophila chromosome. *Cell*, Vol.58, No.4, Aug 25, pp. 791-801

Levis, R.W.; Ganesan, R.; Houtchens, K.; Tolar, L.A. & Sheen, F.M. (1993). Transposons in place of telomeric repeats at a Drosophila telomere. *Cell*, Vol.75, No.6, Dec 17, pp. 1083-1093

Li, C.; Vagin V.V.; Lee S.; Xu J.; Ma S.; Xi H.; Seitz H.; Horwich M.D.; Syrzycka M.; Honda B.M. et al. 2009. Collapse of germline piRNAs in the absence of Argonaute3 reveals somatic piRNAs in flies. *Cell*, Vol.137, No.3, May 1, pp. 509-521

Lim, A.K.; Tao, L. & Kai, T. (2009). piRNAs mediate posttranscriptional retroelement silencing and localization to pi-bodies in the Drosophila germline. *J Cell Biol*, Vol.186, No.3, Aug 10, pp. 333-342

Liu, Y.; Mochizuki, K. & Gorovsky, M.A. (2004). Histone H3 lysine 9 methylation is required for DNA elimination in developing macronuclei in Tetrahymena. *Proc Natl Acad Sci U S A*, Vol.101, No.6, Feb 10, pp. 1679-1684

Luan, D.D.; Korman, M.H.; Jakubczak, J.L. & Eickbush, T.H. (1993). Reverse transcription of R2Bm RNA is primed by a nick at the chromosomal target site: a mechanism for non-LTR retrotransposition. *Cell*, Vol.72, No.4, Feb 26, pp. 595-605

Malone, C.D.; Brennecke J.; Dus M.; Stark A.; McCombie W.R.; Sachidanandam R. & Hannon G.J. 2009. Specialized piRNA Pathways Act in Germline and Somatic Tissues of the Drosophila Ovary. *Cell*, May 1, pp. 522-535

Mason, J.M.; Konev, A.Y.; Golubovsky, M.D. & Biessmann, H. (2003). Cis- and trans-acting influences on telomeric position effect in Drosophila melanogaster detected with a subterminal transgene. *Genetics*, Vol.163, No.3, Mar, pp. 917-930

Maxwell, P.H.; Belote, J.M. & Levis, R.W. (2006). Identification of multiple transcription initiation, polyadenylation, and splice sites in the Drosophila melanogaster TART family of telomeric retrotransposons. *Nucleic Acids Res*, Vol.34, No.19, pp. 5498-5507

Melnikova, L. & Georgiev, P. (2002). Enhancer of terminal gene conversion, a new mutation in Drosophila melanogaster that induces telomere elongation by gene conversion. *Genetics*, Vol.162, No.3, Nov, pp. 1301-1312

Melnikova, L.; Biessmann, H. & Georgiev, P. (2004). The vicinity of a broken chromosome end affects P element mobilization in Drosophila melanogaster. *Mol Genet Genomics*, Vol.272, No.5, Dec, pp. 512-518

Melnikova, L.; Biessmann, H. & Georgiev, P. (2005). The Ku protein complex is involved in length regulation of Drosophila telomeres. *Genetics*, Vol.170, No.1, May, pp. 221-235

Mikhailovsky, S.; Belenkaya, T. & Georgiev, P. (1999). Broken chromosomal ends can be elongated by conversion in Drosophila melanogaster. *Chromosoma*, Vol.108, No.2, May, pp. 114-120

Mochizuki, K. & Gorovsky, M.A. (2005). A Dicer-like protein in Tetrahymena has distinct functions in genome rearrangement, chromosome segregation, and meiotic prophase. *Genes Dev*, Vol.19, No.1, Jan 1, pp. 77-89

Myung, K.; Ghosh, G.; Fattah, F.J.; Li, G.; Kim, H.; Dutia, A.; Pak, E.; Smith, S. & Hendrickson, E.A. (2004). Regulation of telomere length and suppression of genomic instability in human somatic cells by Ku86. *Mol Cell Biol*, Vol.24, No.11, Jun, pp. 5050-5059

Nugent, C.I. & Lundblad, V. (1998). The telomerase reverse transcriptase: components and regulation. *Genes Dev*, Vol.12, No.8, Apr 15, pp. 1073-1085

Oikemus, S.R.; McGinnis, N.; Queiroz-Machado, J.; Tukachinsky, H.; Takada, S.; Sunkel, C.E. & Brodsky, M.H. (2004). Drosophila atm/telomere fusion is required for telomeric localization of HP1 and telomere position effect. *Genes Dev*, Vol.18, No.15, Aug 1, pp. 1850-1861

Okazaki, S.; Ishikawa, H. & Fujiwara, H. (1995). Structural analysis of TRAS1, a novel family of telomeric repeat-associated retrotransposons in the silkworm, Bombyx mori. *Mol Cell Biol*, Vol.15, No.8, Aug, pp. 4545-4552

Olovnikov, A.M. (1971). [Principle of marginotomy in template synthesis of polynucleotides]. *Dokl Akad Nauk SSSR*, Vol.201, No.6, pp. 1496-1499

Olovnikov, A.M. (1973). A theory of marginotomy. The incomplete copying of template margin in enzymic synthesis of polynucleotides and biological significance of the phenomenon. *J Theor Biol*, Vol.41, No.1, Sep 14, pp. 181-190

Osanai, M.; Kojima, K.K.; Futahashi, R.; Yaguchi, S. & Fujiwara, H. (2006). Identification and characterization of the telomerase reverse transcriptase of Bombyx mori (silkworm) and Tribolium castaneum (flour beetle). *Gene*, Vol.376, No.2, Jul 19, pp. 281-289

Palm, W. & de Lange, T. (2008). How shelterin protects mammalian telomeres. *Annu Rev Genet*, Vol.42, pp. 301-334

Pane, A.; Wehr K. & Schupbach T. 2007. zucchini and squash encode two putative nucleases required for rasiRNA production in the Drosophila germline. *Dev Cell*, Vol.12, No.6, Jun, pp. 851-862

Perrini, B.; Piacentini, L.; Fanti, L.; Altieri, F.; Chichiarelli, S.; Berloco, M.; Turano, C.; Ferraro, A. & Pimpinelli, S. (2004). HP1 controls telomere capping, telomere elongation, and telomere silencing by two different mechanisms in Drosophila. *Mol Cell*, Vol.15, No.3, Aug 13, pp. 467-476

Raffa, G.D.; Cenci, G.; Siriaco, G.; Goldberg, M.L. & Gatti, M. (2005). The putative Drosophila transcription factor woc is required to prevent telomeric fusions. *Mol Cell*, Vol.20, No.6, Dec 22, pp. 821-831

Raffa, G.D.; Siriaco, G.; Cugusi, S.; Ciapponi, L.; Cenci, G.; Wojcik, E. & Gatti, M. (2009). The Drosophila modigliani (moi) gene encodes a HOAP-interacting protein required for telomere protection. *Proc Natl Acad Sci U S A*, Vol.106, No.7, Feb 17, pp. 2271-2276

Raffa, G.D.; Raimondo, D.; Sorino, C.; Cugusi, S.; Cenci, G.; Cacchione, S.; Gatti, M. & Ciapponi, L. (2010). Verrocchio, a Drosophila OB fold-containing protein, is a component of the terminin telomere-capping complex. *Genes Dev*, Vol.24, No.15, Aug 1, pp. 1596-1601

Rangan, P.; Malone, C.D.; Navarro, C.; Newbold, S.P.; Hayes, P.S.; Sachidanandam, R.; Hannon, G.J. & Lehmann, R. (2011). piRNA Production Requires Heterochromatin Formation in Drosophila. *Curr Biol*, Vol.21, No.16, Aug 23, pp. 1373-1379

Rashkova, S.; Karam, S.E.; Kellum, R. & Pardue, M.L. (2002). Gag proteins of the two Drosophila telomeric retrotransposons are targeted to chromosome ends. *J Cell Biol*, Vol.159, No.3, Nov 11, pp. 397-402

Rashkova, S.; Athanasiadis, A. & Pardue, M.L. (2003). Intracellular targeting of Gag proteins of the Drosophila telomeric retrotransposons. *J Virol*, Vol.77, No.11, Jun, pp. 6376-6384

Ronsseray, S.; Josse, T.; Boivin, A. & Anxolabehere, D. (2003). Telomeric transgenes and trans-silencing in Drosophila. *Genetica*, Vol.117, No.2-3, Mar, pp. 327-335

Saito, K.; Nishida, K.M.; Mori, T.; Kawamura, Y.; Miyoshi, K.; Nagami, T.; Siomi, H. & Siomi, M.C. (2006). Specific association of Piwi with rasiRNAs derived from retrotransposon and heterochromatic regions in the Drosophila genome. *Genes Dev*, Vol.20, No.16, Aug 15, pp. 2214-2222

Sarot, E.; Payen-Groschene G.; Bucheton A. & Pelisson A. 2004. Evidence for a piwi-dependent RNA silencing of the gypsy endogenous retrovirus by the Drosophila melanogaster flamenco gene. *Genetics*, Vol.166, No.3, Mar, pp. 1313-1321

Savitsky, M.; Kravchuk, O.; Melnikova, L. & Georgiev, P. (2002). Heterochromatin protein 1 is involved in control of telomere elongation in Drosophila melanogaster. *Mol Cell Biol*, Vol.22, No.9, May, pp. 3204-3218

Savitsky, M.; Kwon, D.; Georgiev, P.; Kalmykova, A. & Gvozdev, V. (2006). Telomere elongation is under the control of the RNAi-based mechanism in the Drosophila germline. *Genes Dev*, Vol.20, No.3, Feb 1, pp. 345-354

Schoeftner, S. & Blasco, M.A. (2009). A 'higher order' of telomere regulation: telomere heterochromatin and telomeric RNAs. *Embo J*, Vol.28, No.16, Aug 19, pp. 2323-2336

Sheen, F.M. & Levis, R.W. (1994). Transposition of the LINE-like retrotransposon TART to Drosophila chromosome termini. *Proc Natl Acad Sci U S A*, Vol.91, No.26, Dec 20, pp. 12510-12514

Shpiz, S.; Kwon, D.; Uneva, A.; Kim, M.; Klenov, M.; Rozovsky, Y.; Georgiev, P.; Savitsky, M. & Kalmykova, A. (2007). Characterization of Drosophila telomeric retroelement TAHRE: transcription, transpositions, and RNAi-based regulation of expression. *Mol Biol Evol*, Vol.24, No.11, Nov, pp. 2535-2545

Shpiz, S.; Kwon, D.; Rozovsky, Y. & Kalmykova, A. (2009). rasiRNA pathway controls antisense expression of Drosophila telomeric retrotransposons in the nucleus. *Nucleic Acids Res*, Vol.37, No.1, Jan, pp. 268-278

Shpiz, S.; Olovnikov, I.; Sergeeva, A.; Lavrov, S.; Abramov, Y.; Savitsky, M. & Kalmykova, A. (2011). Mechanism of the piRNA-mediated silencing of Drosophila telomeric retrotransposons. *Nucleic Acids Res*, Vol.39, No.20, Nov 1, pp. 8703-8711

Silva, E.; Tiong, S.; Pedersen, M.; Homola, E.; Royou, A.; Fasulo, B.; Siriaco, G. & Campbell, S.D. (2004). ATM is required for telomere maintenance and chromosome stability during Drosophila development. *Curr Biol*, Vol.14, No.15, Aug 10, pp. 1341-1347

Siriaco, G.M.; Cenci, G.; Haoudi, A.; Champion, L.E.; Zhou, C.; Gatti, M. & Mason, J.M. (2002). Telomere elongation (Tel), a new mutation in Drosophila melanogaster that produces long telomeres. *Genetics*, Vol.160, No.1, Jan, pp. 235-245

Smogorzewska, A. & de Lange, T. (2004). Regulation of telomerase by telomeric proteins. *Annu Rev Biochem*, Vol.73, pp. 177-208

Song, K.; Jung, D.; Jung, Y.; Lee, S.G. & Lee, I. (2000). Interaction of human Ku70 with TRF2. *FEBS Lett*, Vol.481, No.1, Sep 8, pp. 81-85

Song, Y.H.; Mirey, G.; Betson, M.; Haber, D.A. & Settleman, J. (2004). The Drosophila ATM ortholog, dATM, mediates the response to ionizing radiation and to spontaneous DNA damage during development. *Curr Biol*, Vol.14, No.15, Aug 10, pp. 1354-1359

Sugiyama, T.; Cam, H.; Verdel, A.; Moazed, D. & Grewal, S.I. (2005). RNA-dependent RNA polymerase is an essential component of a self-enforcing loop coupling heterochromatin assembly to siRNA production. *Proc Natl Acad Sci U S A*, Vol.102, No.1, Jan 4, pp. 152-157

Sugiyama, T.; Cam, H.P.; Sugiyama, R.; Noma, K.; Zofall, M.; Kobayashi, R. & Grewal, S.I. (2007). SHREC, an effector complex for heterochromatic transcriptional silencing. *Cell*, Vol.128, No.3, Feb 9, pp. 491-504

Takahashi, H.; Okazaki, S. & Fujiwara, H. (1997). A new family of site-specific retrotransposons, SART1, is inserted into telomeric repeats of the silkworm, Bombyx mori. *Nucleic Acids Res*, Vol.25, No.8, Apr 15, pp. 1578-1584

Todeschini, A.L.; Teysset, L.; Delmarre, V. & Ronsseray, S. (2010). The epigenetic trans-silencing effect in Drosophila involves maternally-transmitted small RNAs whose production depends on the piRNA pathway and HP1. *PLoS ONE*, Vol.5, No.6, pp. e11032

Torok, T.; Benitez, C.; Takacs, S. & Biessmann, H. (2007). The protein encoded by the gene proliferation disrupter (prod) is associated with the telomeric retrotransposon array in Drosophila melanogaster. *Chromosoma*, Vol.116, No.2, Apr, pp. 185-195

Vagin, V.V.; Klenov, M.S.; Kalmykova, A.I.; Stolyarenko, A.D.; Kotelnikov, R.N. & Gvozdev, V.A. (2004). The RNA interference proteins and vasa locus are involved in the silencing of retrotransposons in the female germline of Drosophila melanogaster. *RNA Biol*, Vol.1, No.1, May, pp. 54-58

Vagin, V.V.; Sigova, A.; Li, C.; Seitz, H.; Gvozdev, V. & Zamore, P.D. (2006). A distinct small RNA pathway silences selfish genetic elements in the germline. *Science*, Vol.313, No.5785, Jul 21, pp. 320-324

Villasante, A.; Abad, J.P.; Planello, R.; Mendez-Lago, M.; Celniker, S.E. & de Pablos, B. (2007). Drosophila telomeric retrotransposons derived from an ancestral element that was recruited to replace telomerase. *Genome Res*, Vol.17, No.12, Dec, pp. 1909-1918

Volpe, T.A.; Kidner, C.; Hall, I.M.; Teng, G.; Grewal, S.I. & Martienssen, R.A. (2002). Regulation of heterochromatic silencing and histone H3 lysine-9 methylation by RNAi. *Science*, Vol.297, No.5588, Sep 13, pp. 1833-1837

Wallrath, L.L. & Elgin, S.C. (1995). Position effect variegation in Drosophila is associated with an altered chromatin structure. *Genes Dev*, Vol.9, No.10, May 15, pp. 1263-1277

Yin, H. & Lin, H. (2007). An epigenetic activation role of Piwi and a Piwi-associated piRNA in Drosophila melanogaster. *Nature*, Vol.450, No.7167, Nov 8, pp. 304-308

3

The Regulation of Telomerase by Alternative Splicing of TERT

Jiří Nehyba, Radmila Hrdličková and Henry R. Bose, Jr.
University of Texas at Austin
USA

1. Introduction

1.1 Telomerase canonical function

Telomeric DNA consists of tandem oligonucleotide repeats that serve to protect ends of linear eukaryotic chromosomes against chromosome end-to-end fusion. The sequence of the repeat differs among distinct groups of eukaryotes and, with the exception of several Fungi species, is usually 5 to 8 nucleotides-long (Gomes et al., 2010; Watson & Riha, 2010). Since DNA polymerase cannot replicate the ends of linear chromosomes, chromosomal end shorten after each cell cycle in the absence of telomerase (Olovnikov, 1971; Watson, 1972). This gradual loss of telomeric repeats limits the potential lifespan of cells since cells with critically short telomeres undergo senescence (Bodnar et al., 1998). Rapidly proliferating cells activate the telomerase to synthesize telomeric DNA repeats in order to protect telomeres from shortening as a result of DNA replication and oxidative damage (Cech, 2004; Osterhage & Friedman, 2009; von Zglinicki, 2002). Telomerase is a multisubunit enzymatic ribonucleoprotein complex consisting of the telomerase reverse transcriptase (TERT), the telomerase RNA subunit (TR or TERC) which acts as the template, as well as other associated proteins (Blackburn & Collins, 2011).

1.1.1 Domain structure of TERT and TR

Ciliate, yeast, plant and vertebrate TERT protein contains four conserved domains, the telomerase essential N-terminal (TEN) domain, the telomerase RNA binding domain (TRBD), the reverse transcriptase (RT), and the C-terminal extension (CTE) domains (for reviews see (Blackburn & Collins, 2011; Mason et al., 2011; Podlevsky & Chen, 2012; Sekaran et al., 2010; Wyatt et al., 2010)). In vertebrates and plants the TEN and TRBD domains are connected by a linker of variable length which may have a conformational function as a hinge. Certain species apparently lost some of the TERT domains during their evolution. Insect species lack the TEN domain, and nematodes the CTE domain. Each of the TERT domains contain several important conserved motifs which are engaged in the formation of tertiary structures that permit the binding of the telomeric template and telomerase RNA subunit. The TEN domain contains 'anchor' sites which bind single-stranded DNA and also the RNA interacting domain 1 (RID1) which binds to TR with low affinity. The TRBD domain contains RNA interacting domain 2 (RID2) which has a high affinity for TR. The RT domain contains seven motifs conserved between all conventional RTs (1, 2, A, B, C, D, and E). The TERT polymerase active sites are formed by three conserved aspartic acids, with one located in motif A and two in motif C. The CTE domain binds telomeric DNA and contributes to stabilization of the RNA-DNA heteroduplex in the active site of the enzyme. Crystallographic studies reveal a tertiary structure of core TERT protein which resembles a right hand (Gillis et al., 2008). The protein is folded into a ring shaped structure by interactions between the N- and C-terminal domains. The telomerase primer (telomeric DNA) and template are positioned in the center of this ring.

TR is the RNA component of the telomerase holoenzyme and serves as the template for extension. In contrast to the TERT gene, TR is much less conserved during evolution and its size ranges from 300 to 2200 nucleotides. However, several TR domains are essential for its function and their general plan is conserved. The TR molecules of most species contain the pseudoknot/template core domain and the trans-activating domain (CR4/CR5) which are necessary and sufficient for telomerase enzymatic activity *in vitro* and *in vivo*. Moreover, vertebrate TR contains a box H/ACA domain at the 3′ end, which binds two copies of the protein complexes formed from dyskerin, NOP10, NHP2 and GAR1 proteins that are important for biogenesis, localization, transport and stability of the functional RNA molecule. In the 3′ stem-loop of the H/ACA domain is the Cajal body localization sequence (CAB) for binding the Cajal body protein 1 (TCAB1).

Telomerase biogenesis begins with TERT mRNA transcription, maturation and translation. The TERT protein is trafficked from the cytoplasm to nucleoli and then to Cajal bodies for assembly with TR and other proteins of the telomerase complex. The TR precursor is transcribed, bound in the nucleus by accessory proteins which perform the processing and internal modifications of the RNA molecule. The binding of the TCAB1 protein facilitates transport of the mature TR to Cajal bodies where it is assembled with TERT protein into the functional telomerase ribonucleoprotein complex. At least two chaperone proteins (hsp90 and p23) are added before the telomerase complex can be localized to telomere ends.

1.1.2 Telomerase enzymatic function

The telomerase complex is a specialized reverse transcriptase with the ability to produce a long track of telomeric DNA repeats using a short RNA template provided by the TR subunit. This repetitive addition processivity contrasts with the prototypical RT which copies large RNA genomes into DNA. The telomerase catalytic cycle has two phases: nucleotide addition to the 3' end of the telomeric DNA primer and the template translocation for the synthesis of additional repeats. The translocation involves realignment of the RNA template to the new DNA 3′ end (Lewis & Wuttke, 2012; Podlevsky & Chen, 2012). Vertebrate telomerases add six nucleotides (5′-GGTTAG-3′) at the end of the DNA primer. The base-pair binding between the 3′ region of the TR template and 3′ end of the DNA primer is dependent on template length and the presence of several DNA-binding motifs in the TERT molecules. Mutations in these TR and TERT motifs (in motifs 3, 'insertion in fingers' domain (IFD) in the RT domain as well as TEN and CTE domains) alter the rate and processivity of the telomerase reaction (Autexier & Lue, 2006; Christodoulou et al., 2010; Podlevsky & Chen, 2012; Xie et al., 2010). Moreover, POT1 (protection of telomeres 1) and TPP1 (TIN2 and POT1-interacting protein 1), which are components of the telomere DNA-binding protein complex, shelterin, also enhance repeat addition processivity (Latrick & Cech, 2010; Wang, 2007).

1.1.3 Diseases associated with telomere shortening

The regulation of telomere length is the sum of two balanced processes - telomere erosion and telomere synthesis. Therefore, both accelerated telomere shortening and insufficient telomerase function can erode telomeres. Insufficient telomerase function has been implicated in several diseases that are referred to as syndromes of telomere shortening (for reviews (Armanios, 2009; 2012)). Mutations responsible for these conditions were mapped to several components of the telomerase complex (hTERT, hTR, dyskerin, NOP10, NHP2, and TCAB1). Moreover, it was recently described that mutations in the shelterin component, TINF2, and and in conserved telomere maintenance component 1, CTC1, are also implicated in the pathogenesis of one of these diseases (Alter et al., 2012; Keller et al., 2012). Most of these mutations compromise catalytic activity and alter processivity of the telomerase complex that eventually result in telomere shortening. However, the specific mechanism of some remains unknown (Robart & Collins, 2010).

Telomere shortening may manifest in several different diseases depending on the severity of the defect. Dyskeratosis congenita (DC) disease has the X-linked form known to be associated with mutations in dyskerin (Nelson & Bertuch, 2012). Several autosomal forms of DC are associated with mutations in hTERT, hTR and other components of the telomerase ribonucleoprotein complex as well as in TINF2 and CTC1 (Armanios, 2009; Keller et al., 2012; Nelson & Bertuch, 2012; Walne et al., 2012). Patients with DC suffer from abnormal skin pigmentation, nail dystrophy, and oral mucosal leukoplakia. The disease causes premature death as a result of aplastic anemia due to bone marrow failure. Idiopathic pulmonary fibrosis (IPS) is another disease which strongly correlates with telomere shortening due to mutations in telomerase components (Armanios, 2012). This disease has a much higher prevalence than DC and causes a progressive, severe degeneration of lung tissue that leads to respiratory failure. Additionally, several other syndromes were linked to short telomeres, including liver disease and type 2 diabetes (Armanios, 2012; Salpea et al., 2010; Zee et al., 2010). Many of these syndromes occur in different combinations, dependent on the type of mutations, time of disease onset and interaction with environmental factors. DC and other patients with telomere shortening syndromes are more prone to develop three forms of cancer: myelodysplastic syndrome, acute myeloid leukemia and chronic lymphocytic leukemia. Shortened telomeres are implicated in the development of other neoplasias, including lung, pancreatic, and glioma cancers (Baird, 2010). The shortening of telomeres to critical levels increases the risk of chromosomal instability which, in turn, leads to re-arrangements and the acquisition of new oncogenic mutations.

The length of telomeres is in part inherited (Chiang et al., 2010; Jeanclos et al., 2000; Kappei & Londoño-Vallejo, 2008; Nawrot et al., 2004; Njajou et al., 2007; Nordfjäll et al., 2005; Slagboom et al., 1994). However, many environmental factors, especially those related to lifestyle, also have a strong impact (Lin et al., 2012). These include chronic psychological stress, diet, uptake of food, vitamins, aerobic exercise, and obesity. All these factors strongly correlate with telomere length. Other environmental factors, such as smoking, were shown to interact with genetic predispositions in determining the age of onset of diseases of shortened telomeres as has been demonstrated for emphysema (Armanios, 2012).

1.2 Telomerase non-canonical function

In addition to telomere DNA synthesis, there is an accumulating body of evidence which indicates that telomerase has additional activities (Majerská et al., 2011; Parkinson et al., 2008). These non-canonical activities include stimulation of cell proliferation, protection against oxidative damage, inhibition of apoptosis, modulation of global gene expression, activation of stem cells, and tumor promotion (Bollmann, 2008; Cong & Shay, 2008). Some of these functions, such as the protection of mitochondria against oxidative stress, and modulation of the DNA damage response, require the enzymatic activity of TERT. On the other hand, stimulation of proliferation, inhibition of apoptosis and the regulation of gene expression are independent of TERT enzymatic activity. The cell proliferation and anti-apoptotic functions may be mediated by TERT's ability to induce the expression of genes that promote cell proliferation while simultaneously suppressing pro-apoptotic genes (Smith et al., 2003). TERT promotes the proliferation of hair follicle stem cells in the absence of the TR subunit, providing compelling evidence that this function is independent of telomerase canonical function (Sarin et al., 2005). Interestingly, TERT interacts with the chromatin remodeling factor, BRG1, and as a component of a TCF/β-catenin transcription complex, binds to promoters of Wnt target genes and activates their transcription (Park et al., 2009). The catalytic activity of TERT for Wnt activation is also not required.

1.3 Telomerase transcriptional regulation

Telomerase is downregulated during development in most somatic tissues. Telomerase activity may be reactivated during the immune response and also during tumorigenesis. Several experiments in which the expression profile of a reporter gene under control of the hTERT promoter in transgenic mice simulated the specific expression profile of telomerase activity in human tissues demonstrated that transcriptional regulation of TERT plays a key role in the regulation of telomerase activity (Horikawa et al., 2005; Ritz et al., 2005). The TERT promoter is regulated by several transcription factors (for reviews see (Cifuentes-Rojas & Shippen, 2012; Zhu et al., 2010)). Human as well as the TERT promoter of many other vertebrates contains E-boxes, which are bound by the transcription factor c-Myc which activates TERT transcription. In the proximal human promoter there are also binding sites for other activators such as AP-1, HIF-1 (hypoxia-inducible factor 1), SP1, Ets, E2Fs, NF-κB, PAX-5, and IRF-4 (Interferon regulatory factor 4). Distal promoter elements contain estrogen receptor binding sites which are responsible for the activation of TERT transcription by sex hormones. The repression of the TERT promoter is primarily mediated by competition of USF1 (upstream stimulatory factor 1) and Mad1 with c-Myc for E-boxes. Other repressors of TERT activation are WT1 (Wilms tumor protein 1), Smad3, p53 and MZF2 (myeloid zinc finger protein 2).

Epigenetic regulation of the human *TERT* locus through chromatin modifications may preclude binding of transcriptional activators and repressors to their respective cis sites (Gladych et al., 2011; Zhu et al., 2010). The *hTERT* locus is located in a chromosomal domain (at least 100 kb) which normally has a condensed chromatin structure in most somatic cells (Wang & Zhu, 2004). Only after acetyltransferases modify histone proteins to facilitate the relaxation of the *hTERT* locus may transcription factors actively bind the *TERT* locus and regulate TERT transcription. Histone methylation also plays a role in the activation of TERT since one histone methyltransferase, SMYD3, has been shown to activate TERT transcription in tumor cells by methylation of histone H3 at lysine 4 (Liu et al., 2007). In addition to histone modifications, CpG methylation and demethylation also play an important role in the transcriptional regulation of TERT. Demethylation of the *hTERT* locus in telomerase-positive cell lines results in a decrease in telomerase activity. CpG methylation in these cell lines is thought to block telomerase repressors from accessing the TERT promoter (Guilleret & Benhattar, 2003). On the other hand, methylation in other cell lines results in transcriptional silencing suggesting that the effect of CpG methylation on hTERT expression is cell type-specific (Devereux et al., 1999).

1.4 Alternative splicing of TERT

Alternative splicing is a common mechanism that increases the transcriptome complexity in higher eukaryotes. Alternatively spliced variants of TERT are abundant and have been cloned from many vertebrate and plant species (Sýkorová & Fajkus, 2009). However, in depth analysis of their expression, evolution and function is limited. The human TERT gene is expressed principally as alternatively spliced (AS) forms in both normal cells and tumor cells (Hisatomi et al., 2003; Hrdličková et al., 2012a; Saebøe-Larssen et al., 2006; Ulaner et al., 1998; Ulaner et al., 2001; Ulaner et al., 2000; Wick et al., 1999). The chicken is the only other species in which alternative splicing of TERT has been extensively characterized and a large number of AS variants have been identified (Amor et al., 2010; Chang & Delany, 2006; Hrdličková et al., 2012a; Hrdličková et al., 2006).

AS TERT variants can be divided into two groups - the first group retains the original open reading frame (ORF), while the second group of transcripts contains premature termination codons (PTCs). The AS variants which maintain the original ORF have the potential to be translated into functional proteins and contribute to proteome diversification (Nilsen & Graveley, 2010). A frequent human AS variant with a small deletion in the reverse transcriptase (RT) domain retains the original TERT ORF, lacks telomerase activity and has been proposed to function as a dominant-negative mutant (Colgin et al., 2000; Yi et al., 2000). Recently, we have described another abundantly expressed human AS variant, which maintains the original TERT ORF, but has deleted exons 4 through 13 (Hrdličková et al., 2012a). This variant also lacks telomerase activity, but in contrast to the dominant-negative variant retains the ability to stimulate cell proliferation. Similarly, two frequently expressed chicken variants that maintain an original TERT ORF stimulated cell proliferation in the absence or reduction of telomerase activity. We also isolated an AS TERT variant similar to one of these chicken variants from platypus, suggesting that this specific splicing event has been conserved during evolution (Hrdličková et al., 2012b). In contrast to the AS variants which can be translated into protein, the AS variants with PTCs are predicted to be degraded by nonsense mediated decay (NMD) during the first round of translation (Lewis et al., 2003). Nevertheless, two-thirds of the human and chicken AS TERT variants are spliced out-of frame and expressed at levels similar to AS variants that retain an original ORF. These observations suggest that at least some of these TERT AS variants escape NMD and may provide an important though unrecognized function. In conclusion, the alternative splicing of TERT mRNA transcripts is a mechanism which decreases the level of telomerase activity, however, AS TERT variants may retain at least some of the non-canonical functions of TERT.

1.5 Telomerase regulation in different species

Telomerase activity is downregulated in adult tissues of most vertebrates. However, the levels of repression differ among vertebrate species. There are large differences in telomerase activity between cold-blooded fish and amphibians, and warm-blooded mammals and birds. The expression of TERT in all adult organs of fish and frogs remains at high levels through their lifespan (Bousman et al., 2003; Hartmann et al., 2009; Pfennig et al., 2008; Yap et al., 2005). By contrast, in most mammalian and avian adult organs, the expression of TERT is severely repressed (Greenberg et al., 1998; Kim et al., 1994; Prowse & Greider, 1995; Taylor & Delany, 2000). Early studies suggested that even among mammals there are significant differences in telomerase levels in adult tissues (Gomes et al., 2010; Greenberg et al., 1998; Prowse & Greider, 1995). In rodents telomerase activity inversely correlates with body mass (Gorbunova & Seluanov, 2009). Recently, an exhaustive analysis of telomerase activity and telomere length in mammals has been reported (Gomes et al., 2011). This analysis revealed striking differences among major mammalian groups. High telomerase activity tends to correlate with low body mass extending the previous observation in rodents. However, whether similar differences in telomerase activity are present in avian species and the mechanism leading to these differences remains unknown.

1.6 Telomerase regulation in chicken and quail

The goal of this analysis was to determine whether differences in telomerase activity also exist in birds, an independently evolved warm-blooded branch of vertebrates, and to explore if TERT transcription or alternative splicing of TERT may account for these differences. We took advantage of two closely related avian species, the quail (*Coturnix japonica*) and chicken (*Gallus gallus*) from the Galliformes order, which differ substantially in their body mass, in their lifespan, and time when they reach reproductive maturity. Quail is a small bird (0.09 kg) with a lifespan between 2-3 years. By contrast, the closely related chicken is on average 10 times larger and can reach 15 and 20 years (30 years maximum). We expected that the TERT genes of these species would encode highly related proteins, but that quail and chicken cells would express different levels of telomerase activity. We cloned both the quail and chicken TERT genes and their AS variants, determined the steady-state levels of TERT transcripts, the patterns of alternative splicing, and correlated it with telomerase activity in various tissues in these two species. We also isolated a partial TERT clone of a more distantly related species, the duck, and performed a similar analysis. Body mass and lifespan (1-1.4 kg, 10-15 years, 29 maximum) of ducks resemble chicken more closely than quail. Therefore, including this species in analysis allows the correlations possibly drawn from comparison of quail and chicken to be extended.

The results of this analysis revealed that despite a high degree of similarity between the quail and chicken TERT gene (94% of identity), these genes differ greatly in their expression of alternatively spliced forms. In contrast to chicken and duck TERT, where 37 and 10 AS variants were identified, respectively, only three quail AS variants were detected. All three of the quail TERT variants were also present in chicken tissues, consistent with their close evolutionary origin. While the total levels of all TERT transcripts in quail organs were similar to levels in chicken or duck cells, quail tissues principally express full-length TERT transcripts. By contrast, in the chicken and duck, most of the TERT transcripts are alternatively spliced. At least some of the differences in the frequency of the AS variants between chicken and quail were determined by different splicing sequences in the TERT locus. The frequency and complexity of AS variants of TERT correlated with telomerase activity in quail and chicken cells. The lower frequency of TERT AS variants in quail tissues relative to the frequency in chicken and duck tissues was associated with a significantly (5×) higher levels of telomerase activity. Interestingly, these differences in telomerase activity were also discernible in early embryonic tissues. Telomerase activity is downregulated approximately 1,000 times in adult organs of all three species but remains significantly higher in quail. In addition, *in vitro* analysis of embryonic fibroblasts demonstrated that while quail retain high levels of telomerase activity and telomere length, chicken and duck cells rapidly repressed telomerase levels and their telomeres shorten during cell replication. Quail embryonic fibroblasts are at least three times more sensitive to oxidative stress than chicken and duck cells suggesting that relatively high telomerase levels may compensate for this deficiency. In conclusion, the results of these studies suggest a role for the regulation of TERT through alternative splicing as one of mechanisms for determining interspecies differences in telomerase activity.

2. Material and methods

2.1 Cloning of quail TERT and its variants

The chicken TERT (chTERT) gene was cloned previously (Delany & Daniels, 2004; Hrdličková et al., 2006). The quail and duck TERT genes (qTERT and dTERT) were cloned using cDNA obtained from 8 and 12 day-old quail and duck embryos using sets of primers against chicken TERT. Quail genomic sequences were cloned by PCR from genomic DNA of QT6 cells.

2.2 GenBank accession numbers

Newly determined nucleotide sequences were deposited in GenBank (DQ681292 [quail TERT intronic sequences], DQ681293 [duck TERT cDNA], DQ681294 [quail TERT cDNA], JF896279, DQ681295 to DQ681313 [alternatively spliced forms of quail, chicken and duck TERT]).

2.3 Sequence analysis

The full ORF sequence of quail (*Coturnix japonica*) TERT and partial sequence of duck (*Anas platyrhynchos*) TERT were determined in the course of these studies. The TERT protein sequences of chicken (*Gallus gallus* - NP_001026178.1) and Muscovy duck (*Cairina moschata* - ABO65149.1) were retrieved from GenBank. TERT sequences of turkey (*Meleagris gallopavo* - ENSMGAP00000007237), zebra finch *(Taeniopygia guttata* - ENSTGUP00000008676), and green anole (*Anolis carolinensis* - ENSACAP00000001407) were obtained from the Ensembl database (www.ensembl.org). Ensembl models were checked against genomic DNA sequence and minor modifications were introduced where the models did not conform to the evolutionary conserved exon-intron structure of the vertebrate TERT genes. Sequence homology (percentage of identical and similar amino acids) was determined using GeneDoc computer program (http://www.nrbsc.org/gfx/genedoc/). Amino acid similarity was calculated based on BLOSUM62 matrix. Protein sequence alignments were constructed by the ClustalX program (Larkin et al., 2007). All columns containing either gap or unidentified amino acid were removed using Gapstreeze tool (Los Alamos HIV Sequence Database; http://www.hiv.lanl.gov/content/sequence/GAPSTREEZE/gap.html). Evolutionary trees were constructed by Bayesian inference phylogenetic method performed by MrBayes 3.1.2 program using fixed-rate amino acid substitution model Jones (Ronquist & Huelsenbeck, 2003). Two Bayesian analyses each consisting of four Metropolis-coupled Markov chains Monte Carlo were run in parallel for 200,000 generations and sampled every 100th generation. Convergence of both analyses was assessed using a plot of the generations versus the log probability of the data. The consensus tree was created with burn-in value set to 500. The tree was plotted by the tree-drawing program Dendroscope (Huson et al., 2007).

2.4 Animals, cell lines, and tissue culture

Quail (*Coturnix japonica*) embryonated eggs and birds were obtained from University of Texas, Austin. Embryonated duck eggs (Khaki Campbell) were obtained from McMurray hatchery (Webster City, IA). Embryonated eggs from pathogen-free White Leghorn chickens (the SPF-SC strain) were obtained from Charles River SPAFAS, North Franklin, CT. Adult chickens and a Peking duck were obtained from a local vendor. Quail, chicken, and duck embryonic fibroblasts (QEF, CEF, and DEF) were prepared from 8, 10, and 12 day-old embryos, respectively. Tissue culture procedures were carried out as described previously (Hrdličková et al., 2006). QT6 is a quail sarcoma cell line (Moscovici et al., 1977). The duck embryonic cell line (DCL) was obtained from ATCC (ATCC Number: CCL-141) (Marcovici & Prier, 1968).

2.5 Telomere Repeat Amplification Protocol (TRAP)

The level of telomerase activity was evaluated using the TRAP assay as described previously (Hrdličková et al., 2006). Briefly, cells were extracted with CHAPS buffer and protein concentrations were determined by the Bradford method with Bio-Rad Protein Assay Reagent (Bio-Rad Laboratories, Hercules, CA). Protein extracts (20 µg of total protein or less) were first incubated with 0.5 µg of the TS primer and all four dNTPs (1 mM each) in TRAP reaction buffer, 0.8 mM spermidine, 5 mM β-mercaptoethanol in a total reaction volume of 50 µl for 30 minutes at 37°C. The reaction was stopped by incubation at 94°C for 2 minutes. Aliquots of synthesis (2.5 µl) were then PCR amplified as described (Hrdličková et al., 2006). The TRAP PCR products were separated on 7.5% acrylamide gels (ratio of acrylamide to bis-acrylamide 19:1) in 0.5 × TBE (TBE is 0.09 M Tris-borate, 2 mM EDTA pH 8.0) and gels were stained with VISTRA Green (GE Healthcare, Piscataway, NJ). For molecular weight determination a 10 bp ladder (Invitrogen, Carlsbad, CA) was used.

2.6 Terminal restriction fragment (TRF) length analysis

TRF analysis was performed as described previously (Hrdličková et al., 2006). High-molecular-weight genomic DNA (0.2 µg) was digested with a cocktail of restriction enzymes (HinfI, HaeIII, MspI, and RsaI) and separated in TBE in a 0.6% agarose gel. Undigested λ phage DNA mixed with λ digested with EcoRI and HindIII was used as marker. DNA was Southern transferred to a Hybond-N+ membrane (GE Healthcare) and hybridized to the telomeric probe $(CCCTAA)_6$ end-labeled with [γ-^{32}P]-ATP at 42°C using Ultrahyb solution (Ambion, Austin, TX). Blots were washed under stringent conditions. Subsequently, the blots were rehybridized with a λ probe to visualize the position of the markers.

2.7 Identification of TERT and its alternatively spliced variants by semiquantitative RT-PCR

Total RNA was isolated by RNAwiz (Ambion) and cDNA synthesis and RT-PCR were carried out as described previously (Hrdličková et al., 2006). The expression of avian TERT, its AS variants, and GAPDH was detected by RT-PCR using primers specific for TERT and GAPDH genes (Table 1).

Name[a]	Gene	Sequence
Q14F	qTERT	5′-CTGATACTGCTTCATGCTGCTATTATATCC-3′
Q16B	qTERT	5′-GATGGTTCCGTCACTGTCTTCAGCAGTTC-3′
C14F	chTERT	5′-CTGATACTGCTTCATGCTGCTATTTATCC-3′
C16B	chTERT	5′-GATGGTTCCGTCACCGTCTTCAGCAGTTC-3′
D14F	dTERT	5′-CTGAGAATGCATCGTGCTGCTATTCTATGC-3′
D16B	dTERT	5′-GATGGTTCTGTCACTGTCTTCAGTAGTGC-3′
qGAPDH1	qGAPDH	5' -ATTATCTCAGCCCCCTCAGCTGATGC-3'
qGAPDH2	qGAPDH	5' -CACAACTTCCCAGAGGGGCCGTCCAC-3'
chGAPDH1	chGAPDH	5'-ATCATCTCAGCTCCCTCAGCTGATGC-3'
chGAPDH2	ch/dGAPDH	5'-CACAGCTTCCCAGAGGGGCCATCCAC-3'
dGAPDH1	dGAPDH	5′-ATCATCTCCGCCCCCTCAGCTGATGC-3′
QKbSpWT	qTERT	5′-AGTGAATGACTGCGTATGGCTTCGTCTAG-3′
QKbSpA	qTERT	5′-CATGCTGGTTCCCCCAAGTAACTGTTACCAGGTAATC-3′
T6.2	qTERT	5'-CCACACCATGAGATCAAACGACAATCTGG-3'
KbSpWT	chTERT	5'-AGTGAATGACTGCGTATGGCTTCGTCTGG-3'
KbSpA	chTERT	5'-CAGCCTTCTGCAAAAGTGAACTTTCAAGCAGGTAATC-3'
T6	chTERT	5'-CCACACCATGAGATCAAGCGACAATCTGG-3'
D3F	dTERT	5′- GCTGATGGATACGTATGTTGTTCAGTTGCTCAGATC -3′

[a] Primer pairs Q14F and Q16B (quail), C14F and C16B (chicken), D14F and D16B (duck) were used for RT-PCR determination of TERT mRNA levels. Primers pairs qGAPDH1 and qGAPDH2, chGAPDH1 and chGAPDH2, dGADPH1 and chGADPH2 were used for determination of the levels of quail, chicken, and duck GAPDH, respectively. Primers T6.2, QKbSpWT, and QKbSpA were used for cloning the quail TERT isoforms, primers T6, KbSpWT, and KbSpA were used for cloning the chicken TERT isoforms. KbSpWT/QKbSpWT and T6/T6.2 primers detect only TERT transcripts lacking alternative splicing A/qA2 because the KbSpWT/QKbSpWT primer is located in the region which is deleted by this splicing event. KbSpA/QKbSpA and T6/T6.2 primers detect only the alternative splicing A/qA2 form of TERT because the KbSpA/QKbSpA primer binds to the junction created by alternative splicing A/qA2 and is, therefore, incapable of priming the synthesis of wild type TERT. Finally, primers D3F and D16B were used for cloning duck TERT mRNAs from different tissues.

Table 1. Oligonucleotide primers used for RT-PCR analyses

2.8 Determination of cell resistance to oxidative challenge

Exponentially growing cells (0.5×10^6) were seeded into 60 mm plates one day before the experiment. Freshly diluted H_2O_2 (Sigma, St. Louis, MO) was added and cells were counted after 24 hours. The dead cells were excluded by trypan-blue staining.

3. Results

To perform comparative analysis of TERT proteins of three avian species, quail, chicken, and duck, we cloned quail and duck TERT, compared their sequences with the chicken TERT sequence and defined their evolutionary distances. We also cloned alternatively spliced TERT variants from these species and determined their expression in different tissues. We defined the telomere length in embryos and telomerase activity in tissues of these species and correlated them with the frequency and complexity of alternatively spliced variants. Analysis of *in vitro*-cultivated embryonic fibroblasts established the differences in cell growth, telomerase activity, and telomere length during continuous cell passage and compared them with the sensitivity of these cells to oxidative challenge. Finally, to evaluate the role of transcription in the regulation of telomerase activity, we measured the steady-state levels of total TERT transcripts in tissues of these species.

3.1 Quail and chicken TERT have a very similar protein primary structure

Quail and chicken *TERT* genes encode very similar proteins (Fig. 1). The quail reverse transcriptase gene is 1344 amino acids, which is two amino acids shorter than the chicken protein as a result of four single amino acid indel differences. The proteins of both species contain the same conserved regions which encode the structural domains of TERT and represent 70% of the molecule. The amino acid sequences are 94% identical and percentage of identity reaches 97% (100% if similar amino acids are considered) in some of the conserved regions. The majority (65%) of the differences between the quail and chicken TERT protein are concentrated in the less conserved regions of the N-terminus and three linker regions (L1-L3).

To further characterize the similarities of quail and chicken TERT and compare them with the TERT proteins of related species, the best characterized TERT sequences of the sauropsid amniots were aligned. The group Sauropsida includes all living reptiles and birds and their extinct reptilian predecessors and represents one of the two evolutionary branches of amniotes (Benton, 2005). The other amniotic branch, Synapsida, includes mammals and their extinct reptilian grade ancestors. The amino acid homologies of seven sauropsid proteins were then compared in each functional domain/motif (Table 2). Quail TERT exhibited the highest sequence homology with chicken and turkey TERT in all regions. Even in the three linker regions (L1-L3), quail and chicken proteins were 85-91% identical which contrast with the lower conservation over longer evolutionary distances (e.g., 9-19% for quail and anole). The TERT proteins of ducks (both Mallard and Muscovy) are significantly more dissimilar to quail TERT, with the levels of similarities not much different from zebra finch TERT.

The evolutionary tree of these seven sauropsid TERT proteins confirmed the close relationship among the three proteins of the galliform birds - quail, chicken, and turkey (Fig. 2). Apparently TERTs of quail and chicken retained high level of similarity despite that the last common ancestor of the two species lived 30-40 million years ago (MYA) (van Tuinen & Dyke, 2004). The TERT proteins of anseriform birds, ducks, are much more distant even

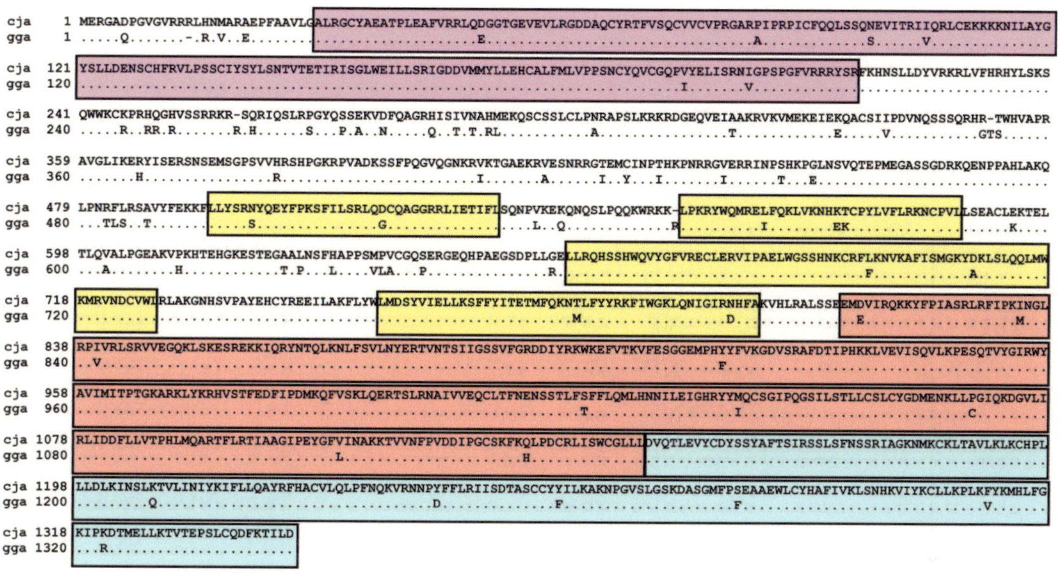

Regions broadly conserved among vertebrate TERTs are color-coded: TEN domain (purple), TRBD motifs v-II/VSR, v-III/CP, QFP, and T (yellow), RT domain (red), CTE-terminal domain (blue). Three linkers of less conserved sequence are situated: L1 between TEN and v-II, L2 between v-II and v-III, and L3 between v-III and QFP. Alignment gaps are indicated by dashes. In chicken TERT, only amino acids that are different from quail TERT are shown.

Fig. 1. Comparison of quail (*Coturnix japonica* - cja) and chicken (*Gallus gallus* - gga) TERT protein sequences though the tree agrees with the joining of both Galliformes and Anseriformes in a one monophyletic group of Galloanserae (Chubb, 2004). Interestingly, the TERT gene of Neoaves (zebra finch) is equally evolutionarily distant from Galliformes and duck TERT. The TERT of Lepidosaurs (green anole) is significantly more distant from two basal avian branches (Neoaves and Galloanserae) than these branches are from each other.

In conclusion, the three avian TERT genes of quail, chicken, and duck exhibit different level of sequence similarity of their protein products. The primary structures of quail and chicken TERT proteins are closely related suggesting high degree of similarity in function and regulation at the protein level while the duck TERT protein is significantly more distant.

Domain/	Percentage of identical amino acids[a]						Percentage of similar amino acids					
motif	gga	mga	cmo	apl	tgu	aca	gga	mga	cmo	apl	tgu	aca
TEN	96.8	ND	73.3	ND	74.9	52.9	99.5	ND	85.6	ND	84.0	72.7
L1	87.8	83.5	45.3	ND	41.7	17.6	92.4	89.9	60.8	ND	60.1	36.7
v-II	94.4	91.7	66.7	ND	72.2	41.7	97.2	97.2	83.3	ND	88.9	72.2
L2	90.5	90.5	71.4	ND	61.9	19.0	100.0	95.2	85.7	ND	90.5	47.6
v-III	91.4	88.6	62.9	ND	65.7	62.9	97.1	97.1	80.0	ND	77.1	80.0
L3	84.5	80.3	39.4	ND	38.0	8.5	87.3	88.7	53.5	ND	56.3	26.8
QFP	97.1	97.1	82.9	ND	80.0	78.6	98.6	98.6	92.9	ND	94.3	90.0
T	95.7	97.9	83.0	78.7	87.2	74.5	97.9	97.9	91.5	93.6	93.6	89.4
RT	97.3	97.0	78.6	78.0	78.3	62.2	99.7	99.4	90.2	89.0	89.6	78.6
CTE	97.0	ND	81.2	81.7	75.6	64.5	98.5	ND	90.4	91.4	84.3	79.7
TERT	93.9	ND	67.9	ND	66.5	48.2	96.8	ND	80.0	ND	79.2	65.8

[a] Animals: gga (*Gallus gallus*) - domestic chicken, mga (*Meleagris gallopavo*) - turkey, cmo (*Cairina moschata*) - Muscovy duck, apl (*Anas platyrhynchos*) - domestic (Mallard) duck, tgu (*Taeniopygia guttata*) - zebra finch, aca (*Anolis carolinensis*) - green anole. Domains and motifs are described in the Fig. 1. TERT indicates the entire protein. ND - not determined, because the complete sequence was not available. The highest numbers for each region are shown in red.

Table 2. Comparison of the functional domains and motifs of quail TERT with six other sauropsid TERT proteins

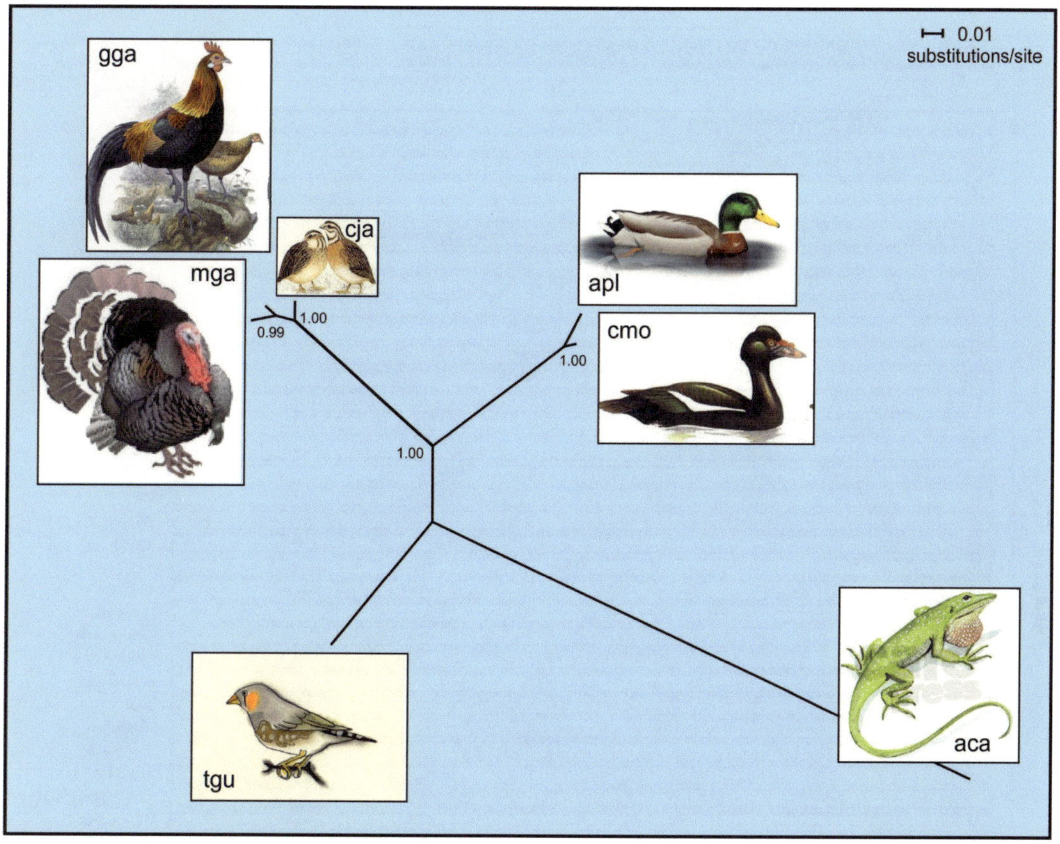

The tree is built on the alignment consisting of 592 columns of amino acid sequences where all seven proteins were aligned without any gaps. The bar represents 0.01 substitutions per site. Species abbreviations are shown in the legend to Table 1. Posterior probabilities are indicated at each node except the node that connects the selected outgroup species - anole.

Fig. 2. Bayesian phylogenetic tree of sauropsid TERT proteins.

3.2 Quail and chicken differ greatly in the number of alternatively spliced variants

Fifty alternatively spliced variants of chicken, duck, and quail TERT were cloned (Fig. 3). Sixty percent of the alternative splicing events of avian TERT introduced novel stop codons which would lead to prematurely terminated proteins during translation and their RNAs would likely be subject to nonsense-mediated mRNA decay (Green et al., 2003). The remaining forty percent were spliced in-frame. In most of these cases, alternative splicing eliminated or modified functional domains or motifs important for telomerase activity. The highest number of alternatively spliced variants was identified in chicken (37), followed by 10 AS variants identified in duck. This number is likely an underestimate since we didn't obtain the N-terminal region of the duck sequence where several alternative splicing events occur in chicken, human, platypus, and one in quail. Also, a variety of TERT mRNA molecules which contain multiple AS events in many combinations were detected in chicken and duck, thereby creating even higher diversity of AS isoforms in these species. In contrast, only three alternatively spliced variants were identified in quail despite screening various

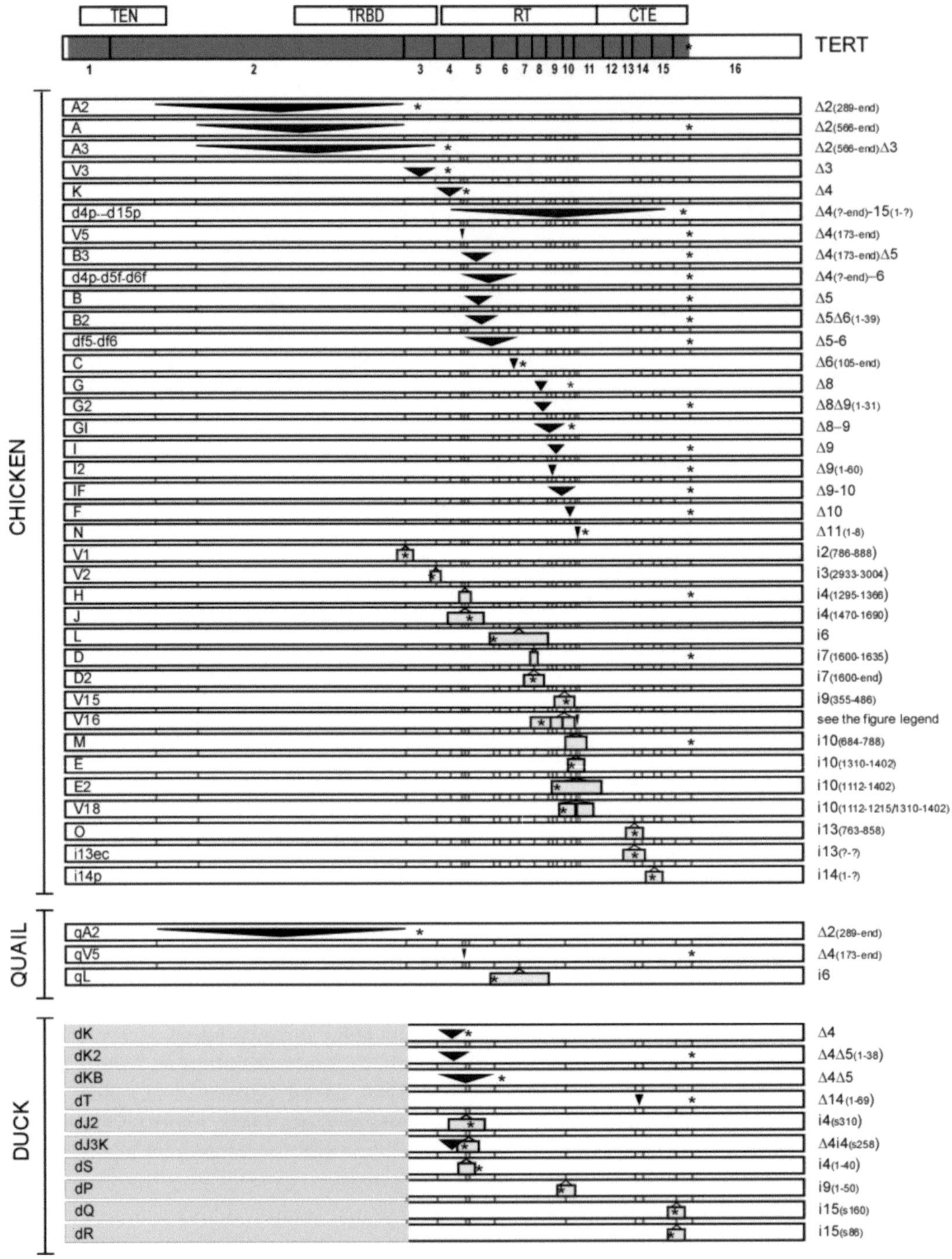

A large number of single AS event variants of avian TERT were identified. Many of the chicken variants were described previously (Amor et al., 2010; Chang & Delany, 2006; Hrdličková et al., 2006). The structure of wild-type (WT) TERT mRNA is shown at the top with the TERT ORF shaded. The positions of exons and the functional domains (TEN - telomerase essential N-terminal domain, TRBD - telomerase

RNA binding domain, RT - reverse transcriptase domain, CTE - C-terminal domain) of avian TERT are indicated. In a set of variants, deletions (triangle) and insertions (gray rectangles) resulting from splicing events are indicated. Asterisks identify the location of stop codons. The trivial names of the TERT AS variants are shown at the left. The descriptive names ("Δ" indicates deletion of exon-derived and "i" insertion of intron-derived sequences) are shown in the right margin. The numbers in parentheses indicate positions within exon or intron. Some of the duck AS variants are described only by the size of the insertion indicated by the preceding letter s. Two complex chicken variants, V16 and V18, likely arose through combinations of several single AS events. The descriptive name of the V16 variant is i9 (355-486/926-988/1091-1162)/Δ11(1-3). The sequence of the first two exons of duck TERT was not determined (gray shading).

Fig. 3. Alternative splicing of quail, chicken, and duck TERT

tissues and obtaining over 60 independent clones of qTERT. All three quail AS variants have identical orthologs among chicken variants consistent with their close evolutionary relation. On the other hand, the more distantly related duck share only variant K with chicken, but five other duck variants have certain structural similarity to chicken AS variants (KB, J2, J3K, S, and P). KB is fusion of chicken AS variants K and B, and J3K is fusion of chicken J with K. The AS variants J2, S, and P introduced novel intron cassette sequences from the same intron as the chicken variants.

In conclusion, despite the close sequence homology, quail expresses ten times less alternatively spliced variants than chicken and three times less than the more distantly related duck. While three quail AS variants identified are also expressed in chicken, the duck AS variants have only limited structural similarly with the chicken AS variants.

3.3 Differences in *cis* regulation of species-specific alternative splicing

Comparison of quail (GenBank, DQ681292) and chicken genomic DNA (GenBank, AADN00000000) suggests that many changes in alternative splicing may have evolved as a result of differences within the TERT gene (*cis*) (Fig. 4). These differences include absence of intron-based alternative cassette exons, presence of premature stop codons, and alteration in alternative splice donor sequences. The most obvious difference is the absence of exon 10B and large regions of exons 10A, 10A2 (cassette exons located in chicken intron 10) (Fig. 4A). Consequently quail cannot produce alternative splicing variants E, E2, and M. Further, although the sequence of exon 7A is conserved in quail, it contains a stop codon (Fig. 4B). This stop codon may prevent the production of TERT isoform D by nonsense-mediated suppression of splicing or decrease its level by nonsense-mediated decay (Wachtel et al., 2004). Finally, chicken exon 2 contains two alternative splice donors for the isoforms A and A2 (Fig. 4C). While quail TERT also produces the isoform A2 (qA2), the quail isoform A was not detected. The quail sequence found in the location of chicken splice donor site for variant A does not contain the critical core dinucleotide (GT) normally used in the removal of more than 98% of all introns, but a much weaker sequence (GC), employed in the removal of less than 1% of introns (Abril et al., 2005). This difference between sequences of the two species may favor use of the upstream located splice donor site (*sd*qA2) in quail TERT. Collectively, these results demonstrate that at least some differences in the alternative splicing pattern of the TERT gene between quail and chicken are regulated in *cis*.

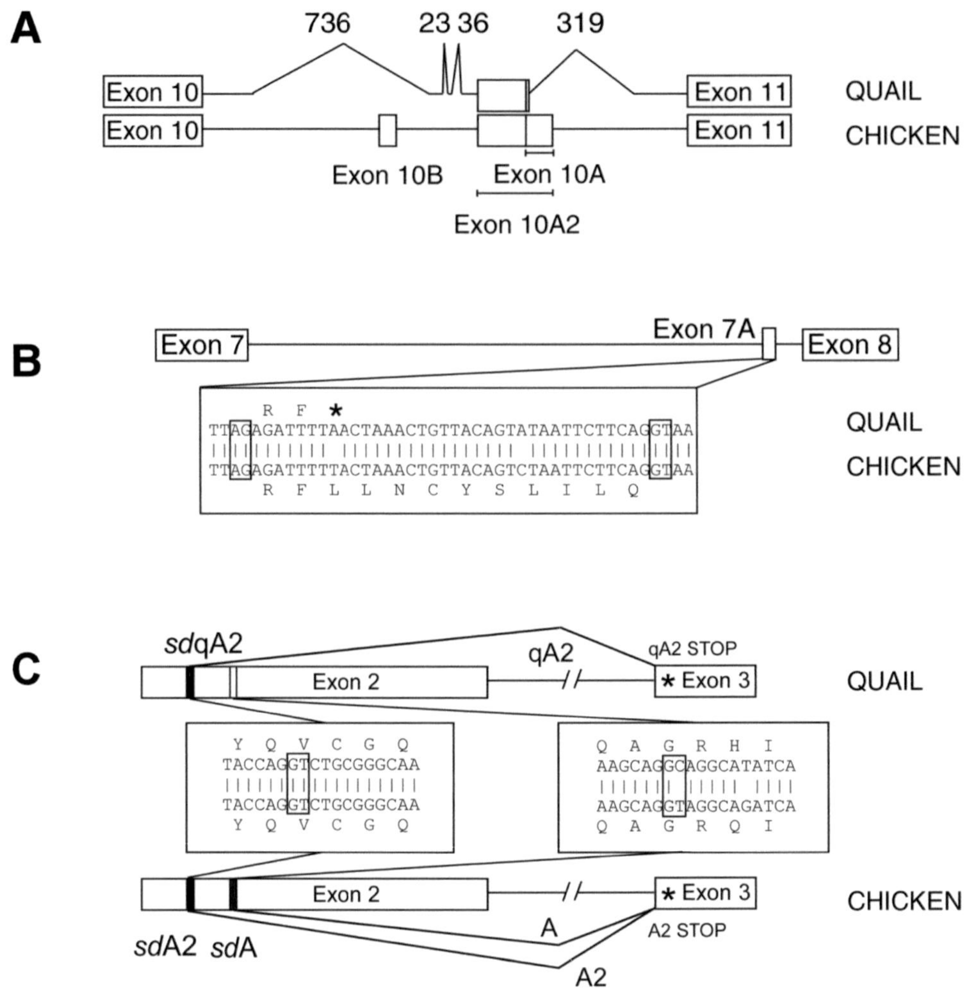

A. Key differences in the sequences of quail and chicken intron 10. Four large regions of DNA present in chicken TERT gene are not found in the corresponding quail intron (736, 23, 36, and 319 nt). B. A stop codon (indicated by asterisk), absent from the chicken cassette exon 7A, is present in the corresponding quail sequence. C. Comparison of splice donor A site in chicken exon 2 (*sd*A) with its quail sequence homolog, and splice donor A2 (*sd*A2) site in the same exon with quail qA2 splice donor site (*sd*qA2). In contrast to the chicken isoform A, chicken isoform A2 and quail isoform qA2 contain stop codons in exon 3 sequences (asterisks).

Fig. 4. *Cis* regulation of species specific alternative splicing

3.4 Quail cells have a reduced frequency and lower complexity of TERT AS variants than do chicken and duck cells

To determine whether the differences in the numbers of AS variants are maintained in different cells and tissues of quail and chicken, large regions of the TERT genes were cloned from each tissue source and 5-20 clones were analyzed by sequencing or by restriction enzyme analysis (Figs. 5 and 6). Differences in alternative splicing were quantified either as a number of distinct isoforms (containing one or more alternative splicing events per molecule) or as a total number of AS events detected in all isoforms (Fig. 5). Analysis of quail cDNAs revealed that TERT AS forms are relatively rare. Only two quail TERT AS variants, qA2 and qV3, were detected in this experiment. The most frequent quail AS variant, qA2, was isolated only from tissues, like embryo and lung, with high proliferation activity. In cells where the qA2 isoform was detected, the isoform was present at much lower levels than were wild-type (WT) TERT transcripts (data not shown). An additional spliced variant (qV3) was detected only once, in lung tissue. In contrast, the analysis of clones from chicken and duck cells revealed the abundance of AS variants with different combinations of AS splicing events. In relatively homogenous cell populations (in embryonic fibroblasts and heart), only one or two spliced variants were detected. In contrast, a great variety of different AS variants were present in cells derived from the brain (5-9 different variants), most likely due to the heterogeneity of cell populations in this tissue. Chicken and duck AS variants contained from one to six splicing events on a single molecule. Generally, measuring AS complexity as either the number of isoforms or the total number of AS events gave very similar results, except in chicken fibroblasts, where one isoform carrying six AS events was detected.

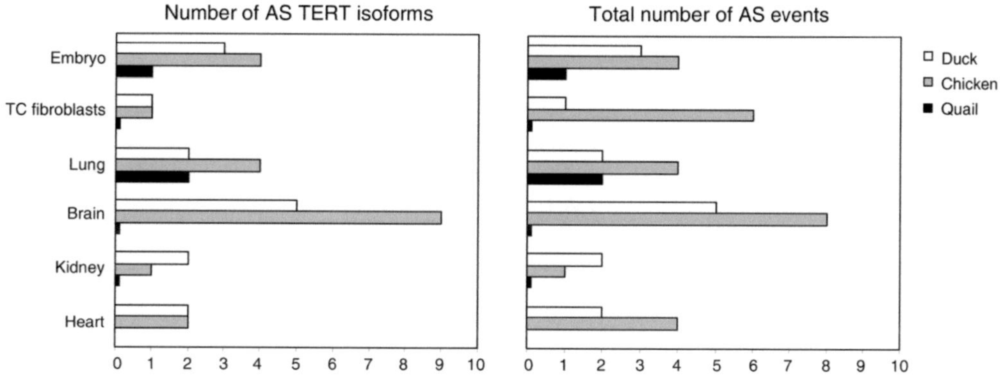

Complexity of TERT alternative splicing is shown as a number of distinct isoforms as well as a total number of alternative splicing events detected in tissues and cells of three galloanserine birds. TC (tissue culture) fibroblasts are embryonic fibroblasts cultivated *in vitro* for 6 days after the establishment of primary cultures. The WT TERT isoform is not included in the number of AS variants. The short columns for quail AS isoforms/AS events in fibroblasts, brain, and kidney indicate that no AS variants (only WT-spliced transcripts) were detected in these cells and tissues. We failed to isolate any TERT clones from quail heart. Identity of AS variants was established by the RT-PCR amplification of several TERT mRNA regions using the primer pairs described in section 2.7. For each tissue (except for chicken fibroblasts) the sequences of 5-18 quail or chicken clones or 3-16 duck clones were determined and the identity of additional 3-11 duck clones was established by restriction analysis. Only two AS chicken TERT clones were obtained from chicken fibroblasts.

Fig. 5. Complexity of TERT alternative splicing

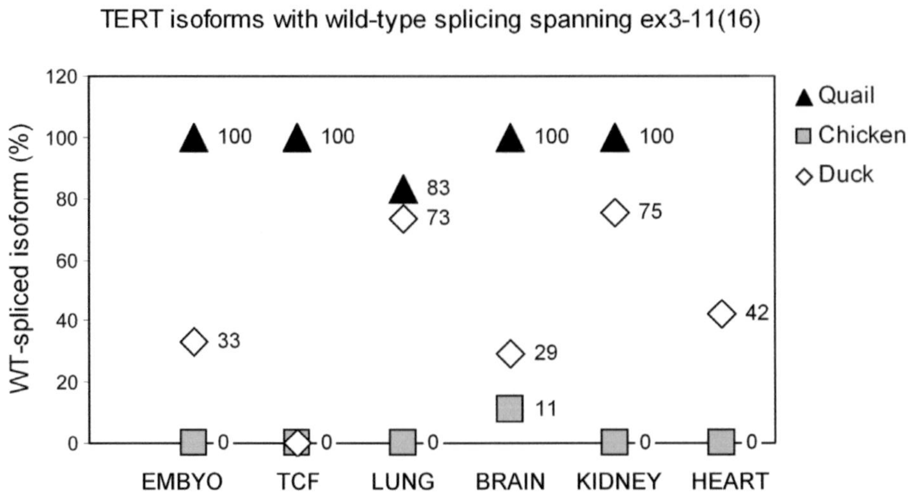

Isolation frequency of WT-spliced clones spanning exons 3-11 (3-16 in duck) cloned from embryo, tissue culture fibroblasts (TCF), lung, brain, kidney, and heart of three galloanserine birds. The RT-PCR amplification used 5' primers complementary to the 3' end of exon 2 (beginning of exon 3 in duck), and 3' primers complementary to the middle of exon 11 (beginning of exon 16 in duck). We failed to isolate any TERT clones from quail heart in any PCR reactions in this study.

Fig. 6. Isolation frequency of WT-spliced clones

The abundance of WT isoforms was estimated by RT-PCR amplification of the specific regions of quail, chicken, and duck TERT (Fig. 6). All AS events identified in this study are located in these regions (except the chTERT AS event O). PCR products were cloned and sequenced. The final percentage was calculated from forms with AS events located between exons 3-11 (3-16 in duck) except the clones from chicken fibroblasts (TCF), lung, and kidney. We failed to isolate any clones from chicken fibroblasts, lung, and kidney with this PCR strategy, suggesting that the both WT and AS isoforms are below the threshold of detection. All clones isolated from these sources contained an A splicing event in the second exon. The analysis revealed that WT-spliced isoforms are frequently expressed in quail tissues, while in chicken tissues WT clones were obtained only from the brain. The frequency of isolation of the WT isoform in duck was intermediate between those in quail and in chicken.

In conclusion, chicken and duck TERT genes produce multiple and abundant AS isoforms in several tissues while the complexity and frequency of AS forms in quail tissues are severely limited. In a complementary manner, the WT-spliced isoform (potentially encoding an enzymatically active protein) is more prevalent in quail tissues than in the tissues of the other two galloanserine birds.

3.5 Quail expresses higher levels of telomerase activity than chicken and duck in all tissues

To investigate whether there are differences in the telomerase activity in quail, chicken, and duck, various organs of these birds were isolated and telomerase activity was determined in tissue extracts by a telomerase repeat amplification protocol (TRAP) assay (Fig. 7A).

Telomerase activity was determined in adult quail (3 month-old), senescent quail (15 month-old), immature chicken (3 month-old), adult chicken (6 month-old), and an immature duck (approximately 5-6 month-old). Telomerase activity was also measured in the corresponding organs from an adult 2 month-old mouse, the prototype of a small mammal with high telomerase activity. Telomerase activity was high in the intestine, ovary, and testes in birds of all ages. In other organs, including the spleen, lung, brain, kidney, and liver, telomerase activity was significantly higher in adult quail (3 month-old) than in the chicken at a comparable developmental stage (6 month-old) and remained high even in the 15 month-old quail. Telomerase activity in duck organs was also lower than in adult quail even though the duck analyzed was not yet sexually mature. The distribution of telomerase activity in the different tissues was similar in all birds with the exception of the duck liver, which had higher activity compared to chicken. Mouse, like quail, had high telomerase activity in several organs but the tissue distribution was strikingly different and telomerase had a lower processivity.

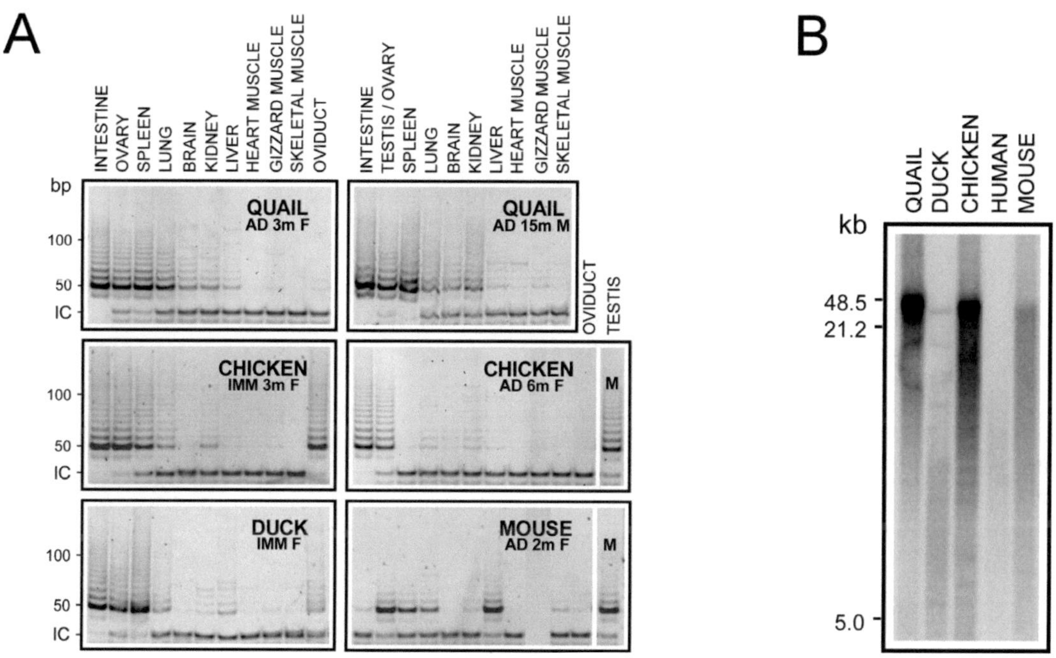

A. Telomerase activity in extracts from different tissues of quail and chicken was determined by the TRAP assay. Sexual maturity (IMMature or ADult), age in months (where known), and sex (F or M) of the experimental animals are indicated. Telomerase activity in the testes from an age matched 6 month-old chicken and 2 month-old mouse are shown on the right. Each lane represents the activity in whole cell extract containing 1 µg of total protein. The position of the PCR internal control (IC) bands is indicated. B. Telomere length was determined by terminal restriction fragment (TRF) length analysis using a 0.6% agarose gel. This analysis included DNA isolated from quail, duck, and chicken embryos, human (BD Biosciences Clontech, Cat. No. S0950), and spleen from a 2 month-old mouse (strain C57BL/6).

Fig. 7. Species-specific differences in telomerase activity and telomere length in quail, chicken, and duck

The detailed study of telomere length of mammals demonstrated that the average length of telomeres ranges from very long (up to 50 kb in some rodents and lagomorphs) to very short (below 10 kb in primates). However, species can be divided into two groups according to their telomere length, one group with the average telomere length below and the second above 20 kb (Gomes et al., 2011). The average length of telomeres in quail, chicken, and duck was determined and compared to human and mouse by terminal restriction fragment (TRF) analysis (Fig. 7B). While quail has slightly longer telomeres than chicken, this difference is only subtle and telomeres of both chicken and quail were above 20 kb (approximately 30-40 kb long) similarly to mouse. In contrast, human and duck had much shorter telomeres (4-10 kb). These results indicate that the length of telomeres only weakly correlates with telomerase activity.

3.6 Quail embryonic fibroblasts express higher levels of telomerase activity than chicken and duck fibroblasts

To further investigate the regulation of telomerase activity in avian cells, telomerase activity was measured in fibroblast cultures of all three avian species (Fig. 8). Quail embryonic fibroblasts (QEFs) underwent senescence after 14 doublings, as determined by β-galactosidase staining, a marker of cellular senescence. In contrast, chicken and duck embryonic fibroblasts (CEFs and DEFs) became senescent after 50 doublings (Fig. 8A).

Telomerase activity was high at the time the cultures were initiated (Fig. 8B). In QEFs, levels of telomerase remained high through the 9th day and then declined slightly, but substantial

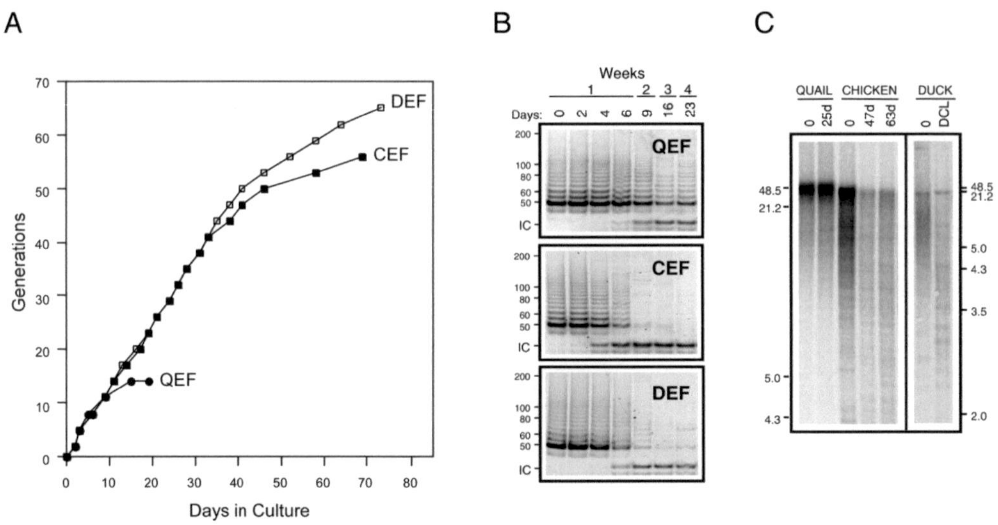

A. The cumulative increase in cell generations with time in culture was determined. Each culture was split 1:8 when it reached confluence. Cells were cultivated until they reached senescence and stopped dividing. This experiment was repeated twice with similar results. B. Telomerase activity was measured by a TRAP assay at various times after establishment of the culture. C. Telomere length in serially passaged quail and chicken fibroblasts at various times after establishment of the cell culture was determined by TRF in a 0.6% agarose gel. Telomere length of freshly prepared DEF (0) was compared to duck embryonic cells cultivated 45 passages (DCL).

Fig. 8. Growth of quail (QEF), chicken (CEF), and duck (DEF) embryonic fibroblasts levels of activity were detected in the senescent cells. By contrast, the telomerase activity in CEFs and DEFs decreased after 6 days in culture and was completely diminished by the 9th day and remained undetectable for additional four weeks. Telomere length did not change significantly in QEFs, while telomeres of CEFs gradually shortened (Fig. 8C). Similarly, telomere length in DEF cells after approximately 45 passages (DCL) is significantly shorter than from freshly prepared DEFs.

These results indicated that telomerase activity is not strongly repressed in quail cells, and telomeres do not shorten, however, these cells underwent early senescence during *in vitro* cultivation. By contrast, in both CEFs and DEFs telomerase activity was strongly repressed, followed by the shortening of telomeres. In conclusion, these results are consistent with the findings that telomerase activity is higher *in vivo* in quail than chicken or duck tissues and suggest that, in contrast to chicken or duck, quail cells do not undergo replicative aging, the process, in which aging is dependent on shortening of telomeres during cell proliferation.

3.7 Telomerase levels inversely correlate with H_2O_2 resistance

Quail embryonic fibroblasts underwent senescence after a relatively short time in tissue culture regardless of high levels of telomerase activity and long telomeres. Previous studies demonstrated that primary embryonic fibroblasts from the short-lived quail are more sensitive to oxidative stress than fibroblasts from long-lived birds such as budgerigar (common pet parakeet), *Melopsittacus undulatus* (Ogburn et al., 2001). It is possible that quail is also more sensitive to oxidative stress than chicken or duck, accounting for its relatively accelerated senescence *in vitro*. To determine whether differences also exist between quail, chicken, and duck cells in their sensitivity to oxidative stress, QEF, CEF, and DEF cultures were exposed to H_2O_2 and their viability determined (Fig. 9). QEFs were at least 3 times more sensitive to H_2O_2 treatment than chicken or duck cells.

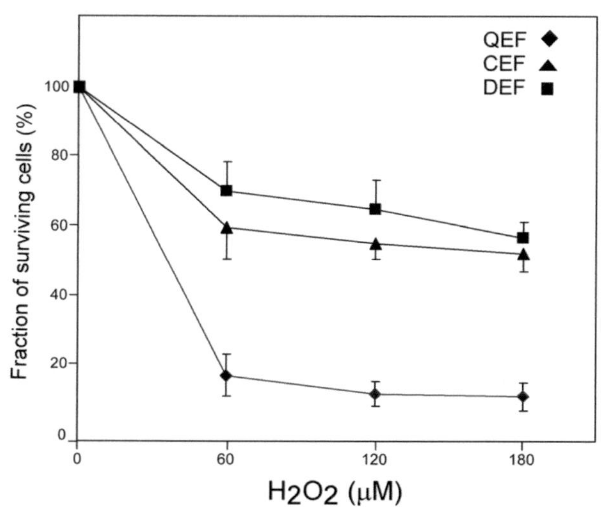

Quail, chicken, and duck fibroblasts were treated with various concentration of hydrogen peroxide for 24 hours and cell number determined. Means and standard errors were calculated from three independent experiments for each cells. Statistically significant differences relative to negative controls are indicated.

Fig. 9. Sensitivity of avian fibroblasts to oxygen radicals

3.8 Telomerase activity is intrinsically higher in quail cells and inversely correlates with frequency and complexity of AS TERT variants

The previous results indicate that the lower frequency and complexity of AS TERT variants correlate with higher telomerase activity in quail cells. However, in samples with high telomerase activity the levels could not be quantitatively measured, because the assay may be saturated. Therefore, to obtain more accurate results, the relative levels of telomerase activity were determined by end-point titration in selected tissues as well as in cultured cells (Fig. 10A). Telomerase activity was approximately 5 times higher in the quail embryo than chicken embryos. In all cases, the activity in adult organs was approximately 1000-fold lower than in the embryonic tissues analyzed. Telomerase activity in adult quail tissues was 2-8 fold higher than chicken or duck tissues (except in heart where telomerase activity is at the threshold of detection). These results indicate that the relative differences in the levels of telomerase activity between quail and chicken or duck are already present in the embryo and are retained in adulthood.

Differences in the levels of telomerase activity between mouse and human cells have been attributed to differential transcription of the TERT gene (Horikawa et al., 2005; Takakura et al., 2005). To determine the contribution of differential transcription of TERT to differences in telomerase activity between quail, chicken, and duck, semiquantitative RT-PCR was performed against the regions of the TERT gene which are not involved in alternative splicing (Fig. 10B). This assay detects the levels of all TERT transcripts, including wild-type TERT as well as the AS TERT variants. The levels of TERT mRNA in some cases mimic the differences in the levels of telomerase activity among the analyzed organs. The cells with the lowest telomerase activity such as heart, and brain had mostly lower amounts of TERT transcripts. However, the levels of TERT mRNA in the corresponding organs of different species did not correlate with the differences in telomerase activity between the species. For example, telomerase activity was approximately five times higher in embryonic cells obtained from quail than in cells from chicken embryo but the levels of TERT mRNA were the same. The levels of TERT mRNA in all analyzed quail tissues were same or lower than in chicken or duck tissues while telomerase activity was always the highest in quail tissues.

In conclusion, these results indicate that there are intrinsic differences in the levels of telomerase activity between quail and chicken or duck, which are already present in embryonic cells and are retained at the same ratio in adult cells. These differences correlate with the frequency and complexity of AS TERT variants expressed in these tissues and not with the steady-state levels of TERT transcripts.

4. Discussion

4.1 The regulation of telomerase activity during ontogenesis and phylogenesis

Telomerase activity is downregulated during ontogenesis in vertebrates. However, poikilothermic animals retain high telomerase activity in all adult organs since their continuous growth throughout their lifespan requires the maintenance of telomere length (Bousman et al., 2003). Homoeothermic animals (mammals and birds) downregulate telomerase activity to a greater extent than poikilotermic animals presumably because they do not grow after they reach sexual maturity and also to decrease the risk of cancer resulting from a higher metabolic rate. However, mammals differ in the extent to which telomerase is

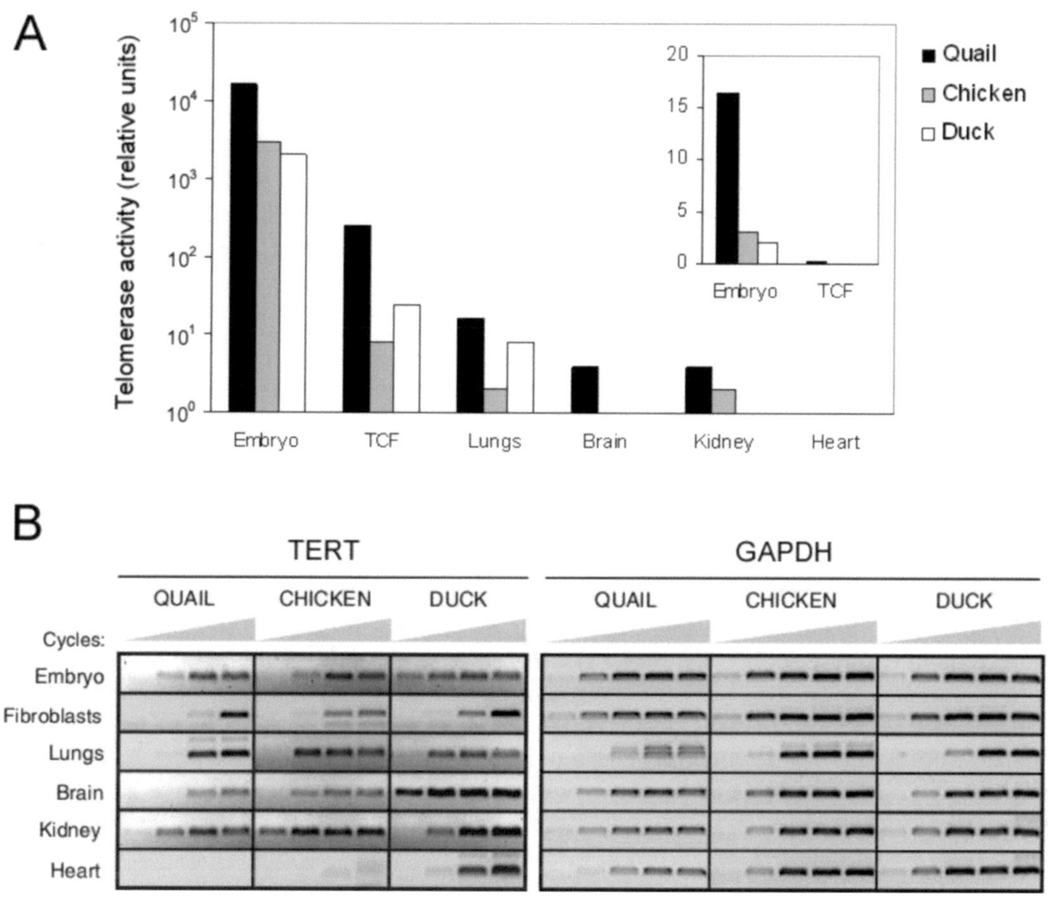

A. Telomerase activity in extracts from different tissues of quail, chicken, and duck was determined by the TRAP assay. CHAPS protein extracts were prepared from quail (4 day-old), chicken (5 day-old), and duck (14 day-old) embryos, embryonic fibroblasts passaged for six days in tissue culture (TCF) and from lung, brain, kidney, and heart of 3 month-old quail, 6 month-old chicken and a sexually immature duck of adult size. Telomerase activity was determined by a TRAP assay in a series of up to 16 two-fold dilutions of the CHAPS extracts. Quail embryo extract where the telomerase activity was detected at the highest dilution (14th dilution) was arbitrarily considered to have 2^{14} relative units per µg of extract and activity in other samples were compared to this standard. B. Steady-state levels of TERT mRNA were determined by RT-PCR. The expression of GAPDH, was analyzed by RT-PCR using primers specific for quail, chicken, and duck GAPDH. Aliquots from the PCR reaction were taken every 5th cycle beginning with cycle 30 for TERT and 20 for GAPDH, PCR products were resolved on agarose gels, and visualized with ethidium bromide. RNA was prepared from the same cells and tissues as at Fig. 10A.

Fig. 10. Interspecies differences in telomerase activity do not correlate with TERT mRNA steady-state levels downregulated. Initial studies indicated that mice maintain higher telomerase activity in a broader spectrum of tissues than humans (Kim et al., 1994; Prowse & Greider, 1995; Taylor & Delany, 2000). The following study of 15 rodent species demonstrated remarkable differences in telomerase activity (Seluanov et al., 2007). In general, the higher levels of telomerase activity correlated with the smaller body mass of the animal. Lastly, the comparative study of more than 60 mammalian species representing all the important mammalian evolutionary groups supported this conclusion (Gomes et al., 2011). Our report demonstrates that the differences in telomerase activity exist not only in mammals but also in other warm-blooded animals - birds. Quail and chicken are closely related species with a significantly different body mass and life expectancy (Pereira & Baker, 2006). Though sequences of quail and chicken TERT proteins are 94% identical, the levels of telomerase activity in quail and chicken cells and organs are strikingly different. Quail embryonic cells express 5 times the level of telomerase activity than chicken embryonic cells. Telomerase activity is downregulated to the same extent (approximately 1000 times) in adult organs of both species but substantially higher levels (about 5 fold) remain in quail relative to chicken tissues. This demonstrates that differences between telomerase activity in adult organs of different species are intrinsic and result of different levels of telomerase activity in their respective embryos.

The downregulation of telomerase activity in the organs of adult homoeothermic vertebrates is believed to provide protection against cancer (Blasco & Hahn, 2003; Shay & Wright, 2005). Quail and mice are short-lived species because they are small, principally terrestrial animals, with limited ability to escape predation (Kirkwood, 2005). Due to the short lifespan of quail and mice, suppression of telomerase activity is not required to protect against tumor development (Prowse & Greider, 1995). The increased sensitivity of quail and mouse cells to spontaneous, carcinogen- or oncogenic virus-induced immortalization is consistent with this hypothesis (Hartl et al., 1995; Moscovici et al., 1977; Prowse & Greider, 1995). However, the question remains whether the high levels of telomerase activity expressed in species with small body mass provides a survival advantage. Quail cells are more sensitive to oxidative stress than chicken or duck cells, and in contrast to chicken or duck cells, they undergo senescence when cultured *in vitro*. Cells from other short-lived mammals are also more sensitive to oxidative stress than cells from long-lived species, and undergo accelerated telomere-length-independent senescence when exposed to higher levels of oxygen during *in vitro* cultivation (Kim et al., 2002; Ogburn et al., 2001; Parrinello et al., 2003). The quail cells stop proliferation and undergo senescence in cell culture in two weeks even though they retain high telomerase activity and long telomeres indicating that the shortening of telomeres is not responsible for cell cycle arrest. Avian TERT, like its mammalian homologs, is able to partially protect cells against apoptosis induced by exposure to oxidative agents (Hrdličková et al., 2006). In conclusion, it is likely that the major role of the higher telomerase activity in cells from quail and other species with small body mass is to partially compensate for their reduced antioxidative defense.

4.2 The mechanism of regulation of telomerase activity during ontogenesis

Transcription rate and alternative splicing of TERT has been proposed as the key mechanisms involved in the developmental regulation of telomerase activity in mammals (Kaneko et al., 2006; Ulaner et al., 2001; Ulaner et al., 1998). Our results suggest that other mechanisms are also likely to be involved in the downregulation of telomerase in the quail, chicken, and duck. Differences in telomerase levels in the embryo relative to adult organs did not strongly correlate with differences in TERT transcription or alternative splicing. Embryos expressed approximately 1000 times higher levels of telomerase activity than adult tissues in all species and expressed similar mRNA levels and numbers of AS variants. In some tissues general transcription of TERT was significantly decreased, however, other non-transcriptional mechanisms likely contribute to the robust downregulation of telomerase activity during differentiation. Likewise, telomerase activity in the quail and mouse are downregulated in tissues where only a limited amount of alternative splicing of TERT transcripts takes place. Other studies also do not support a general role for splicing of TERT during developmental regulation. Like avian species, alternatively spliced TERT forms are present in human gametes and preimplantation embryos (Brenner et al., 1999). If alternative splicing negatively regulates telomerase activity during development one would not expect spliced forms in germinal cells in which telomerase activity is highest.

4.3 The role of alternative splicing in interspecies differences in the regulation of telomerase activity

TERT is the key regulatory component responsible for the regulation of telomerase levels. The most important mechanisms responsible for interspecies differences in the regulation of TERT are probably the structural differences in the regulatory domains encoded by the TERT gene, the level of transcription and alternative splicing. Changes in protein-protein interaction-based regulatory pathways would evolve slowly since only a limited number of mutations in the coding regions of TERT would affect its regulation without complete elimination of the telomerase activity. The downregulation of telomerase by terminating transcription could lead to the methylation of the TERT promoter limiting the possible reactivation of TERT transcription (Devereux et al., 1999). In contrast, changes in alternative splicing sites can be introduced into the genome without interfering with the complex promoter regulation of TERT or its protein structure. Moreover, alternative splicing preserves the transcription of the TERT locus preventing promoter methylation and, thereby, allowing for the rapid reactivation of telomerase when necessary in adult tissues (during immune reaction or healing processes). All these mechanisms of regulation of interspecies differences in the levels of telomerase are used, however, their relative contribution still remains to be evaluated.

The differences in the levels of telomerase activity between the closely related quail and chicken species strongly correlated with differences in alternative splicing. In quail the majority of the TERT transcripts expressed in adult tissue and cells are wild type and telomerase activity levels are high. In contrast, alternatively spliced variants which fail to encode functional TERT proteins, represent nearly all of the TERT transcripts expressed in adult chicken tissue and cells which have low levels of telomerase activity. Our results suggest that alternative splicing of TERT contributes to the establishment of the different levels of telomerase between these two species. Importantly, we demonstrated that these differences are intrinsically present already in embryonic cells. This is consistent with the suggestion that the many changes in the alternative splicing repertoire between quail and chicken are encoded in genomic sequences in the TERT locus.

Recently, differences in the regulation between the human and mouse TERT promoters have been suggested to be responsible for the differences in the levels of telomerase activity in these species (Horikawa et al., 2005; Jia et al., 2011; Takakura et al., 2005; Wang et al., 2009). In our comparison of quail, chicken, and duck, the regulation of transcription did not appear to play a significant role because we did not find differences in the steady-state levels of TERT transcripts (as an approximate measure of TERT transcription) among these species. In contrast, differences in alternative splicing best correlated with differences in levels of telomerase activity between quail and chicken. The probable reason for the preferential use of alternative splicing in quail and chicken is that the evolutionary distance is much smaller between quail and chicken than mouse and human (30 MYA against 75 MYA). Therefore, it is likely that alternative splicing plays the primary role in defining differences in levels of telomerase in these species because the short time window in which quail and chicken diverged. The evolution of new splice donor and acceptor sites for expression of novel AS variants is likely to be more rapid since this does not interfere with existing transcriptional regulation or protein structure. In contrast, more evolutionary distant species, such a duck, which expresses similarly low levels of telomerase like the chicken, has an intermediate number of alternative splice variants, suggesting that other mechanisms are also involved in regulation of telomerase levels among species.

On the other hand, the longer and extremely rapid evolution of the rodent branch of mammals allowed high divergence not only in promoter region, but also resulted in greater structural differences between the mouse and human TERT proteins (mouse/human - 62/74%, quail/chicken - 94/97% identity/similarity of TERT protein sequence). Divergences at the protein level resulted in differences for at least some enzymatic characteristic of telomerase since these differences contribute to their different processivity (Fakhoury et al., 2010). However, it is likely that even between mouse and human the difference in frequency and complexity of TERT alternative splicing plays an important role in differential levels of telomerase in addition to in the promoter and protein structure. Twenty-one AS variants of human TERT have been identified and most of the TERT transcripts in adult human tissue are alternatively spliced (Ulaner & Giudice, 1997). In contrast, mice express only a few AS forms (Sýkorová & Fajkus, 2009) suggesting that alternative splicing of TERT also correlates with levels of telomerase in these two species. In conclusion, alternative splicing of the TERT genes appears to be an important factor in the establishment of the interspecies differences in telomerase activity.

4.4 The co-evolution of alternative splicing of TERT with levels of telomerase in birds and mammals

In many metazoan species TERT transcripts are alternatively spliced. Several AS TERT variants have been reported in a number of species including human, rat, dog, chicken, zebrafish, and plants (Sýkorová & Fajkus, 2009). In the human and chicken, which have been extensively studied, 21 and 37 single-event AS TERT variants have been identified (Amor et al., 2010; Chang & Delany, 2006; Hisatomi et al., 2003; Hrdličková et al., 2012a; Hrdličková et al., 2006; Saebøe-Larssen et al., 2006; Wick et al., 1999). Interestingly, none of the human and chicken AS variants are identical, suggesting that AS TERT variants evolved independently in placental mammals and birds. Results presented in this study offer the explanation for this finding. The evolution of AS splicing may serve as a mechanism in part for the determination of different levels of telomerase activity in homoeothermic species. Apparently, the levels of telomerase activity changed several times in evolution of mammals closely following the respective differences in body mass (Gomes et al., 2011; Seluanov et al.,

2007). We propose that alternative splicing contributes to these changes by reducing the number of AS TERT forms in species with high levels of telomerase activity as a result of the elimination or modifications of splice sites as occurred in quail. In new species that originate from such predecessors, novel AS variants would have evolved by the introduction of new splice sites and enhancers creating structurally different AS variants. Repeated changes in the intrinsic levels of telomerase during evolution of mammals, therefore, resulted in the repeated elimination of AS TERT variants followed by the evolution of new variants, ultimately creating different repertoires of AS variants in birds and mammals. Interestingly, we have exhaustively analyzed alternative splicing of TERT in the platypus and found that this species from the basal branch of the mammalian lineage expresses a limited number of AS variants, which are very closely related to chicken AS variants (Hrdličková et al., 2012b). This suggests that the evolution of levels of telomerase activity and alternative splicing was less dynamic in bird species than in placental mammals. In mammals, the predecessor of placental animals probably evolved after a prolonged period when different species with a small body mass and high levels of telomerase had a reduced number of alternatively spliced TERT variants. This was later followed by the evolution of new repertoire of alternatively spliced forms in placental mammals with a greater body mass.

5. Conclusion

There are great differences in telomerase activity among several groups of mammals indicating that several changes in the regulation of telomerase activity occurred during mammalian evolution (Gomes et al., 2011). However, differences in telomerase activity in birds, an independently evolved branch of homeothermic animals have not been reported. Lastly, the mechanism responsible for these differences in telomerase activity in homeothermic animals is largely unknown. Our comparative analysis of quail, chicken, and duck demonstrated differences in telomerase activity in avian species. Moreover, analysis of the closely related quail and chicken suggested that alternative splicing may play a direct role in determining levels of telomerase expressed in both embryonic and adult tissues of these two species. Elevated telomerase activity in quail tissues correlates with ten times less AS variants. The analysis of the more distantly related duck supports the general conclusion that alternative splicing plays an important role in determining interspecies differences of telomerase activity, but also suggests that other mechanisms are probably involved.

These results suggest that alternative splicing is the key mechanism for differences in telomerase activity in homeothermic animals. We propose that alternative splicing of TERT is a mechanism which contributes to fluctuations in telomerase canonical activity during evolution without losing the non-canonical functions of telomerase and reflects interspecies differences in aging.

Future research will focus on defining the function of alternatively spliced variants, with the emphasis on variants with premature termination codons. Additionally, the identification of AS TERT variants in key mammalian species would further evaluate the role of alternative splicing in evolution of differences in levels in telomerase and will create the precedent for analysis of the role of alternative splicing in evolution of other genes. These studies of alternative splicing from a functional angle would help us understand its role beyond the "stochastic noise" (Melamud & Moult, 2009).

6. Acknowledgment

We thank Addie Dickson for her help with initial TRAP assays and cloning, and Michael P. Domjan and Nicolle Matthews (University of Texas) for quail eggs and adult animals. We thank to W. Bargmann for careful reading of the manuscript. This study was supported by the Public Health Service grants CA33192 and CA098151 from the National Cancer Institute.

7. References

Abril, J.F., Castelo, R., & Guigo, R. (2005). Comparison of splice sites in mammals and chicken. Genome Research, Vol.15, No.1, (January 2005), pp.111-119, ISSN 1088-9051

Alter, B.P., Rosenberg, P.S., Giri, N., Baerlocher, G.M., Lansdorp, P.M., & Savage, S.A. (2012). Telomere length is associated with disease severity and declines with age in dyskeratosis congenita. Haematologica, Vol.97, No.3, (March 2012), pp.353-359, ISSN 1592-8721

Amor, S., Remy, S., Dambrine, G., Vern, Y.L., Rasschaert, D., & Laurent, S. (2010). Alternative splicing and nonsense-mediated decay regulate telomerase reverse transcriptase (TERT) expression during virus-induced lymphomagenesis in vivo. BMC Cancer, Vol.10, No.571, (October 2010), pp.1-12, ISSN 1471-2407

Armanios, M. (2009). Syndromes of telomere shortening. Annual Review of Genomics and Human Genetics, Vol.10, No. 45, (April 2009), pp.1-21, ISSN 1545-293X

Armanios, M. (2012). Telomerase and idiopathic pulmonary fibrosis. Mutation Research, Vol.730, No.1-2, (February 2012), pp.52-58, ISSN 0027-5107

Autexier, C. & Lue, N.F. (2006). The structure and function of telomerase reverse transcriptase Annual Review of Biochemistry, Vol.75, (March 2006), pp.493-517, ISSN 0066-4154

Baird, D.M. (2010). Variation at the TERT locus and predisposition for cancer. Expert Reviews in Molecular Medicine, Vol.12, (May 2010), pp.e16, ISSN 1462-3994

Benton, M.J. (2005). Vertebrate palaeontology (third edition), Blackwell Science Ltd., ISBN 0-632-05637-1, Malden, USA; Oxford, UK; Victoria, Australia.

Blackburn, E.H. & Collins, K. (2011). Telomerase: An RNP enzyme synthesizes DNA. Cold Spring Harbor Perspectives in Biology, Vol.3, No.5, (May 2011), pp.a003558, ISSN 1943-0264

Blasco, M.A. & Hahn, W.C. (2003). Evolving views of telomerase and cancer. Trends in Cell Biology, Vol.13, No.6, (June 2003), pp.289-294, ISSN 0962-8924

Bodnar, A.G., Ouellette, M., Frolkis, M., Holt, S.E., Chiu, C.P., Morin, G.B., Harley, C.B., Shay, J.W., Lichtsteiner, S., & Wright, W.E. (1998). Extension of life-span by introduction of telomerase into normal human cells. Science, Vol.279, No.5349, (January 1998), pp.349-352, ISSN 0036-8075

Bollmann, F.M. (2008). The many faces of telomerase: emerging extratelomeric effects. Bioessays, Vol.30, No.8, (August 2008), pp.728-732, ISSN 1521-1878

Bousman, S., Schneider, G., & Shampay, J. (2003). Telomerase activity is widespread in adult somatic tissues of Xenopus. Journal of Experimental Zoology, Vol.295B, No.1, (February 2003), pp.82-86, ISSN 1552-5007

Brenner, C.A., Wolny, Y.M., Adler, R.R., & Cohen, J. (1999). Alternative splicing of the telomerase catalytic subunit in human oocytes and embryos. Molecular Human Reproduction, Vol.5, No.9, (September 1999), pp.845-850, ISSN 1360-9947

Cech, T.R. (2004). Beginning to understand the end of the chromosome. Cell, Vol.116, No.2, (January 2004), pp.273-279, ISSN 0092-8674

Chang, H. & Delany, M.E. (2006). Complicated RNA splicing of chicken telomerase reverse transcriptase revealed by profiling cells both positive and negative for telomerase activity. Gene, Vol.379, (September 2006), pp.33-39, ISSN 0378-1119

Chiang, Y.J., Calado, R.T., Hathcock, K.S., Landsdorp, P.M., Young, N.S., & Hodes, R.J. (2010). Telomere length is inherited with resetting of the telomere set-point. Proceedings of the National Academy of Sciences of the United States of America, Vol.107, No.22, (June 2010), pp.10148-10153, ISSN 1091-6490

Chubb, A.L. (2004). New nuclear evidence for the oldest divergence among neognath birds: the phylogenetic utility of ZENK (i). Molecular Phylogenetics and Evolution, Vol.30, No.1, (January 2004), pp.140-151, ISSN 1055-7903

Cifuentes-Rojas, C. & Shippen, D.E. (2012). Telomerase regulation. Mutation Research, Vol.730, No.1-2, (February 2012), pp.20-27, ISSN 0027-5107

Colgin, L.M., Wilkinson, C., Englezou, A., Killian, A., Robinson, M.O., & Reddel, R.R. (2000). The hTERT α splice variant is a dominant negative inhibitor of telomerase activity. Neoplasia, Vol.2, No.5, (September-October 2000), pp.426-432, ISSN 1522-8002

Cong, Y. & Shay, J.W. (2008). Actions of human telomerase beyond telomeres. Cell Research, Vol.18, No.7, (July 2008), pp.725-732, ISSN 1748-7838

Delany, M.E. & Daniels, L.M. (2004). The chicken telomerase reverse transcriptase (chTERT): molecular and cytogenetic characterization with a comparative analysis. Gene, Vol.339, (September 2004), pp.61-69, ISSN 0378-1119

Devereux, T.R., Horikawa, I., Anna, C.H., Annab, L.A., Afshari, C.A., & Barret, J.C. (1999). DNA methylation analysis of the promoter region of the human telomerase reverse transcriptase (hTERT) gene. Cancer Research, Vol.59, No.24, (December 1999), pp.6087-6090, ISSN 0008-5472

Fakhoury, J., Marie-Egyptienne, D.T., Londoño-Vallejo, J.-A., & Autexier, C. (2010). Telomeric function of mammalian telomerases at short telomeres. Journal of Cell Science, Vol.123, No.Pt10, (May 2010), pp.1693-1704, ISSN 1477-9137

Gillis, A.J., Schuller, A.P., & Skordalakes, E. (2008). Structure of the Tribolium castaneum telomerase catalytic subunit TERT. Nature, Vol.455, No.7213, (October 2008), pp.633-637, ISSN 1476-4687

Gladych, M., Wojtyla, A., & Rubis, B. (2011). Human telomerase expression regulation. Biochemistry and Cell Biology, Vol.89, No.4, (August 2011), pp.359-376, ISSN 1208-6002

Gomes, N.M.V., Ryder, O.A., Houck, M.L., Charter, S.J., Walker, W., Forsyth, N.R., Austad, S.N., Venditti, C., Pagel, M., Shay, J.W., & Wright, W.E. (2011). Comparative biology of mammalian telomeres: Hypotheses on ancestral states and the roles of telomeres in longevity determination. Aging Cell, Vol.10, No.5, (October 2011), pp.761-768, ISSN 1474-9726

Gomes, N.M.V., Shay, J.W., & Wright, W.E. (2010). Telomere biology in Metazoa. FEBS Letters, Vol.584, No.17, (September 2010), pp.3741-3751, ISSN 1873-3468

Gorbunova, V. & Seluanov, A. (2009). Coevolution of telomerase activity and body mass in mammals: from mice to beavers. Mechanisms of ageing and development, Vol.130, No.1-2, (January-February 2009), pp.3-9, ISSN 0047-6374

Green, R.E., Lewis, B.P., Hillman, R.T., Blanchette, M., Lareau, L.F., Garnett, A.T., Rio, D.C., & Brenner, S.E. (2003). Widespread predicted nonsense-mediated mRNA decay of alternatively-spliced transcripts of human normal and disease genes. Bioinformatics (Oxford, England), Vol.19, Suppl. 1, (February 2003), pp.i118-121, ISSN 1367-4803

Greenberg, R.A., Allsopp, R.C., Chin, L., Morin, G.B., & DePinho, R.A. (1998). Expression of mouse telomerase reverse transcriptase during development, differentiation and proliferation. Oncogene, Vol.16, No.13, (April 1998), pp.1723-1730, ISSN 0950-9232

Guilleret, I. & Benhattar, J. (2003). Demethylation of the human telomerase catalytic subunit (hTERT) gene promoter reduced hTERT expression and telomerase activity and shortened telomeres. Experimental Cell Research, Vol.289, No.2, (October 2003), pp.326-334, ISSN 0014-4827

Hartl, M., Vogt, P.K., & Bister, K. (1995). A quail long-term cell culture transformed by a chimeric jun oncogene. Virology, Vol.207, No.1, (February 1995), pp.321-326, ISSN 0042-6822

Hartmann, N., Reichwald, K., Lechel, A., Graf, M., Kirschner, J., Dorn, A., Terzibasi, E., Wellner, J., Platzer, M., Rudolph, K.L., Cellerino, A., & Englert, C. (2009). Telomeres shorten while Tert expresion increases during ageing of the short-lived fish Nothobranchius furzeri. Mechanisms of ageing and development, Vol.130, No.5, (May 2009), pp.290-296, ISSN 1872-6216

Hisatomi, H., Ohyashiki, K., Ohyashiki, J.H., Nagao, K., Kanamaru, T., Hirata, H., Hibi, N., & Tsukada, Y. (2003). Expression profile of a γ-deletion variant of the human telomerase reverse transcriptase gene. Neoplasia, Vol.5, No.3, (May-June 2003), pp.193-197, ISSN 1522-8002

Horikawa, I., Chiang, Y.J., Patterson, T., Feigenbaum, L., Leem, S.-H., Michishita, E., Larionov, V., Hodes, R.J., & Barret, J.C. (2005). Differential cis-regulation of human versus mouse TERT gene expression in vivo: Identification of a human-specific repressive element. Proceedings of the National Academy of Sciences of the United States of America, Vol.102, No.51, (December 2005), pp.18437-18442, ISSN 0027-8424

Hrdličková, R., Nehyba, J., & H.R.Bose, J. (2012a). Alternatively spliced TERT variants lacking telomerase activity stimulate cell proliferation. Molecular and Cellular Biology, Vol.32, No.21, (November 2012), doi:10.1128/MCB.00550-00512, ISSN 1098-5549

Hrdličková, R., Nehyba, J., Lim, S.L., Grützner, F., & Bose, H.R. (2012b). Insights into the evolution of mammalian telomerase: Platypus TERT shares similarities with genes of birds and other reptiles and localizes on sex chromosomes. BMC Genomics, Vol.13, (June 2012b), pp.216, ISSN 1471-2164

Hrdličková, R., Nehyba, J., Liss, A.S., & Bose, H.R., Jr. (2006). Mechanism of telomerase activation by v-Rel and its contribution to transformation. Journal of Virology, Vol.80, No.1, (January 2006), pp.281-295, ISSN 0022-538X

Huson, D.H., Richter, D.C., Rausch, C., Dezulian, T., Franz, M., & Rupp, R. (2007). Dendroscope: An interactive viewer for large phylogenetic trees. BMC Bioinformatics, Vol.8, (November 2007), pp.460, ISSN 1471-2105

Jeanclos, E., Schork, N.J., Kyvik, K.O., Kimura, M., Skurnick, J.H., & Aviv, A. (2000). Telomere length inversely correlates with pulse presure and is highly familial. Hypertension, Vol.36, No.2, (August 2000), pp.195-200, ISSN 0194-911X

Jia, W., Wang, S., Horner, J.W., Wang, N., Wang, H., Gunther, E.J., DePinho, R.A., & Zhu, J. (2011). A BAC transgenic reporter recapitulates in vivo regulation of human telomerase reverse transcriptase in development and tumorigenesis. The FASEB Journal, Vol.25, No.3, (March 2011), pp.979-989, ISSN 1530-6860

Kaneko, R., Esumi, S., Yagi, T., & Hirabayashi, T. (2006). Predominant expression of rTERTb, an inactive TERT variant, in the adult rat brain. Protein & Peptide Letters, Vol.13, No.1, (January 2006), pp.59-65, ISSN 0929-8665

Kappei, D. & Londoño-Vallejo, J.A. (2008). Telomere length inheritance and aging. Mechanisms of ageing and development, Vol.129, No.1-2, (January-February 2008), pp.17-26, ISSN 0047-6374

Keller, R.B., Gagne, K.E., Usmami, G.N., Asdourian, G.K., Williams, D.A., Hofmann, I., & Agarwal, S. (2012). CTC1 mutations in a patient with dyskeratosis congenita. Pediatric Blood & Cancer, Vol.59, (August 2012), pp.311-314, ISSN 1545-5017

Kim, H., You, S., Farris, J., Kong, B.-W., Christman, S.A., Foster, L.K., & Foster, D.N. (2002). Expression profiles of p53-, p16^{ink4a} -, and telomere-regulating genes in replicative senescent primary human, mouse, and chicken fibroblast cells. Experimental Cell Research, Vol.272, No.2, (January 2002), pp.199-208, ISSN 0014-4827

Kim, N.W., Piatyszek, M.A., Prowse, K.R., Harley, C.B., West, M.D., Ho, P.L.C., Coviello, G.M., Wright, W.E., Weinrich, S.L., & Shay, J.W. (1994). Specific association of human telomerase activity with immortal cells and cancer. Science, Vol.266, No.5193, (December 1994), pp.2011-2015, ISSN 0036-8075

Kirkwood, T.B. (2005). Understanding of odd science of aging. Cell, Vol.120, No.4, (February 2005), pp.437-447, ISSN 0092-8674

Larkin, M.A., Blackshields, G., Brown, N.P., Chenna, R., McGettigan, P.A., McWilliam, H., Valentin, F., Wallace, I.M., Wilm, A., Lopez, R., Thompson, J.D., Gibson, T.J., & Higgins, D.G. (2007). Clustal W and Clustal X version 2.0. Bioinformatics (Oxford, England), Vol.23, No.21, (November 2007), pp.2947-2948, ISSN 1367-4811

Latrick, C.M. & Cech, T.R. (2010). POT1-TPP1 enhances telomerase processivity by slowing primer dissociation and aiding translocation. EMBO Journal, Vol.29, No.5, (March 2010), pp.924-933, ISSN 1460-2075

Lewis, B.P., Green, R.E., & Brenner, S.E. (2003). Evidence for the widespread coupling of alternative splicing and nonsense-mediated mRNA decay. Proceedings of the National Academy of Sciences of the United States of America, Vol.100, No.1, (January 2003), pp.189-192, ISSN 0027-8424

Lewis, K.A. & Wuttke, D.S. (2012). Telomerase and telomere-associated proteins: structural insights into mechanism and evolution. Structure, Vol.20, No.1, (January 2012), pp.28-39, ISSN 1878-4186

Lin, J., Epel, E., & Blackburn, E. (2012). Telomeres and lifestyle factors: Roles in cellular aging. Mutation Research, Vol.730, No.1-2, (February 2012), pp.85-89, ISSN 0027-5107

Liu, C., Fang, X., Ge, Z., Jalink, M., Kyo, S., Bjorkholm, M., Gruber, A., Sjoberg, J., & Xu, D. (2007). The telomerase reverse transcriptase (hTERT) gene is a direct target of the histone methyltransferase SMYD3. Cancer Research, Vol.67, No.6, (March 2007), pp.2626-2631, ISSN 0008-5472

Majerská, J., Sýkorová, E., & Fajkus, J. (2011). Non-telomeric activities of telomerase. Molecular BioSystems, Vol.7, No.4, (April 2011), pp.1013-1023, ISSN 1742-2051

Marcovici, M. & Prier, J.E. (1968). Enhancement of St. Louis arbovirus plaque formation by neutral red. Journal of Virology, Vol.2, No.3, (March 1968), pp.178-181, ISSN 0022-538X

Mason, M., Schuller, A., & Skordalakes, E. (2011). Telomerase structure function. Current Opinion in Structural Biology, Vol.21, No.1, (February 2011), pp.1-9, ISSN 1879-033X

Melamud, E. & Moult, J. (2009). Stochastic noise in splicing machinery. Nucleic Acids Research, Vol.37, No.14, (August 2009), pp.4873-4886, ISSN 1362-4962

Moscovici, C., Moscovici, M.G., Jimenez, H., Lai, M.M., Hayman, M.J., & Vogt, P.K. (1977). Continuous tissue culture cell lines derived from chemically induced tumors of Japanese quail. Cell, Vol.11, No.1, (May 1977), pp.95-103, ISSN 0092-8674

Nawrot, T.S., Staessen, J.A., Gardner, J.P., & Aviv, A. (2004). Telomere length and possible link to X chromosome. Lancet, Vol.363, No.9408, (February 2004), pp.507-510, ISSN 1474-547X

Nelson, N.D. & Bertuch, A.A. (2012). Dyskeratosis congenita as a disorder of telomere maintenance. Mutation Research, Vol.730, No.1-2, (February 2012), pp.43-51, ISSN 0027-5107

Nilsen, T.W. & Graveley, B.R. (2010). Expansion of the eukaryotic proteome by alternative splicing. Nature, Vol.463, No.7280, (January 2010), pp.457-463, ISSN 1476-4687

Njajou, O.T., Cawthon, R.M., Damcott, C.M., Wu, S.-H., Ott, S., Garant, M.J., Blackburn, E.H., Mitchell, B.D., Shuldiner, A.R., & Hsueh, W.-C. (2007). Telomere length is paternally inherited and is associated with parental lifespan. Proceedings of the National Academy of Sciences of the United States of America, Vol.104, No.29, (July 2007), pp.12135-12139, ISSN 0027-8424

Nordfjäll, K., Larefalk, Å., Lindgren, P., Holmberg, D., & Roos, G. (2005). Telomere length and heredity: Indications of paternal inheritance. Proceedings of the National Academy of Sciences of the United States of America, Vol.102, No.45, (November 2005), pp.16374-16378, ISSN 0027-8424

Ogburn, C.E., Carlberg, K., Ottinger, M.A., Holmes, D.J., Martin, G.M., & Austad, S.N. (2001). Exceptional cellular resistance to oxidative damage in long-lived birds requires active gene expression. The journals of gerontology. Series A, Biological sciences and medical sciences, Vol.56, No.11, (November 2001), pp.B468-B474, ISSN 1079-5006

Olovnikov, A.M. (1971). Principles of marginotomy in template synthesis of polynucleotides. Doklady Akademii Nauk SSSR, Vol.201, No.6, (January 1971), pp.1496–1499, ISSN 0002-3264

Osterhage, J.L. & Friedman, K.L. (2009). Chromosome end maintenance by telomerase. The Journal of Biological Chemistry, Vol.284, No.24, (June 2009), pp.16061-16065, ISSN 0021-9258

Park, J.I., Venteicher, A.S., Hong, J.Y., Choi, J., Jun, S., Shkreli, M., Chang, W., Meng, Z., Cheung, P., Ji, H., McLaughlin, M., Veenstra, T.D., Nusse, R., McCrea, P.D., & Artandi, S.E. (2009). Telomerase modulates Wnt signalling by association with target gene chromatin. Nature, Vol.460, No.7251, (July 2009), pp.66-72, ISSN 1476-4687

Parkinson, E.K., Fitchett, C., & Cereser, B. (2008). Dissecting the non-canonical functions of telomerase. Cytogenetic and Genome Research, Vol.122, No.3-4, (July 2008), pp.273-280, ISSN 1424-859X

Parrinello, S., Samper, E., Krtolica, A., Goldstein, J., Melov, S., & Campisi, J. (2003). Oxygen sensitivity severely limits the replicative lifespan of murine fibroblasts. Nature Cell Biology, Vol.5, No.8, (August 2003), pp.741-747, ISSN 1465-7392

Pereira, S.L. & Baker, A.J. (2006). A molecular timescale for galliform birds accounting for uncertainty in time estimates and heterogeneity of rates of DNA substitutions across lineages and sites. Molecular Phylogenetics and Evolution, Vol.38, No.2, (February 2006), pp.499-509, ISSN 1055-7903

Pfennig, F., Kind, B., Zieschang, F., Busch, M., & Gutzeit, H.O. (2008). Tert expression and telomerase activity in gonads and somatic cells of the Japanese medaka (Oryzias latipes). Development, Growth & Differentiation, Vol.50, No.3, (March 2008), pp.131-141, ISSN 1440-169X

Podlevsky, J.D. & Chen, J.J.-L. (2012). It all comes together at the ends: Telomerase structure, function, and biogenesis. Mutation Research, Vol.730, No.1-2, (February 2012), pp.3-11, ISSN 0027-5107

Prowse, K.R. & Greider, C.W. (1995). Developmental and tissue-specific regulation of mouse telomerase and telomere length. Proceedings of the National Academy of Sciences of the United States of America, Vol.92, (May 1995), pp.4818-4822, ISSN 0027-8424

Ren, J.-G., Xia, H.-L., Tian, Y.-M., Just, T., Cai, G.-P., & Dai, Y.-R. (2001). Expression of telomerase inhibits hydroxyl radical-induced apoptosis in normal telomerase negative human lung fibroblasts. FEBS Letters, Vol.488, No.3, (January 2001), pp.133-138, ISSN 0014-5793

Ritz, J.M., Kühle, O., Riethdorf, S., Sipos, B., Deppert, W., Englert, C., & Günes, C. (2005). A novel transgenic mouse model reveals humanlike regulation of an 8-kbp human TERT gene promoter fragment in normal and tumor tissues. Cancer Research, Vol.65, No.4, (February 2005), pp.1187-1196, ISSN 0008-5472

Robart, A.R. & Collins, K. (2010). Investigation of human telomerase holoenzyme assembly, activity and processivity using disease-linked subunit variants. Journal of Biological Chemistry, Vol.285, No.7, (February 2010), pp.4375-4386, ISSN 1083-351X

Ronquist, F. & Huelsenbeck, J.P. (2003). MrBayes 3: Bayesian phylogenetic inference under mixed models. Bioinformatics (Oxford, England), Vol.19, No.12, (August 2003), pp.1572-1574, ISSN 1367-4803

Saebøe-Larssen, S., Fossberg, E., & Gaudernack, G. (2006). Characterization of novel alternative splicing sites in human telomerase reverse transcriptase (hTERT): analysis of expression and mutual correlation in mRNA isoforms from normal and tumour tissues. BMC Molecular Biology, Vol.7, No.26, (August 2006), pp.26, ISSN 1471-2199

Salpea, K.D., Talmud, P.J., Cooper, J.A., Maubaret, C.G., Stephens, J.W., Abelak, K., & Humphries, S.E. (2010). Association of telomere length with type 2 diabetes, oxidative stress and UCP2 gene variation. Atherosclerosis, Vol.209, No.1, (March 2010), pp.42-50, ISSN 1879-1484

Sarin, K.Y., Cheung, P., Gilison, D., Lee, E., Tennen, R.I., Wang, E., Artandi, M.K., Oro, A.E., & Artandi, S.E. (2005). Conditional telomerase induction causes proliferation of hair follicle stem cells. Nature, Vol.436, No.7053, (August 2005), pp.1048-1052, ISSN 1476-4687

Sekaran, V.G., Soares, J., & Jarstfer, M.B. (2010). Structures of telomerase subunits provide functional insights. Biochimica and Biophysica Acta, Vol.1804, No.5, (May 2010), pp.1190-1201, ISSN 0006-3002

Seluanov, A., Chen, Z., Hine, C., Sasahara, T.H.C., Ribeiro, A.A.C.M., Catania, K.C., Presgraves, D.C., & Gorbunova, V. (2007). Telomerase activity coevolves with body mass, not lifespan. Aging Cell, Vol.6, No.1, (February 2007), pp.45-52, ISSN 1474-9718

Shay, J.W. & Wright, W.E. (2005). Senescence and immortalization: role of telomeres and telomerase. Carcinogenesis, Vol.26, No.5, (May 2005), pp.867-874, ISSN 0143-3334

Slagboom, P.E., Droog, S., & Boomsma, D.I. (1994). Genetic determination of telomere size in humans: a twin study of three age groups. American Journal of Human Genetics, Vol.55, No.5, (November 1994), pp.876-882, ISSN 0002-9297

Smith, L.L., Coller, H.A., & Roberts, J.M. (2003). Telomerase modulates expression of growth-controlling genes and enhances cell proliferation. Nature Cell Biology, Vol.5, No.5, (May 2003), pp.474-479, ISSN 1465-7392

Sýkorová, E. & Fajkus, J. (2009). Structure-function relationships in telomerase genes. Biological Cell, Vol.101, No.7, (July 2009), pp.375-392, ISSN 1768-322X

Takakura, M., Kyo, S., Inoue, M., Wright, W.E., & Shay, J.W. (2005). Function of AP-1 in transcription of the telomerase reverse transcriptase gene (TERT) in human and mouse cells. Molecular and Cellular Biology, Vol.25, No.18, (September 2005), pp.8037-8043, ISSN 0270-7306

Taylor, H.A. & Delany, M.E. (2000). Ontogeny of telomerase in chicken: Impact of downregulation on pre- and postnatal telomere length in vivo. Development, Growth & Differentiation, Vol.42, No.6, (December 2000), pp.613-621, ISSN 0012-1592

Ulaner, G.A. & Giudice, L.C. (1997). Developmental regulation of telomerase activity in human fetal tissues during gestation. Molecular Human Reproduction, Vol.3, No.9, (September 1997), pp.769-773, ISSN 1360-9947

Ulaner, G.A., Hu, J.-F., Vu, T.H., Giudice, L.C., & Hoffman, A.R. (1998). Telomerase activity in human development is regulated by human telomerase reverse transcriptase (hTERT) transcription and by alternate splicing of hTERT transcripts. Cancer Research, Vol.58, No.18, (September 1998), pp.4168-4172, ISSN 0008-5472

Ulaner, G.A., Hu, J.-F., Vu, T.H., Giudice, L.C., & Hoffman, A.R. (2001). Tissue-specific alternate splicing of human telomerase reverse transcriptase (hTERT) influences telomere lengths during human development. International Journal of Cancer, Vol.91, No.5, (March 2001), pp.644-649, ISSN 0020-7136

Ulaner, G.A., Hu, J.-F., Vu, T.H., Oruganti, H., Giudice, L.C., & Hoffman, A.R. (2000). Regulation of telomerase by alternate splicing of human telomerase reverse transcriptase (hTERT) in normal and neoplastic ovary, endometrium and myometrium. International Journal of Cancer, Vol.85, No.3, (February 2000), pp.330-335, ISSN 0020-7136

van Tuinen, M. & Dyke, G.J. (2004). Calibration of galliform molecular clocks using multiple fossils and genetic partitions. Molecular Phylogenetics and Evolution, Vol.30, No.1, (January 2004), pp.74-86, ISSN 1055-7903

von Zglinicki, T. (2002). Oxidative stress shortens telomeres. Trends in Biochemical Sciences, Vol.27, No.7, (July 2002), pp.339-344, ISSN 0968-0004

Wachtel, C., Li, B., Sperling, J., & Sperling, R. (2004). Stop codon-mediated suppression of splicing is a novel nuclear scanning mechanism not affected by elements of protein synthesis and NMD. RNA, Vol.10, No.11, (November 2004), pp.1740-1750, ISSN 1355-8382

Walne, A., Bhagat, T., Kirwan, M., Gitaux, C., Desquerre, I., Leonard, N., Nogales, E., Vulliamy, T., & Dokal, I. (2012). Mutations in the telomere capping complex in bone marrow failure and related syndromes. Haematologica, (August 2012), pp.doi:10.3324/haematol.2012.071068, ISSN 1592-8721

Wang, S., Zhao, Y., Hu, C., & Zhu, J. (2009). Differential repression of human and mouse TERT genes during cell differentiation. Nucleic Acids Research, Vol.37, No.8, (May 2009), pp.2618-2629, ISSN 1362-4962

Wang, S. & Zhu, J. (2004). The hTERT gene is embedded in a nuclease-resistant chromatin domain. Journal of Biological Chemistry, Vol.279, No.53, (December 2004), pp.55401-55410, ISSN 0021-9258

Watson, J.D. (1972). Origin of concatemeric T7 DNA. Nature New Biology, Vol.239, No.94, (October 1972), pp.197-201, ISSN 0090-0028

Watson, J.M. & Riha, K. (2010). Comparative biology of telomeres: Where plants stand. FEBS Letters, Vol.584, No.17, (September 2010), pp.3752-3759, ISSN 1873-3468

Wick, M., Zubov, D., & Hagen, G. (1999). Genomic organization and promoter characterization of the gene encoding the human telomerase reverse transcriptase (hTERT). Gene, Vol.232, No.1, (May 1999), pp.97-106, ISSN 0378-1119

Wyatt, H.D.M., West, S.C., & Beattie, T.L. (2010). InTERTpreting telomerase structure and function. Nucleic Acids Research, Vol.38, No.17, (September 2010), pp.5609-5622, ISSN 1362-4962

Xie, M., Podlevsky, J.D., Qi, X., Bley, C.J., & Chen, J.J. (2010). A novel motif in telomerase reverse transcriptase regulates telomere repeat addition rate and processivity. Nucleic Acids Research, Vol.38, No.6, (April 2010), pp.1982-1996, ISSN 1362-4962

Yap, W.H., Yeoh, E., Brenner, S., & Venkatesh, B. (2005). Cloning and expression of the reverse transcriptase component of pufferfish (Fugu rubripes) telomerase. Gene, Vol.353, No.2, (July 2005), pp.207-217, ISSN 0378-1119

Yi, X., White, D.M., Aisner, D.L., Baur, J.A., Wright, W.E., & Shay, J.W. (2000). An alternate splicing variant of the human telomerase catalytic subunit inhibits telomerase activity. Neoplasia, Vol.2, No.5, (September-October 2000), pp.433-440, ISSN 1522-8002

Zee, R.Y.L., Castonguay, A.J., Barton, N.S., Germer, S., & Martin, M. (2010). Mean leukocyte telomere length shortening and type 2 diabetes mellitus: a case-control study. Translational Research, Vol.155, No.4, (April 2010), pp.166-169, ISSN 1878-1810

Zhu, J., Zhao, Y., & Wang, S. (2010). Chromatin and epigenetic regulation of the telomerase reverse transcriptase gene. Protein & Cell, Vol.1, No.1, (January 2010), pp.22-32, ISSN 1674-8018

Section 2

Telomeres and Human Diseases

4

Telomere and Telomerase in Cancer: Recent Progress

Güvem Gümüş-Akay and Ajlan Tükün
Ankara University
Turkey

1. Introduction

Telomeres are specialized structures at the ends of all eukaryotic chromosomes and have special biological functions. They protect chromosomes from nucleolytic degradation, end-to-end fusions, and to be recognized as damaged DNA. Telomeres also contribute to the functional organizations of the chromosomes within the nucleus, participate in the regulation of gene expression, and most importantly, they serve as a molecular clock that controls the replicative capacity of the cells (Allsopp et al., 1992; Bailey et al., 2006; Chan & Blackburn, 2004; Hahn, 2005; O'sullivan & Karlseder, 2010).

In the last decade substantial progress has been made in human telomere biology. Humans, like other vertebrates, have telomeres composed of repetitive 5'-TTAGGG-3' sequences (Meyne et al., 1989; Moyzis et al., 1988). Human telomeres end in a 3' overhang composed of TTAGGG track which is 50-500 nucleotides long (Huffman et al., 2000; Makarov et al., 1997; Wright et al., 1997). Electron microscopy studies of the psoralen cross-linked human telomeres have revealed that telomeres terminate in a lariat-like structure termed a t-loop. Binding of TRF1 and single stranded binding protein suggested that this structure is formed by invasion of the 3' telomeric overhang into the duplex telomeric repeat array (Griffith et al., 1999) (Figure 1A and 1B). The fundamental aspect of the t-loop is thought to be the sequestration of the chromosome ends thereby providing a solution for the telomere end protection problem (de Lange, 2006; Grifith et al., 1999). Indeed, disruption of t-loop can result in telomere dysfunction and induce DNA damage response (d'Adda di Fagagna et al., 2003). Human telomeric DNA is found as associated with nucleosomes, six-subunit protein complex called shelterin, and a number of other chromosomal factors that are not part of the shelterin (de Lange, 2005, 2006; Diotti & Loayza, 2011).

1.1 Shelterin

Shelterin complex represses DNA damage signaling responses at the chromosome ends. It also participates in the formation of t-loops and regulation of telomere length (de Lange, 2005, 2006; Palm & de Lange, 2008) (Figure 1A and 1B). This complex consists of six subunits including TRF1, TRF2, TIN2, Rap1, POT1, and TPP1. The expression of shelterin is ubiquitous and it is present at telomeres throughout cell cycle. It is estimated that hundreds of copies of shelterin are found throughout the double stranded telomeric DNA and unlike other telomere associated non-shelterin proteins; its function is limited only to telomeres (de Lange, 2005, 2006; Takai et al., 2010).

Shelterin binds to double stranded telomeric DNA via its DNA binding proteins TRF1 (TTAGGG-repeat-binding factor 1) and TRF2 (TTAGGG-repeat-biding factor 2) (Broccoli et al., 1997; Chong et al., 1995). TRF1 is the first identified subunit of shelterin complex that particularly binds to the double stranded telomeric DNA mainly as a dimer form that is mediated by its TRF homology (TRFH) domain (Bianchi et al., 1997; Zhong et al., 1992). The TRFH domain also participates in the recruitment of other proteins to the telomere (Y. Chen et al., 2008). In the shelterin complex TRF1 interacts only with TIN2 (S.H. Kim et al., 1999). In telomerase-positive mammalian cells, TRF1 works as a negative regulator of telomere length (Iwano et al., 2004; Okamoto et al., 2008) and supporting of this, the absence of TRF1 from telomeres results in telomere elongation (Iwano et al., 2004; Smith & de Lange, 2000; Smogorzewska et al., 2000; van Steensel & de Lange, 1997).

TRF2, which is a 500 amino acid protein, shows sequence similarity to TRF1. Like TRF1, TRF2 also has a TRFH domain allowing its homodimerization (Broccoli et al., 1997; Fairall et al., 2001). It has been demonstrated that the TRF2 facilitates the t-loop formation *in vitro* (Stansel et al., 2001). TRF2 interacts with other three members of the shelterin complex,TIN2, Rap1, and POT1, and behaves as a negative regulator of telomere length (Smogorzewska et al., 2000; Smogorzewska & de Lange, 2004; Palm & De Lange, 2008). Both TRF1 and TRF2 are subject to post-translational modifications including phosphorylation, SUMOylation, and PARsylation; however, the functional consequences of these modifications have yet to be clarified (Palm & de Lange, 2008).

TIN2 (TRF1-interacting nuclear protein), which is a relatively small protein molecule, associates with TRF1 via its innermost region and at the same time it interacts with TRF2 and TPP1 through its amino terminal domain (S.H. Kim et al., 1999; Palm & de Lange, 2008). Since TIN2 is located in the middle part of the shelterin complex, it can function as a bridge that connects the double stranded telomeric DNA binding proteins to those bind to the single stranded telomeric DNA (S.H. Kim et al., 1999, 2004; Ye et al., 2004a). Rap1 (repressor / activator protein 1) is incorporated to the shelterin complex through binding to the TRF2 in approximately 1:1 ratio, and therefore, its presence on telomeres is TRF2 dependent (B. Li et al., 2000; Takai et al., 2010). Rap 1 plays an important role in telomere length regulation and it is thought that the Rap1 may be important for protective function of shelterin (de Lange, 2005, 2006).

TPP1 (POT1-TIN2 organizing protein, PTOP, PIP1,TINT1), both increases DNA binding activity of POT1 and it also connects POT1 to TIN2 by means of both its POT1 interaction and TIN2 interaction domains (Hockemeyer et al., 2007; D. Liu et al., 2004; Loayza et al., 2004; Ye et al, 2004a; Ye et al., 2004b). The last member of the shelterin complex called POT1 (protection of telomeres 1) was identified in the database through its homology with the DNA binding domain of TEBPα. Similar to TEBPα, POT1 binds to single stranded telomeric sequences by its two OB fold domains (Baumann & Cech, 2001). It has been shown that the POT1binds to single stranded TTAGGG, and it has been predicted that it can bind telomeric sequences both at the 3′ single stranded end and the displaced TTAGGG repeats at the base of the t-loop, called D-loop (Loayza et al., 2004). POT1 has a fundamental role in telomere length regulation, since it functions as a terminal transducer of telomere length control (Loayza & de Lange et al, 2003).

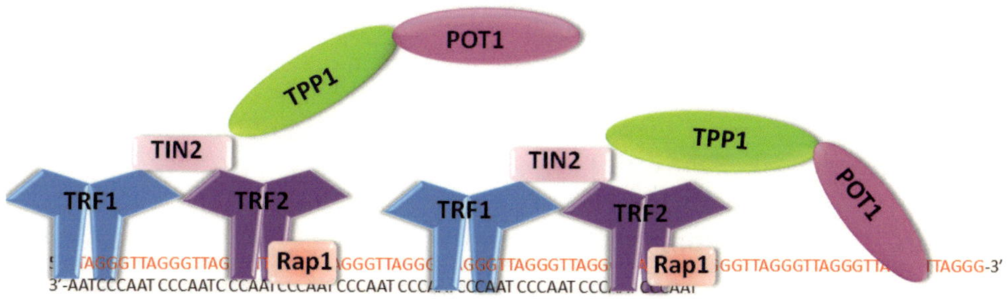

A

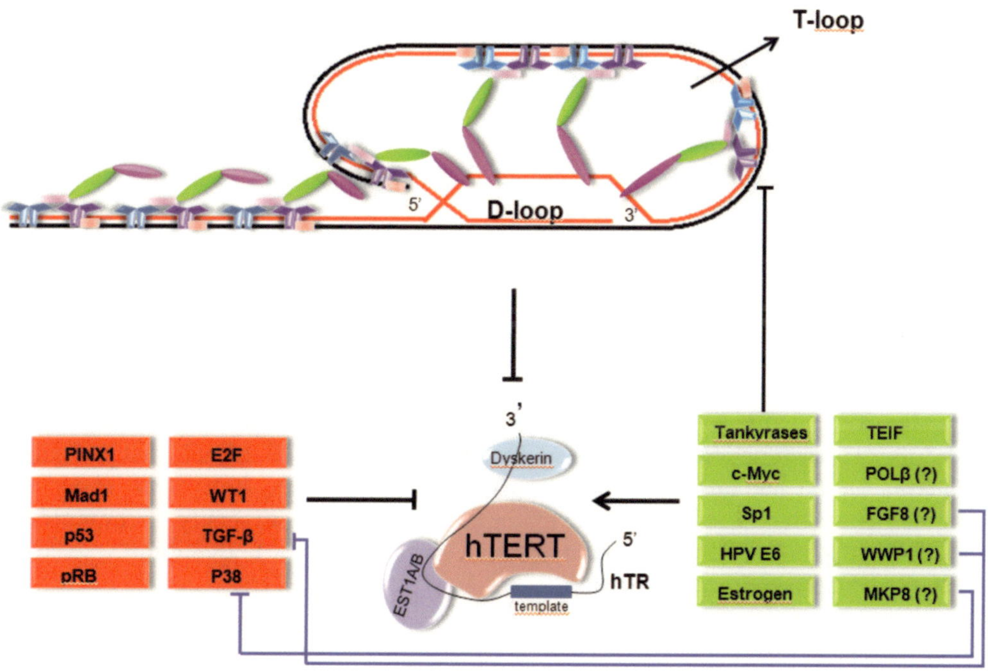

B

Fig. 1. A. Schematic representation of human shelterin complex composed of six protein subunits: TRF1, TRF2, Rap1, TIN2, TPP1 and POT1. B. Illustration of t-loop structure of human telomeres accomplished by shelterin complex. Known/candidate negative and positive regulators of the human telomerase enzyme are shown as red and green rectangulars, respectively. Blue lines show the possible effects of candidate proteins determined in our study (Gümüş-Akay et al., 2009).

1.2 Non-shelterin telomeric proteins

In addition to the shelterin complex, human telomeres consists of a large number of other proteins including Ku70/80, XPF/ERCC1, Apollo, the MRN complex, RecQ helicases, Tankyrase, and PINX1. Unlike shelterin complex that is located at telomeres throughout the cell cycle, these non-shelterin proteins only transiently associate with chromosome ends (Palm & de Lange, 2008). These proteins interact with the shelterin complex mainly by associating with TRF1 and TRF2. All of the non-shelterin telomere associated factors mediate telomere function in chromosome stability and contribute to telomere length regulation (de Lange, 2006; Palm & de Lange, 2008).

2. Structure of human telomerase enzyme

In human somatic cells, telomeres are approximately 10 kb long (Allshire et al., 1989; de Lange et al., 1990; Harley et al., 1990; Moyzis et al., 1988) and gradually shorten ~50-300 bp per cell division because of the end replication problem and post replicational processing by exonuclease that degrades telomere strand at the 5′-end (Huffman et al., 2000; Makarov et al., 1997; Olovnikov, 1973). If this telomere erosion is not balanced by elongation, telomeres will progressively shorten; eventually lead to genomic instability and cell death. Hence, the long-term proliferation of human cells requires mechanisms to counteract telomere attrition that occurs in each cell division. The most widely used way for telomere maintenance is based on the enzyme called telomerase which was discovered by Carol Greider and Elizabeth Blackburn in 1984 (Greider & Blackburn, 1985). Nobel Prize in Physiology or Medicine 2009 was awarded to Elizabeth Blackburn, Carol Greider and Jack Szostak for the discovery of how chromosomes are protected by telomeres and the enzyme telomerase (http://nobelprize.org/nobel_prizes/medicine/laureates/2009/).

Telomerase is a specialized reverse transcriptase that uses its RNA template to elongate the telomeres by addition of 5′-TTAGGG-3′ repeats to the terminal 3′ overhang (Greider & Blackburn, 1985). Human telomerase enzyme is composed of two core subunits involving RNA subunit (hTR) and catalytic telomerase reverse transcriptase (hTERT). In addition to these main components, studies have identified several telomerase-associated proteins required for proper functioning *in vivo*; such as dyskerin, hNop10, hGar1, that are potential components of the holoenzyme complex (Cristofari & Lingner, 2006; Shay et al., 2001). Telomerase components show significant size and sequence diversity among different species especially in the RNA moiety. However, certain parts of both subunits seem to be functionally conserved during evolution.

2.1 hTR

Human telomerase uses single stranded RNA as a template for *de novo* telomeric repeat synthesis. hTR is encoded by the *hTERC* gene located on chromosomal region 3q26 (Feng et al., 1995; Soder et al., 1997) . This gene is transcribed by RNA pol II. hTR is 451 nucleotide long RNA and shows unique secondary structure with four special structural and functional domains, namely the pseudoknot domain, the CR4/CR5 domain, the H/ACA scaRNA domain, and CR7 domain. These domains have discrete functions such as RNA binding, dimerization, and recruitment of telomerase to the telomeres. Moreover, they mediate interactions between the hTR and catalytic subunit, hTERT, and other telomerase-associated proteins. Among functional domains only the core domain and CR4/CR5 domains are required for *in vitro* reconstitution of catalytically active telomerase with hTERT. The template region of hTR is about 1.5-2 times the TTAGGG repeat length allowing both its annealing of the 3′ overhang and addition of telomeric repeats at the ends of chromosomes. Boundary element prevents reverse transcription beyond the 5′ boundary of the template (J.L. Chen et al., 2000; J.L.Chen & Greider, 2006; Cristofari & Lingner, 2006; Zhang et al., 2011).

2.2 hTERT

hTERT is encoded by *hTERT* gene located at 5p15.33 (Bryce et al., 2000). This gene spans approximately 40 kb of the genome and contains 16 exons (Cong et al., 1999). *hTERT* gene produces alternative transcript variants with unknown biological functions (Kilian et al., 1997). Unlike the hTR, sequence of the catalytic subunit of the human telomerase enzyme is conserved across species. hTERT has functional regions that can be grouped into four distinct domains: TERT N-terminal domain (TEN), TERT RNA binding domain (TRBD), the reverse transcriptase domain (RT), and the C-terminal extension (Mason et al., 2011). The TEN domain ,also known as the anchor domain of telomerase, potentially facilitates processivity of the enzyme by preventing enzyme-DNA dissociation during translocation and to promote realignment events that accompany each round of telomere synthesis (Wyatt et al., 2007). TRBD domain, located between TEN and RT domains, is implicated in telomerase ribonucloprotein assembly and RNA binding. This domain contains evolutionarly conserved CP, QFP, T, and VSR motifs required for CR4/5 binding in vertebrates (Bley et al., 2011) The central RT domain is the catalytic part of the enzyme and has seven evolutionarily-conserved RT motifs including 1, 2, A, B′, C, D, E motifs. This domain is organized as two subdomains namely fingers and palm. The TERT active site contains three conserved aspartic acids, one of which resides in motif A and the other two within motif C. These residues form a catalytic triad contributing directly in nucleotide addition (Lingner et al., 1997; Nakamura et al., 1997). The motifs located at the C-terminal domain are not well conserved and telomerase specific (Autexier & Lue, 2006; J.L. Chen and Greider, 2006; Cristofari & Lingner, 2006; Mason et al., 2011; Wyatt et al., 2010). This domain is essential for human telomerase function *in vivo*. It has been shown that the C-terminal domain plays an important role in the catalytic activity and processivity of the telomerase (Huard et al., 2003).

3. Regulation of human telomerase activity

During normal human development, telomerase activity should be strictly regulated to meet proliferative needs of specific cellular functions such as tissue repair, while at the same time preserving proliferative barriers against tumorigenesis. Significant research effort in the last two decades has provided important data for our understanding of the complex processes of the telomere length homeostasis and telomerase regulation. Telomerase activity is regulated at many levels including transcription, mRNA splicing, maturation, processing and nuclear localization of both hTR and hTERT subunits, post-translational modifications and correct folding of hTERT, assembly of ribonucleoprotein complex, and accessibility of the telomeres to the holoenzyme (Cong et al., 2002; Ćukušić et al., 2008).

However, regulation at the *hTERT* level, particularly at the transcription level, seems to be the primary and rate limiting step in the telomerase activity control (L. Liu et al. 2004; Shay et al., 2001)

Several positive and negative regulators of the *hTERT* gene have been identified (Figure 1B). Some of the positive regulators of the *hTERT* promoter are oncogene *c-myc* , the transcription factor Sp1, the human papillomavirus 16 (HPV 16) protein E6, and steroid hormones (e.g. estrogen) (Cong et al., 2002; Ćukušić et al., 2008; L. Liu et al., 2004). By means of microcell-mediated chromosome transfer studies, it has been shown that the normal somatic cells have transcriptional repressors that inhibits *hTERT* transcription. The chromosomal regions that contain genes encoding these repressors have been determined as 3p21.3 in renal cancer cell line RCC23, 3p12-21.1 in breast cancer cell line 21NT (Oshimura & Barrett, 1997), 10p15.1 in hepatocellular carcinoma cell line (Nishimoto et al., 2001), and 6p in human papilloma virus immortalized keratinocyte cell line and cervical cancer cell line (Steenbergen et al., 2001; L. Liu et al., 2004). In addition to these chromosomal regions, certain factors have been demonstrated to repress telomerase activity including antiproliferation factors such as transcription factor Mad1, the tumor suppressor proteins p53, pRb, E2F, the Wilms' tumor 1, the myeloid cell-specific zinc finger protein 2, and differentiation factors, such as interferon-gamma and transforming growth factor β (Cong et al., 2002; Ćukušić et al., 2008; L. Liu et al., 2004). In addition to the transcription factors, *hTERT* expression is also regulated epigenetically (Cong et al., 2002; L. Liu et al., 2004).

Apart from the mechanisms summarized above, telomerase is also regulated by the shelterin and non-shelterin proteins localized at the telomeres. This type of regulation based on the accessibility of telomere substrates to the enzyme, telomerase. Several studies have shown that shelterin may affect the telomerase action, particularly, as a negative regulator (Smogorzewska & de Lange, 2004; de Lange, 2005, 2006; Palm & de Lange, 2008) (Figure 1B). Shelterin recognizes telomere length via its ability to accumulate all along the double stranded telomeric DNA. The longer the telomeric DNA, the more shelterin complex associated with it. This results in a t-loop formation and decreases the chance of the telomerase to reach the telomeric end (de Lange, 2006; Smogorzewska & de Lange, 2004). All of the shelterin subunits behave as a telomere length regulator and their amount at telomeric DNA affects elongation of telomeres. For example, the absence of TRF1 from telomeres results in telomere elongation (Iwano et al., 2004; van Steensel & deLange, 1997), whereas increased amount of TRF1 on telomeres leads them to become shorter (van Steensel & deLange, 1997). Similarly, as telomeres get longer, the number of TRF2 on telomeres increases. It has been shown that the overexpression of TRF2 results in telomere shortening, implying TRF2 also can modulate telomere length (Smogorzewska et al., 2000).

Since telomerase ribonucleoprotein functions on the single stranded 3′ overhang, shelterin complex should perform its negative regulatory functions at this place (de Lange, 2005, 2006). POT1, which is the only member binding to the single stranded telomeric sequences plays an important role in the effect of shelterin on telomerase (de Lange, 2005, 2006). According to the counting model for telomere length regulation, POT1 is the key player that functions as a terminal transducer of telomere length control (Loayza & de Lange, 2003). When telomeres become elongated, they are occupied with more shelterin, thereby the chance of POT1 to associate with single stranded 3′ overhang also increases, which in turn leads to blockage of telomerase (Figure 1B).

While shelterin complex seems to be responsible for negative telomerase regulation (Smogorzewska & de Lange, 2004; de Lange, 2005; Palm & de Lange, 2008), unexpected results showed that the POT1–TPP1 complex may activate telomerase processivity (Tejera et al., 2010; Wang et al., 2007). In order to explain the two opposit functions of the TPP1-POT1 complex, three-state model of telomere length regulation has been proposed by Wang et al. (2007). When POT1–TPP1 coat the 3′ end of the G-overhang, it makes the telomeres inaccesible to the telomerase. On the other hand, it has been suggested that the TPP1-POT1 complex probably function together to positively recruit telomerase to telomeric ssDNA through the TPP1 OB fold (Xin et al., 2007). At second state, TPP1-POT1 are removed from their binding sites by an as yet unidentified mechanism such as post-translational modification and disruption of the shelterin complex. The POT1–TPP1 complex then act as a telomerase processivity factor during telomere elongation. As the telomere length reaches a certain threshold, the newly synthesized repeats bind shelterin complexes, and the 3′ end of the G-overhang is again bound by POT1–TPP1, thereby preventing telomerase action (Bianchi & Shore, 2008; Wang et al., 2007).

As mentioned before, non-shelterin telomere associated factors mediate telomere function in chromosome stability and contributes to telomere length regulation. For example, poly-ADP-ribose polymerase called tankyrase binds to TRF1 and adds ADP-ribose chain to the Glu residues located at the N-terminal domain of the protein. This post-translational modification leads to separation of TRF1 from telomeres. Therefore, tankyrase acts as a positive regulator of telomere length (Hsiao & Smith, 2008; Smith & de Lange, 2000). Another shelterin accessory factor PINX1, for instance, functions as a telomerase inhibitor and participates in TRF-1 mediated telomere length control (Soohoo et al., 2010; Zhou et al., 2001).

Unfortunately, the mechanisms involved in control of telomerase activity seem to be a big puzzle. It is clear that the understanding the mechanisms involved in telomere length and telomerase regulation, and identification of novel candidate molecules would certainly have implications for understanding the molecular basis and management of human cancers. We have determined the chromosomal localizations of putative unidentified telomerase activator(s) and/or repressor(s) by high resolution comparative genomic hybridization (HR-CGH) in highly telomerase expressing gastric tumor samples. We have found that genomic imbalances including 1q+, 8p+, 8q+, 10q+, 17p-, and 20p+ are associated with the higher telomerase activity. Our results suggest that 1q24, 8p21-p11.2, 8q21.1-q23, 10q21-qter and 20pter-p11.2 may contain putative telomerase activator(s), whereas the 17p12 region may harbor candidate telomerase suppressor(s) (Gümüş-Akay et al., 2009).

WWP1 (WW domain containing E3 ubiquitin protein ligase 1) gene located at 8q21 seems to be a candidate telomerase regulator. It is known that the TGF-β (beta), inhibits positive regulatory effect of c-Myc on *hTERT* promoter by increasing Smad3 phosphorylation (H. Li et al., 2006a, 2006b). Komuro et al. (2004) have shown that WWP1 protein could block the transcriptional activities of TGF-β by inducing nuclear export of Smad7 and eventually enhancing degradation of TGF- β type I receptor through ubiquitination. Our results have suggested that increase in WWP1 gene copy number could have caused blockage of TGF-β-mediated hTERT repression. We have suggested that the *POLB* and *MKP8* genes located at 8p11.2 and 8p12, respectively, might be putative telomerase activators (Gümüş-Akay et al., 2009). *POLB* encodes a DNA repair enzyme called β-pol which is an error-prone polymerase (Bergoglio et al., 2001; Canitrot et al., 2000). TEIF (Telomerase Transcriptional Element Interacting Factor) is one of the newly identified transcriptional activators of *POLB* gene. This transcription factor can also bind to the promoter region of *hTERT* and activates its expression. Transcriptional regulation of both *POLB* and *hTERT* by the same transcription factor and increased activity of these two enzymes in cancers suggest a functional link between β-pol and telomerase (Tang et al., 2004; Zhao et al., 2005). The *MKP8* gene at 8p12 encodes a mitogen-activated protein kinase phosphatase-8 that inhibits P38 by dephosphorylation (Vasudevan et al., 2005). It has been shown that the P38 bind to the *hTERT* promoter and repress its transcription (Chang et al., 2005). Therefore, MKP8 might be another putative telomerase activator. *FGF8* encoding Fibroblast Growth Factor 8 is located at 10q24. Repression of FGF8 protein has been reported to be necessary for TGF- β mediated transcriptional suppression (Takayashiki et al., 2005). Our results have insinuated that the FGF8 might regulate telomerase activity via TGF- β pathway.

4. Telomeres and telomerase in cancer

Telomerase activity is undetectable in most normal human somatic cells. However, it is expressed during early development and remains fully active in specific germ-line/embryonic stem cells and cancer cells (Hahn et al., 2005; N.W. Kim et al., 1994). In addition, modest levels of telomerase activity are determined in proliferative tissues with high renewal potential such as the bone marrow, skin, gastrointestinal tract and testis as well as in activated lymphocytes (Yui et al., 1998; K. Liu et al., 1999). Normal human somatic cells have a limited replicative potential and after 50-70 doublings they become senescent. This is known as the Hayflick limit (Hayflick & Moorhead, 1961). This raises the question of what is the mechanism accounting for the finite division capacity of normal somatic cells? Although the whole mechanism has yet to be understood, one of the main determinants of cellular replicative capacity is the progressive loss of telomeric repeats occurs in each cell division (Allsopp et al., 1992; Harley et al., 1990).

At the Hayflick limit one or a few critically shorten telomeres, which lose their capping function and activate DNA damage checkpoints, trigger an irreversible growth arrest known as a Mortality stage 1 (M1). Senescence involves p53 and pRb pathways and leads to the termination of cell proliferation (Wright et al., 1989; Shay et al., 1991). Senescence, therefore, can be accepted as a tumor suppressor mechanism (Campisi, 2005). Cells that can bypass this replicative senescence by inactivation of important cell cycle checkpoint genes (e.g. p53) continue to divide and lose their telomeres further until reaching the crisis stage or Mortality stage 2 (M2) (Wright et al., 1989; Shay et al., 1991; Zou et al., 2004). Cells that are able to reactivate/up-regulate their telomerase enzyme can escape from crisis and become immortalized, which is generally believed to be a critical step in cancer progression (Counter et al., 1992; N.W. Kim et al., 1994; Shay & Bacetti, 1997; Shay & Wright, 2010) (Figure 2). Although most cancer cells (80-90%) express a high level of telomerase activity, the remaining uses alternative lengthening of telomeres (ALT) by recombination to maintain their immortality (Bryan & Reddel, 1997).

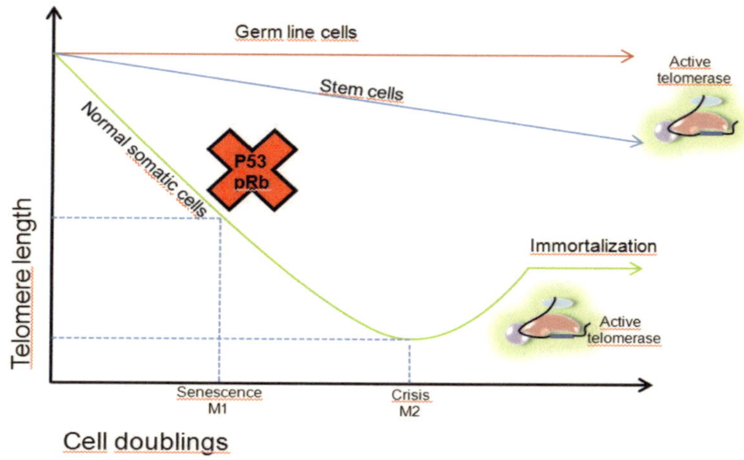

Fig. 2. The telomere hypothesis of replicative senescence and cancer.
Telomere length is maintained in germ cells and stem cells by active telomerase. In the absence of active telomerase enzyme one or a few critically shorten telomeres trigger an irreversible growth arrest known as a Mortality stage 1 (M1). Cells that can bypass this replicative senescence by inactivation of important cell cycle checkpoint genes (e.g. p53) continue to divide and lose their telomeres further until reaching the crisis stage or Mortality stage 2 (M2). Cells those are able to reactivate/upregulate their telomerase enzyme can escape from crisis and become immortalized.

The pivotal role of telomere and telomerase biology in cancer has been well documented by means of cellular and animal models (Artandi & Depinho, 2000). In 1994, N.W. Kim et al. showed that telomerase could be detected in about 90% of all human tumors examined, and a couple of years later other groups have demonstrated that the *hTERT* transfected cells never show a growth arrest (Bodnar et al., 1998; Counter et al., 1998). After that time, the number of articles on telomeres, telomerase and cancer has increased tremendously. All of the studies indicate that telomerase activity is almost universally an essential requirement for cellular immortalization and unlimited proliferative characteristic of cancer cells. In many human primary cancers increased or up-regulated telomerase activity have been reported, and increased telomerase activity has also been demonstrated to be related to poor prognosis. Thus telomerase activity emerges as an attractive target for both cancer diagnosis and treatment (Artandi & Depinho, 2010; Donate & Blasco, 2011; Granger et al., 2002).

4.1 Telomere dysfunction and its consequences in carcinogenesis

As mentioned above, telomeres are critical for maintenance, protection and stabilization of linear chromosomes, enabling continuous cell division. In the absence of telomere maintenance mechanisms progressive telomere shortening is thought to be the major cause of replicative senescence. Critically shortened telomeres lose the protection of telomere-binding proteins, leading to telomere uncapping, and this is known as telomere dysfunction. In normal cells, telomere dysfuntion activates DNA damage checkpoint pathways, particularly p53 and RB pathways, leading to stable growth arrest or programmed cell death called apoptosis (d'Adda di Fagagna et al., 2003; d'Adda di Fagagna et al., 2004; Zou et al., 2004).

On the contrary, cells derived from tumors can divide indefinitely in culture by means of their tumor maintenance mechanisms, most prominently by telomerase. It has been shown that the dysfunctional telomeres can lead to chromosome fusions before the reactivation/upregulation of telomerase, which has been proposed as a mechanism of chromosome instability in cancers (Gisselson et al., 2001; Maser & Depinho, 2002; Murnane, 2010). Comparative genomic hybridization techniques have demonstrated extensive focal amplifications and deletions in human cancers which are now known to harbor oncogenes and tumor suppressor genes, respectively. This raises the question whether these chromosomal loci contain genes that induce carcinogenesis or they are the consequences of the genomic instability seen in cancer cells. Copy number alterations comes from aCGH analyses of tumors from telomerase-deficient mice (TERC -/- p53+/-) have suggested that chromosome breakage-fusion-bridge process caused by telomere dysfunction might provide a major mechanism driving amplifications and deletions in human cancer genomes (reviewed in Artandi & Depinho, 2010).

4.2 Telomerase as diagnostic and prognostic marker in cancer

Even though morphological assessment remains the gold standard for cancer diagnosis, there has been continuous seeking for new molecular markers that are less subjected to evaluation bias (E. Hiyama & K. Hiyama, 2003). Given that both of its crucial role in the carcinogenesis process and its uniqueness to all types of cancers, analysis of telomerase activity has been anticipated as a diagnostic and/or prognostic marker for this disease.

After the development of PCR-based telomerase assay called telomeric repeat amplification protocol (TRAP) by N.W. Kim et al. (1994), investigation of telomerase activity in different tumor tissues and their normal counterparts has become easier. TRAP assay can detect as few as 10 telomerase positive cells (Wright et al., 1995) in a variety of biological samples, including solid tissue samples (Gümüş-Akay et al., 2007), blood, urine (Hess & Highsmith, 2002), fine needle asprites (E. Hiyama & K. Hiyama, 2004), ascites, and peritoneal washing fluids (Hess & Highsmith, 2002; Ozmen et al., 2008). In its original form, TRAP assay was not able to measure the telomerase activity quantitatively, and serial dilutions of the tissue extracts and use of internal control were recommended in each assay. However, modified and more user-friendly versions of this method have been developed to improve its sensitivity and quantitative detection of telomerase activity, including TRAP-ELISA (enzyme-linked immunosorbent assay) (Gonzalez-Quevedo et al., 2000; Wu et al., 2000), TRAP-ELIDA (enzymatic luminometric inorganic pyrophosphate detection assay) (Xu et al., 2001), and real-time TRAP assay (Shim et al., 2005). The main disadvantages of detecting telomerase activity by TRAP assay are the contamination of telomerase expressing normal cells with the tissue of tested and the possibility of presence of PCR inhibitors in some tissue extracts (E. Hiyama & K. Hiyama, 2002, 2003, 2004). To avoid false–positive results due to contamination of cell samples with lymphocytes, K. Hiyama et al. (1995) suggested using of 1000 cell equivalents of cell lysate per assay, since proteins extracted from 1000 adult lymphocytes do not show detectable telomerase activity. Nevertheless, this assay is an indispensable method enabling sensitive and quantitative measurement of the telomerase activity.

In addition to the TRAP assay that directly assesses the enzymatic activity, detection of transcript levels of *hTERT* or *hTR* by RT-PCR and detection of hTERT and hTR by *in situ* hybridization techniques are also used in telomerase investigations (Heaphy & Meeker, 2011; E. Hiyama and K. Hiyama, 2002, 2003, 2004). Expression studies of both *hTERT* and *hTR* via RT-PCR allow quantitative measurement of these subunits, although mRNA levels of *hTERT* may not always correlate with telomerase activity due to alternative splicing variants and post-translational modifications of this subunit and *hTR* is constitutively expressed in most of the cell types (Cong et al., 2002; Heaphy & Meeker, 2011). *In situ* hybridization studies of both hTERT and hTR enable detection and visualization of these subunits at single cell level, however, detection of transcripts does not always correlate with telomerase activity and quantitative analysis is almost imposable (Heaphy & Meeker, 2011; E. Hiyama and K. Hiyama, 2004).

The increase in telomerase in cancer cells generally occurs very early during tumorigenesis; i.e. at the preneoplastic or *in situ* stage, telomerase activity may be useful for early detection of cancer, particularly in cytology samples. In some instances telomerase activity might not be very high, but it could show correlation with the tumor progression. Due to space limitations, here we focus predominantly on two types of malignancies that we had experiences: gastric and ovarian cancer. Readers who are interested in the clinical utility of telomerase in other types of cancer can find well-written articles in the literature.

4.2.1 Telomerase in gastric cancer

The prevalence of telomerase activity in gastric cancer has been reported as 70-98% (C.H. Chen and R.J. Chen, 2011). Telomerase activity in gastric lavage fluid has been suggested as a potential tumor marker that might help for early diagnosis of gastric cancer rate (S.C. Wong et al., 2006). Telomerase activity has also been reported in the peritoneal lavage of patients with gastric cancer and shown to be associated with advanced stages of the disease or peritoneal metastasis (Hu et al., 2009; Mori et al., 2000). Clinicopathological significance of telomerase activity in human gastric cancer is controversial. Some investigators have indicated that the telomerase activity in tumor tissues correlates well with depth of invasion and tumor differentiation (Usselmann et al., 2001; Yoo et al., 2003). On the other hand, other groups, similar to us, have shown no relation between clinical or histological factors and telomerase activity (Furugori et al., 2000; Gümüş-Akay et al., 2007; Kameshima et al., 2000).

As mentioned before, although telomerase is repressed in most somatic cells, it can be detected in highly proliferative tissues. We have shown that in addition to the tumor samples (98%), normal gastric mucosa samples (95%) also show appreciable telomerase activity (Gümüş-Akay et al., 2007). According to our results, we suggest that if someone has to study the telomerase activity in tumors of such proliferative/regenerative tissues, care must be taken in order to make correct evaluations and telomerase activity should be tested in both tumor sample and their corresponding normal tissue sample obtained from the same patient. Moreover, we have experienced that the telomerase activity in tumor/normal tissues show great inter-individual variability. Therefore, it is difficult to set a general cut-off level of telomerase activity for gastric adenocarcinoma.

The expression of catalytic subunit hTERT and the methylation status of its promoter have also been investigated in gastric cancer samples. Although it is highly expressed in tumor tissues, there is a disagreement between the studies evaluating the usefulness of *hTERT* expression as a prognostic factor (Gigek et al., 2009; W. Li et al., 2008; Suzuki et al., 2000). It could be concluded that there is no a strict association between telomerase activity and staging or grading of disease with regard to all of information obtained by different research groups. This may explain why detection of telomerase activity have not reached the clinic in terms of predicting outcome for patients with gastric cancer.

4.2.2 Telomerase in ovarian cancer

In ovarian tumors, telomerase activity has been widely investigated among malignant, borderline, and benign lesions (Datar et al., 1999; Zheng et al. 1997). Studies have shown that telomerase activity is increased in about 74-100% of ovarian cancer subjects (C.H. Chen and R.J. Chen, 2011). Rate of telomerase activity in benign and borderline ovarian tumors have produced diverse results. It has been reported that the majority of cystadenomas do not show telomerase activity, while all borderline tumors express this enzyme (Wan et al., 1997). In contrast, Yokoyama et al. (1998) have found that 40% of ovarian cystadenomas have telomerase activity. We have investigated the applicability of telomerase activity in detecting early recurrences of epithelial ovarian cancer after first-line chemotherapy (Ozmen et al., 2008). We have found that although mean telomerase activity was statistically higher in epithelial ovarian cancer patients than patients with benign disease, there was no relation between telomerase activity levels at second-look surgery and early recurrences of epithelial ovarian cancer.

Buttitta et al (2003) have reported that an immunohistochemical study on archival tissue sections showing a moderate to strong nuclear hTERT staining in 86% of serous epithelial ovarian cancers. A significant correlation between hTERT expression and response to platinum-based chemotherapy has been documented in advanced epithelial ovarian cancer patients. However, the prognostic significance of hTERT in epithelial ovarian cancer is still uncertain. Similar to gastric cancer studies, some authors have reported that hTERT expression does not reflect the clinical outcome (Wisman et al., 2003 as cited in Gadducci et al., 2009; Widschwendter et al., 2004), whereas others have showed a poor survival for patients whose tumors displayed moderate to strong hTERT immunostaining (Brustmann, 2005). It has been suggested that telomerase activity might only be used as a supplementary diagnostic procedure beside conventional pathological diagnosis.

4.3 Telomerase as a target for cancer therapy

Since most of the cancer cells and putative cancer stem or stem-like cells have appreciable telomorase activity (E. Hiyama & K. Hiyama, 2003; N.W. Kim et al., 1994; Shay & Bacchetti, 1997; Shay & Wright, 2010) to circumvent the telomere-dependent cellular senescence, inhibiting the telomerase activity by means of different approaches has emerged as potential cancer therapeutics. When compared to other cancer therapy strategies, anti-telomerase approaches seem to be more promising because of the following three main reasons. Firstly, unlike other molecular genetic changes, which show great differences in different types of cancers, telomerase can be accepted as a hallmark of all cancer types. Secondly, it is thought that cancer cells are less likely to develop resistance to anti-telomerase approaches than they are to other cancer targets. Finally, telomerase is a relatively specific cancer/cancer stem cell target because normal somatic cells show slight or diminished telomerase activity and generally have longer telomeres. This reduces the probability of therapy- related toxicity to normal tissues. At present, two main telomerase targeting methodologies are presently in clinical trials: A direct inhibition of telomerase, and a number of active immunotherapy targeting against catalytic protein subunit hTERT. In addition to these strategies, agents blocking telomerase expression and biogenesis, telomere disrupting agents, and suicide gene therapy are also understudy (H. Chen et al., 2009; Harley, 2008).

There has been several strategies that seek to inhibit telomerase activity at its expression and biogenesis levels, including, single-stranded antisense oligonucleoties and small-interfering RNAs that target hTERT mRNA and hTR (Folini et al., 2005; Glukhov et al., 1998; Kraemer et al., 2003; You et al., 2006), ribozyme cleavage of hTERT mRNA and hTR (Hao et al., 2003, 2005; Lu et al., 2011) , expression of dominant-negative hTERT protein (Hahn et al., 1999), and Hsp90 inhibitors (Lee and Chung, 2010). However, agents belonging to this category may be more leaky, or less efficient than direct inhibitors. In addition, similar to the gene-therapy based methodologies, this group of agents also has delivery and stability problems (Harley, 2008).

Telomerase activity can also be inhibited by stabilizing the G-quadruplex structure of telomeres by G-quadruplex-interacting agents, like telomestatin (M.Y. Kim et al., 2002). This group of agents inhibits telomerase activity by fixing the single-stranded telomere substrate into a quadruplex structure so as to blocking telomere accessibility. Although several compounds in this class have demonstrated relatively rapid activity in human tumor xenograft studies in mice, their safety is under question, because they can also target endogenous telomeric sequences or G-rich sequences, which might be lethal for normal cells (Ogenasian & Bryan, 2007). Another telomerase based approach in cancer treatment is the *hTERT* promoter-driven cancer cell suicide. Because of its higher tumor specificity, stronger activity, and universal presence in cancel cells have made the *hTERT* promoter encouraging over other known promoters (Gu & Fang, 2003). Bax, caspase 8, and cytosine deaminase (CD) are among the suicide genes that have been used in *hTERT* promoter-driven cancer cell suicide (Gu et al., 2000; Komata et al., 2002; Yu et al., 2011). However, this methodology has not yet received clinical development support (Harley, 2008).

Although gene therapy and antisense strategies have remarkable potential for the treatment of many human diseases, the practicability and clinical utility of these methodologies remain to be confirmed. One of the anti-telomerase approaches that seems to be more practical is the use of small-molecule inhibitors, such as reverse transcriptase inhibitors (Strahl & Blackburn, 1996), BIBR1532 {2-[(E)-3-naphtalen-2-yl-but-2-enoylamino]-benzoic acid}, and BIBR1591 {5-morpholin-4-yl-2-[(E)-3-naphtalen-2-yl-but-2-enoylamino]-benzoic acid} to the catalytic component hTERT (Damm et al., 2001). Another group of direct telomerase inhibitors, namely 2′-deoxy and 2′-substituted N-3′→ P5′ NP oligonucleotides (NPS), have been identified, which binds to their complementary sequences on hTR. These oligonucleotides, unlike hTR antisense counterparts, do not activate RNase-H mediated degradation of the hTR. Instead, they inhibit telomerase activity through functioning as a template antagonist (Gryaznov et al., 2001; Shea-Herbert et al., 2002). GRN163 was developed in 2003 as a competitive telomerase inhibitor. This molecule hybridizes to hTR and represses primer binding to telomere It has been shown that GRN163 suppresses tumor growth without major toxicity (Asai et al., 2003). GRN163 has been further modified by covalent lipid conjugation in order to improve its pharmacological properties, and named GRN163L. This compound is currently in multiple Phase-I and Phase-I/II clinical trials as potential broad-spectrum anticancer agent (Gryaznov, 2010).

Because of its universal expression and fundamental function in cancer cells, TERT has been regarded as a self antigen useful for developing active telomerase immunotherapy/vaccine strategies. In this approach, TERT immunotherapy products are constructed to stimulate the immune system of the organism to damage and kill TERT expressing tumor cells. In order to achieve this, antigen-presenting cells (APCs) are subjected to peptide fragments or TERT coding gene products *ex vivo* or *in vivo*. Then, APCs cause an activation and propagation of TERT-specific T-cells that kill the cells displaying TERT peptides on their surfaces (Harley, 2008; J.P. Liu et al., 2010). Vaccination with dendritic cells transfected with hTERT mRNA has been shown to induce strong immune responses to multiple hTERT epitopes and is therefore accepted as an attractive approach to more potent immunotherapy (Suso et al., 2011). Clinical trials using telomerase immunotherapy/vaccine approaches involving GRNVAC1, GV1001, Vx001 have been very encouraging, and have involved several types of solid tumors and acute myeloid leukemia (Harley, 2008; Kotsakis et al., 2011; Suso et al., 2011; Vetsika et al., 2011; Vonderheide, 2008).

It is thought that in a well-designed clinical trial, if the p53 statuses of the patients are screened and those patients with an intact p53 are selected, better response rates to the telomerase inhibitors might be expected. On the other hand, tumors deficient for p53 would show high levels of genomic instability so as to gain resistance to other therapeutics in the regimen and could acquire ALT mechanism (K. K. Wong et al., 2006). Although ALT seems to be a potential resistance pathway to telomerase inhibitors, it is unlikely to be a major factor limiting the usefulness of telomerase inhibitors in a clinical setting (Shay & Wright, 2006). The telomerase knockout mouse model has also demonstrated that absence of telomerase and associated telomere dysfunction enhance sensitivity to ionizing radiation and chemotherapeutic agents that generate double strand breaks. Therefore, it is suggested that one particularly attractive clinical trial design would be the potentially synergistic combination of telomerase inhibitors and radiation or break inducing agents (K. K. Wong et al., 2006). In support of this Ward & Autexier (2005) have shown that pharmacological inhibition of telomerase catalytic activity by BIBR1532 can sensitize cells to traditional etoposide, melphalan, and doxorubicin treatments in a telomere length-dependent fashion. Similarly, Incles et al. (2003) demonstrated that a G-quadruplex–interacting agent, BRACO-19, sensitized parental and flavopiridol-resistant human colon carcinoma cell lines.

There are several ongoing phase I and II clinical trials targeting telomerase activity, and phase III clinical trial has been recruited for pancreatic cancer. It is interesting that, none of them telomerase activity has not been used for exclusion or inclusion criteria for patient registration. It also reveals that more accurate, sensitive and robust test for telomerase activity has been requested.

5. Conclusion

Telomeres were first discovered in the 1930s, as the ends of linear chromosomes which have unique molecular structure that prevent end-to-end fusion of different chromosomes. Alexey Olovnikov reported in 1973 that the ends of human chromosomes could not replicate by previously known replication machineries. This observation implied that cells had an enzyme that could lengthen telomeres. In 1984, Greider and Blackburn discovered that the enzyme telomerase has the ability to lengthen chromosomal ends by its reverse transcriptase activity. In 2009 Blackburn, Greider and Szostak were awarded the Noble Prize in Physiology or Medicine "for the discovery of how chromosomes are protected by telomeres and the enzyme telomerase".

Thousand studies have been published on telomeres and telomerase, and at the present time it is known that, they are essential for stability of genome as well as regulation of DNA repair pathways. The long and short of it is that they regulate cellular viability and proliferative capacity. Loss of telomerase in differentiated cells limits cell division, while reactivation of telomerase sustains proliferation and transformation. Cancer cells need a mechanism to maintain telomeres if they are going to divide indefinitely, and telomerase solves this problem. This precious function of telomerase causes itself to gain a unique role in cellular immortality and carcinogenesis. In many human primary cancers increased or up-regulated telomerase activity has been reported, and increased telomerase activity has also been demonstrated to be related to prognosis. The discovery of the central role of telomerase in cancer offer entirely new therapy alternatives targeting the telomeres and/or telomerase.

6. Acknowledgement

We apologize to those scientists whose work has not been cited in this chapter due to limited space. Our works cited here were supported by grants from the Ankara University Scientific Research Projects.

7. References

Allshire, R.C.; Dempster, M. & Hastie, N.D. (1989). Human telomeres contain at least three types of G-rich repeat distributed non-randomly. *Nucleic Acids Research,* Vol. 17, No.12, (June 1989), pp. 4611-4627, ISSN 1362-4962

Allsopp, R.C.; Vaziri, H.; Patterson, C.; Goldstein, S.; Younglai, E.V.; Futcher, A.B.; Greider, C.W. & Harley C. (1992). Telomere length predicts replicative capacity of human fibroblasts. *Proceedings of the National Academy of Sciences of the United States of America,* Vol. 89, No. 21, (November 1992), pp. 10114-10118, ISSN 1091-6490

Artandi, S.E. & DePinho, R.A. (2000). Mice without telomerase: what can they teach us about human cancer? *Nature Medicine,* Vol. 6, No. 8, (August 2000), pp. 852-855, ISSN 1078-8956

Artandi, S.E.& Depinho, R.A. (2010). Telomeres and telomerase in cancer. *Carcin ogenesis,* Vol. 31, No.1, (January 2010), pp. 9-18. ISSN 1460-2180

Asai, A.; Oshima, Y.; Yamamoto, Y.; Uochi, T.A.; Kusaka, H.; Akinaga, S.; Yamashita, Y.; Pongracz, K.; Pruzan, R.; Wunder, E.; Piatyszek, M.; Li, S.; Chin, A.C.; Harley, C.B. & Gryaznov, S. (2003). A novel telomerase template antagonist (GRN163) as a potential anticancer agent. *Cancer Research,* Vol. 63, No.14, (July 2003), pp.3931-3939, ISSN 1538-7445

Autexier, C. & Lue, N.F. (2006). The structure and function of telomerase reverse transcriptase. *Annual Review of Biochemistry,* Vol. 75, No. , pp. 493-517, ISSN1545-4509

Bailey, S.M. & Murnane, J.P. (2006). Telomeres, chromosome instability and cancer. *Nucleic Acids Research,* Vol. 34, No.8, (May 2006), pp. 2408-2417, ISSN 1362-4962

Baumann, P. & Cech, T.R. (2001) Pot1, the putative telomere end-binding protein in fission yeast and humans. *Science,* Vol. 292, No. 5519, (May 2001), pp. 1171-1175, ISSN 1095-9203

Bergoglio, V.; Canitrot, Y.; Hogarth, L.; Minto, L.; Howell, S.B.; Cazaux, C. & Hoffman, J.S. (2001). Enhanced expression and activity of DNA polymerase beta in human ovarian tumor cells: impact on sensitivity towards antitumor agents. *Oncogene*, Vol. 20, No. 43, (September 2001), pp. 6181–6187, ISSN 1476-5594

Bianchi, A.; Smith, S.; Chong, L.; Elias, P. & de Lange T. (1997). TRF1 is a dimer and bends telomeric DNA. *The EMBO Journal,* Vol. 16, No. 7, (April 1997), pp. 1785-1794, ISSN 1460-2075

Bianchi, A. & Shore, D. (2008). How telomerase reaches its end: mechanism of telomerase regulation by the telomeric complex. *Molecular Cell,* Vol. 31, No. 2, (July 2008), pp. 153-165, ISSN 1097-4164

Bley, C.J.; Qi, X.; Rand, D.P.; Borges, C.R.; Nelson, R.W. & Chen, J.J. (2011). RNA-protein binding interface in the telomerase ribonucleoprotein. *Proceedings of the National Academy of Sciences of the United States of America,* Vol. 108, No. 51, (December 2011), pp. 20333-20338, ISSN 1091-6490

Bodnar, A.G.; Ouellette, M.; Frolkis, M.; Holt, S.E.; Chiu, C.P.; Morin, G.B.; Harley, C.B.; Shay, J.W.; Lichtsteiner, S. & Wright, W.E. (1998). Extension of life-span by introduction of telomerase into normal human cells. *Science*. Vol. 279, No. 5349, (January 1998), pp.349-352. ISSN 1095-9203

Broccoli, D.; Smogorzewska, A.; Chong, L.& de Lange T. (1997). Human telomeres contain two distinct Myb-related proteins, TRF1 and TRF2. *Nature Genetics,* Vol. 17, No.2, (October 1997), pp. 231-235, ISSN 1061-4036

Brustmann, H. (2005). Immunohistochemical detection of human telomerase reverse transcriptase (hTERT) and c-kit in serous ovarian carcinoma: a clinicopathologic study. *Gynecologic Oncology,* Vol. 98, No. 3, (September 2005), pp. 396–402, ISSN 1095-6859

Bryan, T.M. & Reddel, R.R. (1997). Telomere dynamics and telomerase activity in *in vitro* immortalised human cells. *European Journal of Cancer,* Vol. 33, No. 5, (April 1997), pp. 767-773, ISSN 1879-0852

Bryce, L.; Morrison, N.; Hoare, S.; Muir, S. & Keith, W. (2000). Mapping of the gene for the human telomerase reverse transcriptase, hTERT, to chromosome 5p15.33 by fluorescence in situ hybridization. *Neoplasia,* Vol. 2, No. 3, (May-June 2000), pp. 197–201, ISSN 1476-5586

Buttitta, F.; Pellegrini, C.; Marchetti, A.; Gadducci, A.; Cosio, S.; Felicioni, L.; Barassi, F.; Salvatore, S.; Martella, C.; Coggi, G. & Bosari, S. (2003). Human telomerase reverse transcriptase mRNA expression assessed by real-time reverse transcription polymerase chain reaction predicts chemosensitivity in patients with ovarian carcinoma. *Journal of Clinical Oncology.* Vol. 21, No. 7, (April 2003), pp. 1320-1325, ISSN 1527-7755

Campisi, J. Suppressing cancer: the importance of being senescent. (2005). *Science,* Vol. 309, No. 5736, (August 2005), pp. 886-887, ISSN 1095-9203

Canitrot, Y.; Hoffmann, J.S.; Calsou, P.; Hayakawa, H.; Salles, B. & Cazaux, C. Nucleotide excision repair DNA synthesis by excess DNA polymerase beta: a potential source of genetic instability in cancer cells. (2000). *The FASEB Journal*, Vol. 14, No. 12, (September 2000), pp. 1765–1774, ISSN 1530-6860

Chan, S.R.W.L.& Blackburn, E.H. (2004). Telomeres and telomerase. *Philosophical Transactions of the Royal Society of London. Series B, Biological Sciences,* Vol.359, No. 1441, (January 2004), pp.109-121, ISSN 1471-2970

Chang, J.T.; Yang, H.T.; Wang, T.C. & Cheng, A.J. (2005). Upstream stimulatory factor (USF) as a transcriptional suppressor of human telomerase reverse transcriptase (hTERT) in oral cancer cells. *Molecular Carcinogenesis,*. Vol. 44, No. 3, (November 2005), pp. 183-192, ISSN 1098-2744

Chen, J.L.; Blasco, M.A.& Greider, C.W. (2000). Secondary structure of vertebrate telomerase RNA. *Cell,* Vol.100, No.5, (March 2000), pp. 503-514, ISSN 1097-4172

Chen, J.L. & Greider, C.W. (2006). Telomerase biochemistry and biogenesis, In: *Telomeres*, de Lange, T.; Lundblad, V. & Blackburn, E. (2nd Ed.) pp. 49-79, Cold Spring Harbor Laboratory Press, ISBN 0-87969-734-2, New York, USA

Chen, Y.; Yang, Y.; van Overbeek, M.; Donigian, J.R.; Baciu, P.; et al. (2008). A shared docking motif in TRF1 and TRF2 used for differential recruitment of telomeric proteins. *Science*, Vol. 319, No. 5866, (February 2008), pp.1092–1096, ISSN 1095-9203

Chen, H.; Li, Y. & Tollefsbol, T.O. (2009). Strategies targeting telomerase inhibition. *Molecular Biotechnology,*Vol. 41, No. 2, (February 2009), pp. 194-199, ISSN 1559-0305

Chen, C.H. & Chen, R.J. (2011). Prevalence of telomerase activity in human cancer. *Journal of the Formosan Medical Association,* Vol. 110, No. 5, (May 2011), pp. 275-289, ISSN 0929-6646

Chong, L.; van Steensel, B.; Broccoli, D.; Erdjument-Bromage, H.; Hanish, J.; Tempst, P.& de Lange, T. (1995). A human telomeric protein. *Science,* Vol. 270, No. 5242, (December 1995), pp. 1663-1667, ISSN 0036-8075

Cong, Y.S.; Wen, J.& Bacchetti S. (1999). The human telomerase catalytic subunit hTERT: organization of the gene and characterization of the promoter. *Human Molecular Genetics,* Vol. 8, No. 1, (January 1999), pp. 137–142, ISSN 1460-2083

Cong, Y.S.; Woodring, W.E. & Shay JW. (2002). Human telomerase and its regulation. *Microbiology and Molecular Biology Reviews,* Vol. 66, No. 3, (September 2002), pp. 407-425, ISSN 1098-5557.

Counter, C.M.; Avilion, A.A.; LeFeuvre, C.E.; Stewart, N.G.; Greider, C.W.; Harley, C.B. & Bacchetti, S. (1992). Telomere shortening associated with chromosome instability is arrested in immortal cells which express telomerase activity. *The EMBO J,* Vol. 11, No. 5, (May 1992), pp.1921-1929, ISSN 1460-2075

Counter, C.M.; Hahn, W.C.; Wei, W.; Caddle, S.D.; Beijersbergen, R.L.; Lansdorp, P.M.; Sedivy, J.M. & Weinberg, R.A. (1998). Dissociation among in vitro telomerase activity, telomere maintenance, and cellular immortalization. *Proceedings of the National Academy of Sciences of the United States of America,* Vol. 95, No. 25, (December 1998), pp. 14723-14728, ISSN 1091-6490

Cristofari, G. & Lingner, J. (2006). The telomerase ribonucleoprotein particle, In: *Telomeres,* de Lange, T.; Lundblad, V. & Blackburn, E. (2nd Ed.) pp. 21-47, Cold Spring Harbor Laboratory Press, ISBN 0-87969-734-2, New York, USA

Ćukušić, A.; Škrobot Vidaček, N.; Sopta, M. & Rubelj, I. (2008). Telomerase regulation at the crossroads of cell fate. *Cytogenetics and Genome Resesarch,* Vol.122, No. 3-4, pp. 263–272, ISSN 1424-859X

d'Adda di Fagagna, F.; Reaper, F.M.; Cray-Fallace, L.; Fiegler, H.; Car, P.; Von Zglinicki, T.; Saretzki, G.; Carter, N.P. & Jackson, S.P. (2003). A DNA damage checkpoint response in telomerase-initiated senescence. *Nature,* Vol. 426, No. 6963, (November 2003), pp. 194-198, ISSN 1476-4687

d'Adda di Fagagna, F.; Teo, S.H. & Jackson, S.P. (2004). Functional links between telomeres and proteins of the DNA-damage response. *Genes and Development,* Vol. 18, No. 15, (August 2004), pp. 1781-1799, ISSN 0890-9369

Damm, K.; Hemmann, U.; Garin-Chesa, P.; Hauel, N.; Kauffmann, I.; Priepke, H.; Niestroj, C.; Daiber,C.; Enenkel, B.; Guilliard, B.; Lauritsch, I.; Müller, E.; Pascolo, E.; Sauter, G.; Pantic, M.; Martens, U.M.; Wenz, C.; Lingner, J.; Kraut, N.; Rettig, W.J. & Schnapp, A. (2001). A highly selective telomerase inhibitor limiting human cancer cell proliferation. *The EMBO Journal,* Vol. 20, No. 24, (December 2001), pp. 6958-6968, ISSN 1460-2075

Datar, R.H.; Naritoku, W.Y.; Li, P.; Tsao-Wei, D.; Groshen, S.; Taylor, C.R. & Imam, S.A. (1999). Analysis of telomerase activity in ovarian cystadenomas, low-malignant-potential tumors, and invasive carcinomas. *Gynecologic Oncology,* Vol. 74, No. 3, (September 1999), pp. 338-345, ISSN 1095-6859

de Lange, T.; Shiue, L.; Myers, R.M.; Cox, D.R.; Naylor, S.L.; Killery, A.M. & Varmus, H.E. (1990). Structure and variability of human chromosome ends. *Molecular and Cellular Biology,* Vol. 10, No. 2, (February 1990), pp. 518-527, ISSN 1098-5549

de Lange, T. (2005). Shelterin: the protein complex that shapes and safeguards human telomeres. *Genes and Development,* Vol. 19, No. 18, (September 2005), pp. 2100-2110, ISSN 1549-5477

de Lange, T. (2006). Mammalian telomeres, In: *Telomeres,* de Lange, T.; Lundblad, V. & Blackburn, E. (2nd Ed.) pp. 387-431, Cold Spring Harbor Laboratory Press, ISBN 0-87969-734-2, New York, USA

Diotti, R. & Loayza, D. (2011). Shelterin complex and associated factors at human telomeres. *Nucleus,* Vol. 2, No. 2, (March 2011), pp. 119-135, ISSN 1949-1042

Donate, L.E. & Blasco, M.A. (2011). Telomeres in cancer and aging. *Philosophical Transactions of the Royal Society of London. Series B, Biological Sciences,* Vol. 366, No. 1561, (January 2011), pp. 76-84, ISSN 1471-2970

Fairall, L.; Chapman, L.; Moss, H.; de Lange, T. & Rhodes, D. (2001). Structure of the TRFH dimerization domain of the human telomeric proteins TRF1 and TRF2. *Molecular Cell,* Vol. 8, No. 2, (August 2001), pp. 351-361, ISSN 1097-4164

Feng, J.; Funk, W.D.; Wang, S.S.; Weinrich, S.L.; Avilion, A.A.; Chiu, C.P.; Adams, R.R.; Chang, E.; Allsopp, R.C.; Yu, J.; et al. (1995). The RNA component of human telomerase. *Science,* Vol. 269, No. 5228, (September 1995), pp. 1236-1241, ISSN 1095-9203

Folini, M.; Brambilla, C.; Villa, R.; Gandellini, P.; Vignati, S.; Paduano, F.; Daidone, M.G. & Zaffaroni, N. (2005). Antisense oligonucleotide-mediated inhibition of hTERT, but not hTERC, induces rapid cell growth decline and apoptosis in the absence of telomere shortening in human prostate cancer cells. *European Journal of Cancer,* Vol. 41, No. 4, (March 2005), pp. 624-634, ISSN 1879-0852

Furugori, E.; Hirayama, R.; Nakamura, K.I.; Kammori, M.; et al. (2000). Telomere shortening in gastric carcinoma with aging despite telomerase activation. *Journal of Cancer Research and Clinical Oncology,* Vol. 126, No. 8, (August 2000), pp. 481-485, ISSN 1432-1335

Gadducci, A.; Cosio, S.; Tana, R. & Genazzani, A.R. (2009). Serum and tissue biomarkers as predictive and prognostic variables in epithelial ovarian cancer. *Critical Reviews in Oncology/Hematology,* Vol. 69, No. 1, (January 2009), pp. 12-27, ISSN 1879-0461

Gigek, C.O.; Leal, M.F.; Silva, P.N.; Lisboa, L.C.; Lima, E.M.; Calcagno, D.Q.; Assumpção, P.P.; Burbano, R.R. & Smith Mde, A. (2009). hTERT methylation and expression in gastric cancer. *Biomarkers,* Vol. 14, No. 8, (December 2009), pp. 630-636, ISSN 1366-5804

Gisselsson, D.; Jonson, T.; Petersen, A.; et al. (2001). Telomere dysfunction triggers extensive DNA fragmentation and evolution of complex chromosome abnormalities in human malignant tumors. *Proceedings of the National Academy of Sciences of the United States of America, Vol.* 98, No. 22, (October 2001), pp. 12683–12688, ISSN 1091-6490.

Glukhov, A. I.; Zimnik, O. V.; Gordeev, S. A.; & Severin, S. E. (1998). Inhibition oftelomerase activity of melanoma cells in vitro by antisense oligonucleotides. *Biochemical and Biophysical Research Communications,* Vol. 248, No. 2, (July 1998), pp. 368 –371, ISSN 1090-2104

González-Quevedo, R.; de Juan, C.; Massa, M.J.; Sánchez-Pernaute, A.; Torres, A.; Balibrea, J.L.; Benito, M. & Iniesta, P. (2000). Detection of telomerase activity in human carcinomas using a trap-ELISA method: correlation with hTR and hTERT expression. *International Jiurnal of Oncology,* Vol. 6, No. 3, (March 2000), pp. 623-628, ISSN 1791-2423

Granger, M. P.; Wright, W. E. & Shay, J. W. (2002). Telomerase in cancer and aging. *Crit. Rev. Oncol. Hematol.* Vol. 41, No. 1, (January 2002), pp. 29-40, ISSN 1879-0461

Greider, C.W. & Blackburn, E.H. (1985). Identification of a specific telomere terminal transferase activitiy in Tetrahymena extracts. *Cell.* Vol. 43, No. 4, pp. 405-413, ISSN 1097-4172

Griffith, J.D.; Comeau, L.; Rosenfield, S.; Stansel, R.M.; Bianchi, A.; Moss, H. & de Lange T. (1999). Mammalian telomeres end in a large duplex loop. *Cell,* Vol. 97, No. 4, (May 1999), pp. 503-514, ISSN 1097-4172

Gryaznov, S.; Pongracz, K.; Matray, T.; Schultz, R.; Pruzan, R.; Aimi, J.; Chin, A.; Harley, C.; Shea-Herbert, B.; Shay, J.; Oshima, Y.; Asai, A. & Amashita, Y. (2001). Telomerase inhibitors- oligonucleotide phosphoramidates as potential therapeuticagents. *Nucleosides Nucleotides Nucleic Acids,* Vol. 20, No. 4-7, (April-July 2001), pp. 401-410, ISSN 1532-2335

Gryaznov, S.M.(2010). Oligonucleotide n3'-->p5' phosphoramidates and thio-phoshoramidates as potential therapeutic agents. *Chemistry and Biodiversity,* Vol. 7, No. 3, (March 2010), pp. 477-493, ISSN 1612-1880

Gu, J.; Kagawa, S.; Takakura, M.; Kyo, S.; Inoue, M.; Roth, J.A. & Fang, B. (2000). Tumor-specific transgene expression from the human telomerase reverse transcriptase promoter enables targeting of the therapeutic effects of the Bax gene to cancers. *Cancer Research,* Vol. 60, No. 19, (October 2000), pp. 5359-5364, ISSN 1538-7445

Gu, J. & Fang, B. (2003). Telomerase promoter-driven cancer gene therapy. *Cancer Biol Ther,* Vol. 2, No. 4, Suppl 1, (July-August 2003), pp. S64-S70, ISSN 1555-8576

Gümüş-Akay, G.; Unal, A.E.; Bayar, S.; Karadayi, K.; Elhan, A.H.; Sunguroğlu, A. & Tükün, A. (2007). Telomerase activity could be used as a marker for neoplastic transformation in gastric adenocarcinoma: but it does not have a prognostic significance. *Genetics ans Molecular Research,* Vol. 6, No.1, (February 2007), pp. 41-49, ISSN 1676-5680

Gümüş-Akay, G.; Elhan, A.H.; Unal, A.E.; Demirkazik, A.; Sunguroğlu, A. & Tükün, A. (2009). Effects of genomic imbalances on telomerase activity in gastric cancer: clues to telomerase regulation. *Oncology Research,* Vol. 17, No.10 , pp. 455-462, ISSN 0965-0407

Hahn, W.C.; Stewart, S.A.; Brooks, M.W.; York, S.G.; Eaton, E.; Kurachi, A.; Beijersbergen, R.L.; Knoll, J.H.M.; Meyerson, M. & Weinberg, R.A. (1999). Inhibition of telomerase limits the growth of human cancer cells. *Nature Medicine,* Vol. 5, No.10, (October 1999), pp. 1164 –1170, ISSN 1546-170X

Hahn, W.C. (2005). Telomere and telomerase dynamics in human cells. *Current Molecular Medicine,* Vol. 5, No.2, (March 2005), pp. 227-231, ISSN 1875-5666

Hao, Z.M.; Luo, J.Y.; Cheng, J.; Wang, Q.Y. & Yang, G.X. (2003). Design of a ribozyme targeting human telomerase reverse transcriptase and cloning of it's gene. *World Journal of Gastroenterology,* Vol 9, No. 1, (January 2003), pp. 104-107, ISSN 1007-9327

Hao, Z.M.; Luo, J.Y.; Cheng, J.; Li, L.; He, D.; Wang, Q.Y. & Yang, G.X. (2005). Intensive inhibition of hTERT expression by a ribozyme induces rapid apoptosis of cancer cells through a telomere length-independent pathway. *Cancer Biology and Therapy,* Vol. 4, No. 10, (October 2005), pp. 1098-1103, ISSN 1555-8576

Harley, C.B.; Futcher, A.B. & Greider, C.W. (1990). Telomeres shorten during aging of human fibroblasts. *Nature,* Vol. 345, No.6274 , (May 1990) pp. 458-460, ISSN 0028-0836

Harley, C.B. Telomerase and cancer therapeutics. (2008). *Nature Reviews. Cancer,* Vol. 8, No. 3, (March 2008), pp. 167-179, ISSN 1474-1768

Hayflick, L. & Moorhead, P.S. (1961). The serial cultivation of human diploid cell strains. *Experimental Cell Resesearch,* Vol. 25, (December 1961), pp. 585-621, ISSN 0014-4827

Heaphy, C.M. & Meeker, A,K. (2011). The potential utility of telomere-related markers for cancer diagnosis. *Journal of Cellular and Molecular Medicine,* Vol. 15, No. 6, (June 2011), pp. 1227-1238, ISSN 1582-4934

Hess, J.L. & Highsmith, W.E. Jr. (2002). Telomerase detection in body fluids. *Clinical Chemistry,* Vol. 48, No. 1, (January 2002), pp. 18-24, ISSN 1530-8561

Hiyama, K.; Hirai, Y.; Kyoizumi, S.; Akiyama, M.; Hiyama, E.; Piatyszek, M.A.; Shay, J.W.; Ishioka, S. & Yamakido, M. (1995). Activation of telomerase in human lymphocytes and hematopoietic progenitor cells. *The Journal of Immunology,* Vol. 155, No. 8, (October, 1995), pp.3711-3715, ISSN 1550-6606

Hiyama, E. & Hiyama, K. (2002).Clinical utility of telomerase in cancer. *Oncogene,* Vol. 21, No. 4, (January 2002), pp. 643-649, ISSN 1476-5594

Hiyama, E. & Hiyama, K. (2003). Telomerase as tumor marker. *Cancer Letters,* Vol. 194, No. 2, (May 2003), pp. 221–233, ISSN 1872-7980

Hiyama, E. & Hiyama, K. (2004). Telomerase detection in the diagnosis and prognosis of cancer. *Cytotechnology,* Vol. 45, No. 1-2, (June 2004), pp. 61-74, ISSN 1573-0778

Hockemeyer, D.; Palm, W.; Else, T.; Daniels, J.P.; Takai, K.K.; Ye, J.Z.; Keegan, C.E.; de Lange, T. & Hammer, G.D. (2007). Telomere protection by mammalian Pot1 requires interaction with Tpp1. *Nature Structural and Molecular Biology*, Vol. 14, No.8, (August 2007), pp. 754-761, ISSN 1545-9985

Hsiao, S.J. & Smith, S. (2008). Tankyrase function at telomeres, spindle poles and beyond. *Biochimie*, Vol. 90, No.1, (January 2008), pp. 83-92, ISSN 1638-6183

http://nobelprize.org/nobel_prizes/medicine/laureates/2009/ "The Nobel Prize in Physiology or Medicine 2009". Nobelprize.org. 24 Jun 2011

Hu, X.; Wu, H.; Zhang, S.; Yuan, H. & Cao, L. (2009). Clinical significance of telomerase activity in gastric carcinoma and peritoneal dissemination. *Journal of International Medical Research*, Vol. 37, No. 4, (July-August 2009), pp. 1127-1138, ISSN 1473-2300

Huard, S.; Moriarty, T.J. & Autexier, C. (2003). The C terminus of the human telomerase reverse transcriptase is a determinant of enzyme processivity. *Nucleic Acids Research*, Vol. 31, No. 14, (July 2003), pp. 4059-4070, ISSN 1362-4962

Huffman, K.E.; Levene, S.D.; Tesmer, V.M.; Shay, J.W. & Wright, W.E. (2000). Telomere shortening is proportional to the size of the G-rich telomeric 3'-overhang. *The Journal of Biological Chemistry*, Vol. 275, No. 26, (June 2000), pp.19719-19722, ISSN 1083-351X

Incles, C.M.; Schultes, C.M.; Kelland, L.R. & Neidle, S. (2003). Acquired cellular resistance to flavopiridol in a human colon carcinoma cell line involves up-regulation of the telomerase catalytic subunit and telomere elongation. Sensitivity of resistant cells to combination treatment with a telomerase inhibitor. *Molecular Pharmacology*, Vol. 64, No. 5, (November 2003), pp. 1101–1108, ISSN 1521-0111

Iwano, T.; Tachibana, M.; Reth, M. & Shinkai, Y. (2004). Importance of TRF1 for functional telomere structure. *The Journal of Biological Chemistry*, Vol. 279, No. 2, (January 2004), pp. 1442-1448, ISSN 1083-351X

Kameshima, H.; Yagihashi, A.; Yajima, T.; Kobayashi, D.; Denno, R.; Hirata, K. & Watanabe, N. (2000). Helicobacter pylori infection: augmentation of telomerase activity in cancer and noncancerous tissues. *World Journal of Surgery*, Vol. 24, No.10, (October 2000), pp. 1243-1249, ISSN 1432-2323

Kilian, A.; Bowtell, D.D.; Abud, H.E.; Hime, G.R.; Venter, D.J.; Keese, P.K.; Duncan, E.L.; Reddel, R.R. & Jefferson, R.A. (1997). Isolation of a candidate human telomerase catalytic subunit gene, which reveals complex splicing patterns in different cell types. *Human Molecular Genetics*, Vol. 6, No. 12, (November 1997), pp. 2011–2019, ISSN 1460-2083

Kim, N.W.; Piatyszek, M.A.; Prowse, K.R.; Harley, C.B.; West, M.D.; Ho, P.L.; Coviello, G.M.; Wright, W.E.; Weinrich, S.L. & Shay J.W. (1994). Specific association of human telomerase activity with immortal cells and cancer. *Science*, Vol. 266, No. 5193, (December 1994), pp. 2011-2015, ISSN 0036-8075

Kim, S.H.; Kaminker, P. & Campisi, J. (1999). TIN2, a new regulator of telomere length in human cells. *Nature Genetics*, Vol. 23, No. 4, (December 1999), pp. 405-412, ISSN 1061-4036

Kim, M.Y.; Vankayalapati, H.; Shin-Ya, K.; Wierzba, K. & Hurley, L.H. (2002).Telomestatin, a potent telomerase inhibitor that interacts quite specifically with the human telomeric intramolecular g-quadruplex. *Journal of the American Chemical Society*, Vol. 124, No. 10, (March 2002), pp. 2098-2099, ISSN 1520-5126

Kim, S.H.; Beausejour, C.; Davalos, A.R.; Kaminker, P.; Heo, S.J. & Campisi, J. (2004). TIN2 mediates functions of TRF2 at human telomeres. *The Journal of Biological Chemistry*, Vol. 279, No. 42, (October 2004), pp, 43799–43804, ISSN 1083-351X

Komata, T.; Kondo, Y.; Kanzawa, T.; Ito, H.; Hirohata, S.; Koga, S.; Sumiyoshi, H.; Takakura, M.; Inoue, M.; Barna, B.P.; Germano, I.M.; Kyo, S. & Kondo, S. (2002). Caspase-8 gene therapy using the human telomerase reverse transcriptase promoter for malignant glioma cells. *Human Gene Therapy*, Vol. 13, No. 9, (June 2002), pp.1015-1025, ISSN 1557-7422

Komuro, A.; Imamura, T.; Saitoh, M.; Yoshida, Y.; Yamori, T.; Miyazono, K. & Miyazawa, K. (2004). Negative regulation of transforming growth factor-beta (TGF-beta) signaling by WW domain-containing protein 1 (WWP1). *Oncogene*, Vol. 23, No. 41, (September 2004), pp. 6914-6923, ISSN 1476-5594

Kotsakis, A.; Vetsika, E.K.; Christou, S.; Hatzidaki, D.; Vardakis, N.; Aggouraki, D.; Konsolakis, G.; Georgoulias, V.; Christophyllakis, C.; Cordopatis, P.; Kosmatopoulos, K. & Mavroudis, D. (2011). Clinical outcome of patients with various advanced cancer types vaccinated with an optimized cryptic human telomerase reverse transcriptase (TERT) peptide: results of an expanded phase II study. (2011). *Annals of Oncology*, doi:10.1093/an nonc/mdr 396, Accesses on October 23 2011, ISSN 1569-8041

Kraemer, K.; Fuessel, S.; Schmidt, U.; Kotzsch, M.; Schwenzer, B.; Wirth, M.P. & Meye, A. (2003). Antisense-mediated hTERT inhibition specifically reduces the growth of human bladder cancer cells. *Clinical Cancer Research*,Vol. 9, No. 10 Pt 1, (September 2003), pp. 3794-3800, ISSN 1078-0432

Lee, J.H. & Chung, I.K. (2010). Curcumin inhibits nuclear localization of telomerase by dissociating the Hsp90 co-chaperone p23 from hTERT. *Cancer Letters*,Vol. 290, No. 1, (April 2010), pp. 76-86, ISSN 1872-7980

Li, B.; Oestreich, S. & de Lange, T. (2000). Identification of human Rap1: implications for telomere evolution. *Cell*, Vol. 101, No. 5, (May 2000), pp. 471-483, ISSN 1097-4172

Li, H.; Xu, D.; Toh, B.H. & Liu, J.P. (2006a). TGFβ and cancer: Is Smad3 a repressor of hTERT gene? *Cell Research*,Vol. 16, No. 2, (February 2006), pp. 169-173, ISSN 1748-7838

Li, H.; Xu, D.; Li, J.; Berndt, M.C. & Liu, J,P. (2006b). Transforming growth factor beta suppresses human telomerase reverse transcriptase by smad3 interactions with c-Myc and hTERT gene. *The Journal of Biological Chemistry*,Vol. 281, No.35, (September 2006), pp.25588-25600, ISSN 1083-351X

Li, W.; Li, L.; Liu, Z.; Liu, C.; Liu, Z.; Strååt, K.; Björkholm, M.; Jia, J. & Xu, D. (2008). Expression of the full-length telomerase reverse transcriptase (hTERT) transcript in both malignant and normal gastric tissues. *Cancer Letters*, Vol. 260, No. 1-2, (February 2008), pp. 28-36, ISSN 1872-7980

Lingner,J.; Hughes,T.R.; Shevchenko,A.; Mann,M.; Lundblad,V. & Cech,T.R. (1997). Reverse transcriptase motifs in the catalytic subunit of telomerase. *Science* , Vol. 276, No. 5312, (April 1997), pp. 561–567, ISSN 1095-9203

Liu, K.; Schoonmaker, M.M.; Levine, B.L.; June, C.H.; Hodes, R.J. & Weng, N,P. (1999) Constitutive and regulated expression of telomerase reverse transcriptase (hTERT) in human lymphocytes. *Proceedings of the National Academy of Sciences of the United States of America*, Vol. 96, No. 9, (April 1999), pp. 5147–5152, ISSN 1091-6490

Liu, D.; Safari, A.; O'Connor, M.S.; Chan, D.W.; Laegeler, A.; Qin, J. & Songyang, Z. (2004). PTOP interacts with POT1 and regulates its localization to telomeres. *Nature Cell Biology,* Vol. 6, No. 7, (July 2004), pp. 673–680, ISSN 1476-4679

Liu, L.; Lai, S.; Andrews, L.G. & Tollefsbol, T.O. (2004). Genetic and epigenetic modulation of telomerase activity in development and disease. *Gene,* Vol. 340, No. 1, (September 2004), pp. 1-10, ISSN 1879-0038

Liu, J.P.; Chen, W.; Schwarer, A.P. & Li, H. (2010). Telomerase in cancer immunotherapy. *BBA international journal of biochemistry and biophysics,*Vol. 1805, No. 1, (January 2010), pp. 35-42, ISSN 0006-3002

Loayza, D. & De Lange, T. (2003). POT1 as a terminal transducer of TRF1 telomere length control. *Nature,* Vol. 423, No. 6943, (June 2003), pp. 1013-1018, ISSN 1476-4687

Loayza, D.; Parsons, H.; Donigian, J.; Hoke, K. & de Lange, T. (2004). DNA binding features of human POT1: a nonamer 5'-TAGGGTTAG-3' minimal binding site, sequence specificity, and internal binding to multimeric sites. *The Journal of Biological Chemistry,* Vol. 279, No. 13, (March 2004), pp. 13241-13248, ISSN 1083-351X

Lu, Y.; Gu, J.; Jin, D.; Gao, Y. & Yuan, M. (2011). Inhibition of telomerase activity by HDV ribozyme in cancers. *Journal of Experimental and Clinical Cancer Research,* Vol. 30, No. 1, (January 2011), pp. 1, ISSN 1756-9966

Makarov, V.L.; Hirose, Y. & Langmore, J.P. (1997). Long G tails at both ends of human chromosomes suggest a C strand degradation mechanism for telomere shortening. *Cell,* Vol. 88, No. 5, (March 1997), pp. 657-666, ISSN 1097-4172

Maser, R.S. & DePinho, R.A. (2002). Connecting chromosomes, crisis, and cancer. *Science,* Vol. 297, No. 5581, (July 2002), pp. 565–569, ISSN 1095-9203

Mason, M.; Schuller, A. & Skordalakes, E. (2011). Telomerase structure and function. *Current Opinion In Structural Biology,* Vol. 21, No. 1, (Fbruary 2011), pp. 92-100, ISSN 1879-033X

Meyne, J.; Ratliff, R.L.; Moyzis R.K. (1989). Conservation of the human telomere sequence (TTAGGG)n among vertebrates. *Proceedings of the National Academy of Sciences of the United States of America,* Vol. 86, No. 18, (September 1989), pp. 7049-7053, ISSN 1091-6490

Mori, N.; Oka, M.; Hazama, S.; Iizuka, N.; Yamamoto, K.; Yoshino, S.; Tangoku, A.; Noma, T. & Hirose, K. (2000). Detection of telomerase activity in peritoneal lavage fluid from patients with gastric cancer using immunomagnetic beads. *British Journal of Cancer,* Vol. 83, No. 8, (October 2000), pp. 1026-1032, ISSN 1532-1827

Moyzis, R.K.; Buckingham, J.M.; Cram, L.S.; Dani, M.; Deaven, L.L.; Jones, M.D.; Meyne, J.; Ratliff, R.L. & Wu, J.R. (1988). A highly conserved repetitive DNA sequence, (TTAGGG)n, present at the telomeres of human chromosomes. *Proceedings of the National Academy of Sciences of the United States of America,* Vol. 85, No. 18, (September 1988), pp. 6622-6626, ISSN 1091-6490

Murnane, J.P. (2010). Telomere loss as a mechanism for chromosome instability in human cancer. *Cancer Res*earch, Vol. 70, No. 11, (June 2010), pp. 4255-4259, ISSN 1538-7445

Nakamura,T.M.; Morin,G.B.; Chapman,K.B.; Weinrich,S.L.; Andrews,W.H.; Lingner,J.; Harley,C.B. & Cech,T.R. (1997), Telomerase catalytic subunit homologs from fission yeast and human. *Science* , Vol. 277, No. 5328, (August 1997), pp. 955–959, ISSN 0036-8075

Nishimoto, A.; Miura, N.; Horikawa, I.; Kugoh, H.; Murakami, Y.; Hirohashi, S.; Kawasaki, H.; Gazdar, A.F.; Shay, J. W.; Barrett, J. C. & Oshimura, M. (2001). Functional evidence for telomerase repressor gene on human chromosome 10p15.1. *Oncogene*, Vol. 20, No.7, (February 2001), pp. 828-835, ISSN 1476-5594

Oganesian, L. & Bryan, T. (2007). Physiological relevance of telomeric G-quadruplex formation: a potential drug target. *Bioessays*, Vol. 29, No. 2, (February 2007), pp. 155–165, ISSN 1521-1878

Okamoto, K.; Iwano, T.; Tachibana, M. & Shinkai Y. (2008). Distinct roles of TRF1 in the regulation of telomere structure and lengthening. *The Journal of Biological Chemistry*, Vol. 283, No. 35, (August 2008), pp.23981-23988, ISSN 1083-351X

Olovnikov, A.M. (1973). A theory of marginotomy. The incomplete copying of template margin in enzymic synthesis of polynucleotides and biological significance of the phenomenon. *Journal of Theoretical Biology*, Vol. 41, No. 1, (September 1973), pp. 181-90, ISSN 1095-8541

O'sullivan, R.J. & Karlseder, J. (2010). Telomeres: protecting chromosomes against genome stability. *Nature Reviews Molecular Cell Biology*.Vol. 11, No. 3, (March 2010), pp. 171-81, ISSN 1471-0080

Oshimura, M. & Barrett, J. C. (1997). Multiple pathways to cellular senescence: role of telomerase repressors. *European Journal of Cancer*, Vol. 33, No.5, (April 1997), pp. 710-715, ISSN 1879-085

Ozmen B.; Duvan C.I.; Gümüş G.; Sönmezer M.; Gungor M. & Ortaç F. (2009). The role of telomerase activity in predicting early recurrence of epithelial ovarian cancer after first-line chemotherapy: a prospective clinical study. *European Journal of Gynaecological Oncology*, Vol. 30, No. 3, pp. 303-308, ISSN 0392-2936

Palm, W. & de Lange, T.(2008). How shelterin protects mammalian telomeres. *Annual Reviews of Genetics*,Vol. 42, pp. 301-334, ISSN 1545-2948

Shay, J.W.; Wright, W.E. & Werbin, H. (1991). Defining the molecular mechanisms of human cell immortalization. *BBA International Journal of Biochemistry and Biophysics*, Vol. 1072, No. 1, (April 1991), pp. 1-7, ISSN 0006-3002

Shay, J.W. & Bacchetti, S. (1997). A survey of telomerase activity in human cancer. *European Journal of Cancer*, Vol. 33, No. 5, (April 1997), pp. 787-791, ISSN 1879-085

Shay, J.W.; Zou, Y.; Hiyama, E. & Wright, W.E. (2001). Telomerase and cancer. *Human Molecular Genetics*, Vol. 10, No. 7, (April 2001), pp. 677-685, ISSN 0964-6906

Shay, J.W & Wright, W.E. (2006). Telomerase and human cancer, In: *Telomeres*, de Lange, T.; Lundblad, V. & Blackburn, E. (2nd Ed.) pp. 81-108, Cold Spring Harbor Laboratory Press, ISBN 0-87969-734-2, New York, USA

Shay, J.W. & Wright, W.E. (2010). Telomeres and telomerase in normal and cancer stem cells. *FEBS Letters*, Vol. 584, No. 17, (September 2010), pp. 3819–3825, ISSN 1873-3468

Shea-Herbert, B.; Pongracz, K.; Shay, J. & Gryaznov, S. (2002). Oligonucleotide N3'→P5'phosphoramidates as efficient telomerase inhibitors. *Oncogene*, Vol. 21, No. 4, (January 2002), pp. 638 – 642, ISSN 1476-5594

Shim, W.Y.; Park, K.H.; Jeung, H.C.; Kim, Y.T.; Kim, T.S.; Hyung, W.J.; An, S.H.; Yang, S.H.; Noh, S.H.; Chung, H.C. & Rha, S.Y. (2005). Quantitative detection of telomerase activity by real-time TRAP assay in the body fluids of cancer patients. *International Journal of Molecular Medicine*, Vol. 16, No. 5, (November 2005), pp: 857-863, ISSN 1791-244X

Smith, S. & de Lange, T. (2000). Tankyrase promotes telomere elongation in human cells. *Current Biology,* Vol. 10, No. 20, (October 2000), pp. 1299-1302, ISSN 1879-0445

Smogorzewska, A.;van Steensel, B.; Bianchi, A.; Oelmann, S.; Schaefer, M.R. ; Schnapp, G. & de Lange, T. (2000). Control of human telomere length by TRF1 and TRF2. *Molecular and Cellular Biology,* Vol. 20, No. 5, (March 2000), pp. 1659–1668, ISSN 1098-5549

Smogorzewska, A ; de Lange T. (2004). Regulation of telomerase by telomeric proteins. *Annual Review of Biochemistry,* Vol. 73, pp. 177-208, ISSN 1545-4509

Soder, A.I.; Hoare, S.F.; Muir, S.; Going, J.J., Parkinson, E.K. & Keith, W.N. (1997). Amplification, increased dosage and in situ expression of the telomerase RNA gene in human cancer. *Oncogene,* Vol. 14, No. 9, (March 1997), pp. 1013–1021, ISSN 1476-5594.

Soohoo, C.Y.; Shi, R.; Lee, T.H.; Huang, P.; Lu, K.P. & Zhou, X.Z. (2010). Telomerase inhibitor PINX1 provides a link between TRF1 and telomerase to prevent telomere elongation. *The Journal of Biological Chemistry,* Vol. 286, No. 5, (February 2010), pp. 3894-3906, ISSN 1083-351X.

Stansel, R.M. & de Lange, T. & Griffith, J.D. (2001). T-loop assembly in vitro involves binding of TRF2 near the 3' telomeric overhang. *The EMBO Journal,* Vol. 20, No. 19, (October 2001), pp. 5532-5540, ISSN 1460-2075

Steenbergen, R. D.; Kramer, D.; Meijer, C. J.; Walboomers, J. M.; Trott D.A.; Cuthbert, A. P.; Newbold, R. F.; Overkamp, W. J.; Zdzienicka, M. Z. & Snijders, P. J. (2001). Telomerase suppresion by chromosome 6 in a human papilloma virus type 16-immortalized keratinocyte cell line and in a cervical cancer cell line. *Journal of the National Cancer Institute,* Vol. 93, No.11, (June 2001), pp. 865-872, ISSN 1460-2105

Strahl, C. & Blackburn, E.H. (1996). Effects of reverse transcriptase inhibitors on telomere length and telomerase activity in two immortalized human cell lines. *Molecular and Cellular Biology,* Vol. 16, No. 1, (January 1996), pp. 53-65, ISSN.

Suso, E.M.; Dueland, S.; Rasmussen, A.M.; Vetrhus, T.; Aamdal, S.; Kvalheim, G. & Gaudernack, G. (2011). hTERT mRNA dendritic cell vaccination: complete response in a pancreatic cancer patient associated with response against several hTERT epitopes. *Cancer Immunology and Immunotherapy,* Vol. 60, No. 6, (June 2011), pp. 809-818, ISSN 1432-0851.

Suzuki, K.; Kashimura, H.; Ohkawa, J.; Itabashi, M.; Watanabe, T.; Sawahata, T.; Nakahara, A.; Muto, H. & Tanaka, N. (2000). Expression of human telomerase catalytic subunit gene in cancerous and precancerous gastric conditions. *Journal of Gastroenterology and Hepatology,* Vol. 15, No. 7, (July 2000), pp. 744-751, ISSN 1440-1746

Takai, K.K.; Hooper, S.; Blackwood, S.; Gandhi, R. & de Lange. T, (2010). In Vivo Stoichiometry of Shelterin Components. *The Journal of Biological Chemistry,*Vol. 285, No. 2, (January 2010), pp. 1457–1467, ISSN, 1083-351X

Takayashiki, N.; Kawara, H.; Kamiakito, T.; Tanaka, A. (2005). Transcriptional repression of fibroblast growth factor 8 by transforming growth factor-β in androgen-dependent SC-3 cells. *The Journal of Steroid Biochemistry and Molecular Biology.*Vol. 96, No. 1, (June 2005), pp. 1-12, ISSN 1879-1220

Tang, Z.; Zhao, Y.; Mei, F.; Yang, S.; Li, X.; Lv, J.; Hou, L. & Zhang, B. (2004). Molecular cloning and characterization of a human gene involved in transcriptional regulation of hTERT. *Biochemical and Biophysical Research Communications*, Vol. 324, No. 4, (November 2004), pp. 1324-1332, ISSN 1090-2104

Tejera, A.M.; Stagno d'Alcontres, M.; Thanasoula, M.; Marion, R.M.; Martinez, P.; Liao, C.; Flores, J.M.; Tarsounas, M. & Blasco, M.A. (2010). TPP1 is required for TERT recruitment, telomere elongation during nuclear reprogramming, and normal skin development in mice. *Developmental Cell,* Vol. 18, No. 5, (May 2010), pp.691-702, ISSN 1878-1551.

Usselmann, B.; Newbold, M.; Morris, A.G. & Nwokolo, C.U. (2001). Telomerase activity and patient survival after surgery for gastric and oesophageal cancer. *European Journal of Gastroenterology and Hepatology,* Vol. 13, No. 8, (August 2001), pp. 903-908, ISSN 1473-5687

van Steensel, B. & de Lange, T. (1997). Control of telomere length by the human telomeric protein TRF1. *Nature,* Vol. 385, No. 6618, (February 1997), pp. 740-743, ISSN 0028-0836

Vasudevan, S.A.; Shoko, J.; Wang, K.; Burlingame, S.M.; Patel, P.M.; Lazo, J.S.; Nuchtern, J.G. & Yang, J. (2005). MKP-8, a novel MAPK phosphatase that inhibits p38 kinase. *Biochemical and Biophysical Research Communications,* Vol. 330, No. 2, (May 2005), pp. 511-518, ISSN 1090-2104

Vetsika, E.K.; Konsolakis, G.; Aggouraki, D.; Kotsakis, A.; Papadimitraki, E.; Christou, S.; Menez-Jamet, J.; Kosmatopoulos, K; Georgoulias, V. & Mavroudis, D. (2011). Immunological responses in cancer patients after vaccination with the therapeutic telomerase-specific vaccine Vx-001. *Cancer Immunology and Immunotherapy*. DOI 10.1007/s00262-011-1093-4 , accessed on October 24, 2011, ISSN 1432-0851

Vonderheide, R.H. (2008). Prospects and challenges of building a cancer vaccine targeting telomerase. *Biochimie.* Vol. 90, No. 1, (January 2008), pp. 173-180, ISSN 1638-6183

Wan, M.; Li, W.Z.; Duggan, B.D.; Felix, J.C.; Zhao, Y. & Dubeau, L. (1997). Telomerase activity in benign and malignant epithelial ovarian tumors. *Journal of the National Cancer Institute,* Vol. 89, No. 6, (March 1997), pp. 437–441, ISSN 1460-2105

Wang, F.; Podell, E.R.; Zaug, A.J.; Yang, Y.; Baciu, P.; Cech, T.R. & Lei, M. (2007). The POT1–TPP1 telomere complex is a telomerase processivity factor. *Nature,* Vol. 445, No. 7127, (February 2007), pp. 506–510, ISSN 1476-4687

Ward, R.J. & Autexier, C. (2005). Pharmacological telomerase inhibition can sensitize drug-resistant and drug-sensitive cells to chemotherapeutic treatment. *Molecular Pharmacology,* Vol. 68, No. 3, (September 2005), pp. 779-786, ISSN 1521-0111

Widschwendter, A.; M¨uller, H.M.; Hubalek, M.M.; Wiedemair, A.; Fiegl, H.; Goebel, G.; Mueller-Holzner, E.; Marth, C. & Widschwendter, M. (2004). Methylation status and expression of human telomerase reverse transcriptase in ovarian and cervical cancer. *Gynecologic Oncology,*Vol. 93, No. 2, (May 2004), pp. 407–416, ISSN 1095-6859

Wong, S.C.; Yu, H. & So, J,B. (2006). Detection of telomerase activity in gastric lavage fluid: a novel method to detect gastric cancer. *The Journal of Surgical Research,* Vol. 131, No. 2, (April 2006), pp. 252–255, ISSN 1095-8673.

Wong, K.K., Chang, S. & DePinho, R.A. (2006). Modeling cancer and aging in the telomerease deficient mouse, In: *Telomeres,* de Lange, T.; Lundblad, V. & Blackburn, E. (2nd Ed.) pp. 109-138, Cold Spring Harbor Laboratory Press, ISBN 0-87969-734-2, New York, USA

Wright, W.E.; Pereira-Smith, O.M. & Shay, J.W. (1989). Reversible cellular senescence: implications for immortalization of normal human diploid fibroblasts. *Molecular and Cellular Biology,* Vol. 9, No. 7, (July 1989), pp. 3088-3092, ISSN 1098-5549

Wright W.E., Shay J.W. and Piatyszek M.A. (1995). Modification of a telomeric repeat amplification protocol (TRAP) result in increased reliability, linearity and sensitivity. Nucl. Acid Res. 23: 3794–3795.

Wright, W.E.; Tesmer, V.M.; Huffman, K.E.; Leven, S.D. & Shay, J,W. (1997). Normal human chromosomes have long G-rich telomeric overhangs at one end. *Genes and Development,* Vol. 11, No. 21, (November 1997), pp. 2801-2809, ISSN 1549-5477

Wu, Y.Y.; Hruszkewycz, A.M.; Delgado, R.M.; Yang, A.; Vortmeyer, A.O.; Moon, Y.W.; Weil, R.J.; Zhuang, Z. & Remaley, A.T. (2000). Limitations on the quantitative determination of telomerase activity by the electrophoretic and ELISA based TRAP assays. *Clinica Chimica Acta; International Journal of Clinical Chemistry* Vol. 293, No. 1-2, (March 2000), pp. 199-212, ISSN 1873-3492

Wyatt, H.D.; Lobb, D.A. & Beattie, T.L. (2007). Characterization of physical and functional anchor site interactions in human telomerase. *Molecular and Cellular Biology,* Vol. 27, No. 8, (February 2007), pp. 3226-3240, ISSN 1098-5549

Wyatt, H.D.; West, S.C. & Beattie TL. (2010). InTERTpreting telomerase structure and function. *Nucleic Acids Research,* Vol. 38, No. 17, (September 2010), pp. 5609-5622, ISSN 1362-4962

Xin, H.; Liu, D.; Wan, M.; Safari, A.; Kim, H.; Sun, W.; O'Connor, M.S. & Songyang, Z. (2007). TPP1 is a homologue of ciliate TEBP-ß and interacts with POT1 to recruit telomerase. *Nature,* Vol. 445, 7127, (February 2007), pp. 559-562, ISSN 1476-4687

Xu, S.; He, M.; Yu, H.; Cai, X.; Tan, X.; Lu, B. & Shu, B. (2001). A quantitative method to measure telomerase activity by bioluminescence connected with telomeric repeat amplification protocol. *Analytical Biochemistry,*. Vol. 299, No. 2, (December 2001), pp. 188-193, ISSN 1096-0309

Ye, J.Z.; Donigian, J.R.; van Overbeek, M.; Loayza, D.; Luo, Y.; Krutchinsky, A.N.; Chait, B.T. & de Lange, T. (2004 a). TIN2 binds TRF1 and TRF2 simultaneously and stabilizes the TRF2 complex on telomeres. *The Journal of Biological Chemistry,* Vol. 279, No. 45, (November 2004), pp. 47264-47271, ISSN 1083-351X.

Ye, J.Z.; Hockemeyer, D.; Krutchinsky, A.N.; Loayza, D.; Hooper, S.M.; Chait, B.T. & de Lange, T. (2004b). POT1-interacting protein PIP1: a telomere length regulator that recruits POT1 to the TIN2/TRF1 complex. *Genes and Development,* Vol. 18, No. 14, (July 2004), pp. 1649–1654, ISSN 1549-5477

Yokoyama, Y.; Takahashi, Y.; Shinohara, A.; Lian, Z. & Tamaya, T. (1998). Telomerase activity in the female reproductive tract and neoplasms. *Gynecologic Oncology,* Vol. 68, No. 2, (February 1998), pp. 145–149, ISSN 1095-6859

Yoo, J.; Park, S.Y.; Kang, S.J.; Kim, B.K.; Shim, S.I. & Kang, C.S. (2003). Expression of telomerase activity, human telomerase RNA, and telomerase reverse transcriptase in gastric adenocarcinomas. *Modern Pathology,* Vol. 16, No. 7, (July 2003), pp. 700-707, ISSN 1530-0285

You, Y.; Pu, P.; Huang, Q.; Xia, Z.; Wang, C.; Wang, G.; Yu, C.; Yu, J.J.; Reed, E. & Li, Q.Q. (2006). Antisense telomerase RNA inhibits the growth of human glioma cells in vitro and in vivo. *International Journal of Oncology,* Vol. 28, No. 5, (May 2006), pp. 1225-1232, ISSN 1791-2423

Yu, S.T.; Li, C.; Lü, M.H.; Liang, G.P.; Li, N.; Tang, X.D.; Wu, Y.Y.; Shi, C.M.; Chen, L.; Li, C.Z.; Cao, Y.L.; Fang, D.C. & Yang, S.M. (2011). Noninvasive and real-time monitoring of the therapeutic response of tumors in vivo with an optimized hTERT promoter. *Cancer,* doi: 10.1002/cncr.26476, accessed on October 24, 2011, ISSN 1097-0142

Yui,J; Chiu, C.P. & Lansdorp, P.M. (1998). Telomerase activity in candidate stem cells from fetal liver and adult bone marrow. *Blood,* Vol. 91, No. 9, (May 1998), pp. 3255–3262, ISSN 1528-0020

Zhang, Q.; Kim, N-K. & Feigon J. (2011). Architecture of human telomerase RNA. *Proceedings of the National Academy of Sciences of the United States of America,* www.pnas.org/cgi/doi/10.1073/pnas.1100279108, accessed on October 19, 2011, ISSN 1091-6490

Zhao, Y.; Zheng, J.; Ling, Y.; Hou, L.; Zhang, B. (2005). Transcriptional upregulation of DNA polymerase β by TEIF. Biochem. *Biochemical and Biophysical Research Communication,* Vol. 333, No. 3, (August 2005), pp. 908-916, ISSN 1090-2104

Zheng, P.S.; Iwasaka, T.; Yamasaki, F.; Ouchida, M.; Yokoyama, M.; Nakao, Y.; Fukuda, K.; Matsuyama, T. & Sugimori, H. (1997). Telomerase activity in gynecologic tumors. *Gynecologic Oncology,* Vol. 64, No. 1, (January 1997), pp. 171-175, ISSN 1095-6859

Zhong, Z.; Shiue, L.; Kaplan, S. & de Lange, T. (1992). A mammalian factor that binds telomeric TTAGGG repeats in vitro. *Molecular and Cellular Biology,* Vol. 12, No. 11, (November 1992), pp. 4834-4843, ISSN 1098-5549

Zhou, X.Z. & Lu, K.P. (2001). The Pin2/TRF1-interacting protein PinX1 is a potent telomerase inhibitor. *Cell,* Vol. 107, No. 3, (November 2001), pp. 347-59, ISSN 1097-4172

Zou, Y.; Sfeir, A.; Gryaznov, S.M.; Shay, J.W. & Wright, W.E. (2004). Does a sentinel or a subset of short telomeres determine replicative senescence? *Molecular and Cellular Biology,* Vol. 15, No. 8, (August 2004), pp.3709-3718, ISSN 1098-5549

5

Inhibiting Telomerase Activity and Inducing Apoptosis in Cancer Cells by Several Natural Food Compounds

Didem Turgut Cosan and Ahu Soyocak
Eskisehir Osmangazi University, Medical Faculty, Department of Medical Biology
Turkey

1. Introduction

Today cancer is one of the most important causes of death. Therefore, researches pertinent to diagnosis, prognosis and treatment of cancer increase day by day. A large part of cancer can be treated by surgery, radiotherapy and chemotherapy. Various compounds are used for chemotherapy. Most of these anti-cancer compounds are synthetics that have toxic adverse effects. Therefore, it is crucial to reveal beneficial effects of natural compounds such as milder side effects on normal cells and potential anti-tumour effects. A great number of these compounds also have the potential to be anti-cancerogenic. Thus, importance of natural food-derived anti-cancer compound consumption has recently increased. Researches demonstrate these anti-cancerogenic features through various mechanisms. These mechanisms also include inhibition of telomerase activity and induction of apoptosis. It is presumed that these mechanisms are in interaction with each other. After giving brief information on telomeres, telomerase activity and apoptosis in this chapter, we will address the effects of several compounds on telomerase activity and apoptosis and the possible relationship they have with each other.

Telomeres, which are located at both termini of the chromosomes of eukaryotic organisms, contain DNA and protein. Telomeres are different from other chromosomal DNA sequences in terms of both structural and functional aspects. In vertebrates, telomere is shaped by tandem repetitions of a short pattern which consists of TTAGGG hexanucleotide. The lengths of these repetitions in kilo base vary from one organism to another. The telomeric DNA strand, which is rich in guanine, ends with a single stranded 3'overhang. This single-stranded overhang folds onto the double-stranded telomere and forms the structure called t-loop. Through formation of this t-loop, the capping structure formed at the ends of chromosomes protects the ends from end-to-end fusion, degradation and recombination. Telomere can preserve a certain length or gain or lose length through special proteins and telomerase enzyme. It was demonstrated that these special proteins fulfil certain duties by binding to single and double stranded telomere DNA. Telomeric repeat binding factor 1 (TRF1) and telomeric repeat binding factor 2 (TRF2) are double-strand telomere DNA binding proteins. These proteins and some other proteins related to them are responsible for formation of the telomere complex and t-loop. The telomere is protected through the complex formed by these proteins (Blackburn, 2000; Blackburn, 2001; Celli et al., 2005; Chan & Blackburn, 2002; De Lange, 2002; Griffith et al., 1999; Moyzis et al, 1988;Sfeir et al, 2009; Smogorzewska et al., 2000; van Steensel et al., 1998; van Steensel & de Lange, 1997). The other telomere proteins which compose this complex and their duties are summarized shortly in **Table 1.**

Proteins	**Functions**	**References**
Rap 1 (Repressor activator protein 1)	Mammalian Rap1, whose function is still unclear, TRF2-binding protein, negative regulator of telomere length.	Li & de Lange (2003); Li et al. (2000); Bae & Baumann (2007); O'Connor et al. (2004); Sarthy et al. (2009); Sfeir et al. (2010); Martinez et al. (2010); Diotti & Loayza (2011); Palm & de Lange (2008); de Lange (2009); Martínez & Blasco (2010).
TIN2 (TRF1 Interacting Nuclear protein 2)	TRF1-TRF2 binding protein, negative regulator of telomere length.	Kim et al. (2004); Ye et al. (2004a); Diotti & Loayza (2011); Palm & de Lange (2008); de Lange (2009); Martínez & Blasco (2010).
TPP1 (previously called TINT1 [Houghtaling et al. 2004], PTOP [Liu et al. 2004], and PIP1 [Ye et al. 2004b])	Plays a role in telomere capping by interacting with TIN2 and POT1.	Liu et al. (2004); Ye et al. (2004b); Houghtaling et al. (2004); Diotti &Loayza (2011); Palm &de Lange (2008); de Lange (2009); Martínez &Blasco (2010); Zong et al. (2012); Takai et al. (2011); Wang & Lei (2011).
POT 1 (Protection of telomeres 1)	Binds single-stranded TTAGGG repeats, necessary for telomere-length maintenance and telomere protection.	Baumann & Cech (2001); Loayza & de Lange (2003); Diotti & Loayza (2011); Palm & de Lange (2008); de Lange (2009); Martínez & Blasco (2010).
TANK1 and TANK2 Tankyrase (TANK) telomere-associated poly (ADP-ribose) polymerase (PARP) 1	Positive regulator of telomere length through inhibition of TRF1	Smith et al. (1998); Kaminker et al. (2001).
PINX1 (PIN2-interacting protein X1)	Potential telomerase inhibitor, negatively regulating telomere length by interacting with TRF1.	Zhou & Lu (2001).
Ku86	Negative regulator of telomere length, role in telomere capping, regulation of telomerase recruitment.	Espejel et al. (2002); Pfingsten et al. (2012).
DNA-PK (DNA-dependent protein kinase)	Plays a role in telomere capping, putative role in post-replicative processing of telomeres.	Bailey et al. (2001).

Proteins	Functions	References
ERCC1/XPF (excision repair cross-complementing 1/ xeroderma pigmentosum group F)	Negative mediator of telomere length maintenance.	Zhu et al. (2003); Wu et al. (2008).
Mre11/Rad50/Nbs1	Binds TRF2, DNA-repair complex, possible role in T-loop formation.	Zhu et al. (2000).
PARP-2 (poly (ADP-ribose) polymerase-2)	PARP activity negatively regulates TRF2.	Dantzer et al. (2004).
Apollo (also called SNM1B)	TRF2 interacting, protein absence leads to DNA damage signal at telomeres.	Lenain et al. (2006); van Overbeek & de Lange (2006); Wu et al. (2012).

Table 1. Telomere-binding proteins and their functions

Telomerase, which is a DNA polymerase with special ribonucleoprotein structure, is responsible for synthesis of DNA tandem repeats at chromosomal termini. This enzyme is active in embryonic cells and adult stem cells while inactive or at low level in normal somatic cells. Telomerase, which is a reverse transcriptase, consists of a catalytic subunit (hTERT=Human Telomerase Reverse Transcriptase) and an RNA component (hTR=hTERC=Human Telomerase RNA Complex). Human telomerase enzyme uses a short segment (8-30 bases) of hTR that is complementary to telomeric DNA sequence as the template for extension of 3′ strand of DNA sequence. In this way, telomerase enzyme increases the telomere length and prevents DNA loss known as the end replication problem that occurs at each cell division. When telomere length reaches the critical shortness, the cell cannot divide further and go into senescence. Chromosomal instability, cell senescence and apoptosis can not only be induced by critically short telomeres but also by disruption in telomeric protein complex which is responsible for the loop structure at the chromosome ends (Blackburn, 2000; Bryan & Cech, 1999; Collins, 2006; Cong et al., 2002; Feng et al., 1995; Greider &Blackburn, 1989; Morin, 1997; Shay & Wright, 2005; Wong et al., 2010; Zakian, 1995).

Researches have shown that telomerase is reactivated in most tumour cells. These cells, which have been immortalized, need telomerase activity for ensuring the telomere length required for genetic stability and unlimited proliferative ability. Telomerase reactivation is not sufficient in order to transform a normal cell into a carcinogenic cell, but it is necessary for the cells to preserve effective telomere lengths for providing the cells with unlimited growth capacity and being immortal. Studies show that there is no telomerase activity in benign tumours and that these tumour cells return to early stages as their telomeres get shorter. High telomerase activity is observed in more invasive metastatic tumours. For this reason, the studies conducted recently bring telomerase to the forefront as a target for development of diagnostic, prognostic and therapeutic mechanisms of cancer or even as a potential biomarker (Chatziantoniou, 2001; Hiyama & Hiyama, 2002; Kim, 1997; Lichtsteiner et al. 1999; Shay &Bacchetti, 1997; Shay & Wright, 2011).

Another important cellular event associated with telomere and telomerase is apoptosis. Cells, which lose their functions in the organism or have some disorders, are destroyed through a programmed cell death called apoptosis. Therefore, apoptosis plays an important role in control of normal development in multicellular organisms and regulation of tissue homoeostasis. Through apoptosis, which is a physiological mechanism used for elimination of immortalized cells, in-vitro development of carcinogenesis may be prevented.

Apoptosis is characterized by typical morphological changes that cover many factors which are responsible for DNA fragmentation and protein cleavage. It occurs mainly through pathways activated by extrinsic and intrinsic factors. Extrinsic pathway is induced by activation of Tumour Necrosis Factor (TNF) or Fas receptor in target cell membrane. TNF is released from macrophage sand initiates cell death. Fas ligand is cell surface protein and causes death of cells such as infected cells and tumor cells. Activated TNF and Fas receptors compose complex (DISC) with adapter proteins such as TNF receptor associated death domain (TRADD) and Fas associated death domain (FADD). DISC activates caspases (cysteine-**asp**artic-**a**cid-protea**se**s). Caspases are members of cystein protease family and they are synthesized as an inactive zimogene. Caspases are activated via proteolytic cleavage. In this pathway, caspase-8 is activated. While caspase-8 activates caspase-3, it also directly affects some proapoptotic proteins such as BID. Caspases generally serve as initiator (caspase 2, 8, 9, 10) and effector (caspase 3, 6, 7) in the apoptotic process. Intrinsic pathway is activated by growth factor deprivation, DNA damage, and other stress stimuli. Activated intrinsic pathway is interacted with apoptotic proteins. Bcl-2 family members consist of proapoptotic or antiapoptotic bcl-2 proteins. Among the members of this family, proteins such as Bcl-2, Bcl-X_L and Mcl-1 inhibit apoptosis, while proteins such as Bax, Bad, Bid, Bak, Bim, PUMA, NOXA stimulate apoptosis. These molecules cause to releasing cytochrom c by creating pores. Cytochrom c is localized in intermembrane space of mitochondria. Distruption of the outher mitochondrial membrane leads to releasing of endonuclease G, Smac/DIABLO, Omi/HtrA2, Apoptosis Inducing Factor (AIF) and cytochrom c into cytoplasm. Additionally, proapoptotic proteins such as Bid, Bim, Bad, inhibit Bcl-2 and activate Bax/Bak heterodimer. Together with cytochrom c, Apaf-1 and dATP compose the apoptosome. The apoptosome cleaves procaspase-9 into caspase-9. Similarly caspase-8 and caspase-9 activate caspase-3. Activated caspase-3 causes DNA fragmentation and apoptosis by death substrates such as poly (ADP-ribose) polymerase (PARP), Caspase Activated DNase (CAD)/Inhibitor of Caspase Activated DNase (ICAD) (Bradshaw et al., 2003; Cain et al., 2002; Cory & Adams, 2002; Debatin et al., 2004; Green & Kroemer, 1998; Holdenrieder et al., 2004; Kaufmann & Earnshaw, 2000; Kerr, et al., 1972; Letai, 2008; Nuñez et al., 1998; Parone et al., 2002; Turgut Cosan & Soyocak, 2012; Wyllie, 1992, Wong, 2011). Proteins related with apoptosis in signal pathways and their functions are summarized in **Figure 1** and **Table 2.**

Telomere dysfunction induces two types of cellular response. These cellular responses are cellular senescence and apoptosis. The researches carried out with regard to the relationship among telomere, telomerase and apoptosis report that apoptosis may be induced through different mechanisms by weakening telomere/telomerase activity in cancer cells. In one of these mechanisms, inhibition of telomerase in cancer cells can result in shortening of telomere length and subsequently induce apoptosis. In another telomere/telomerase and apoptosis relationship, inhibition of telomerase can result in apoptosis by causing telomere uncapping. If telomerase is positive, the tumor grows due to survival signals and long telomeres. If telomerase is negative, telomeres are short due to progressive telomere loss. In the telomerase negativity stage, if telomerase becomes positive then tumor regrowth is initiated. If telomerase is still negative then subsequently telomere fusions, p53 activation,

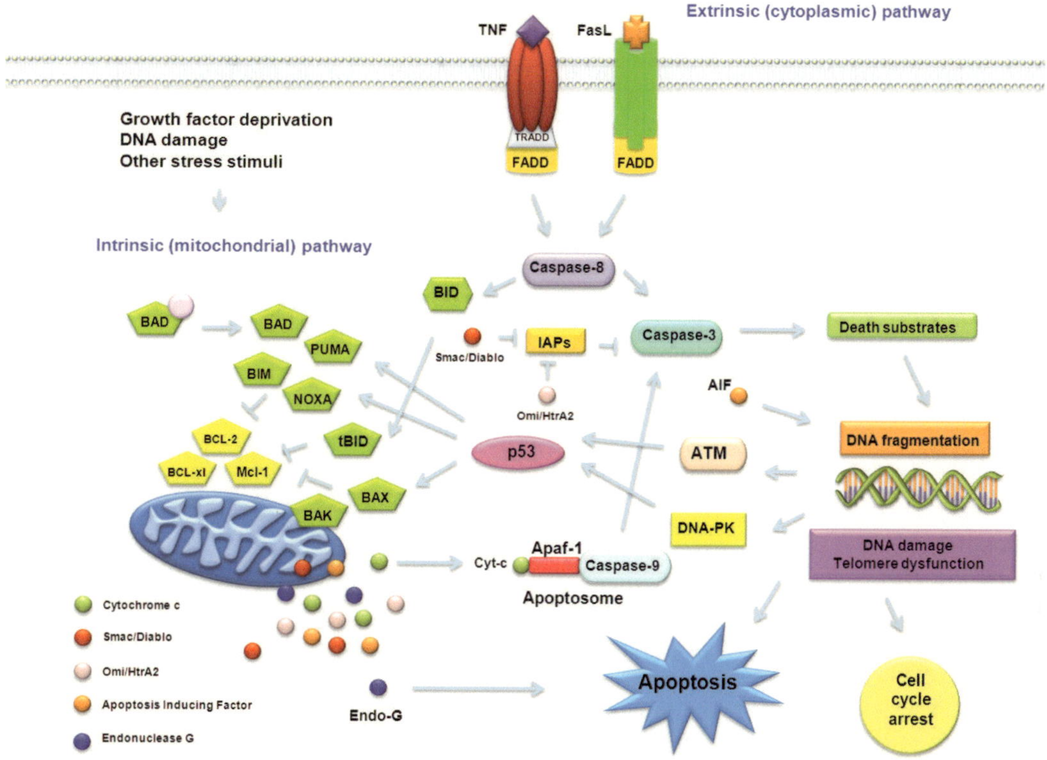

Fig. 1. Proteins related to apoptosis in signal pathways and their functions.

Apoptotic Proteins	Functions	References
Caspase Family (e.g. Caspase 3,6,7,2,8,9,10)	Caspases are members of a cystein protease family and are synthesized in the form of inactive zymogens activated by proteolytic cleavage. The intracellular transmission of the apoptotic signal is regulated by caspase family.	Bradshaw et al. (2003) Holdenrieder et al. (2004) Wong (2011)
Bcl-2 Family (e.g. Bcl-2,Bcl-X_L,Mcl-1,Bax, Bad, Bid, Bak,Bcl-X_S, NOXA, PUMA)	Bcl-2 family proteins can target the mitochondria and regulated membrane permabilization.	Bradshaw et al. (2003) Debatin et al. (2004) Wong (2011)
p53	P53 is a tumor-supressor and transcription factor. It is a critical regulator in many cellular prosesses including cell signal transduction, cellular response to DNA-damage, genomic stability, cell cycle control, and apoptosis.	Aggarwal & Shishodia (2006)
IAPs (Inhibitor of Apoptosis Proteins) (e.g. Survivin, IXAP)	IAPs block activity of caspases and may target active caspases for degradation.	Bradshaw et al. (2003) Debatin et al. (2004) Kroemer et al. (2007) Wong (2011)

Apoptotic Proteins	Functions	References
AIF (Apoptosis Inducing Factor)	AIF induce apoptosis by causing DNA fragmentation and chromatin condensation.	Kroemer et al. (2007) Wong (2011)
Endonuclease G (Endo G)	Endo G is a mitochondrion-specific enzyme and it cleaves chromatin DNA into nucleosomal fragments.	Kroemer et al. (2007)
Smac/DIABLO (secondmitochondria-derived activator of caspase/ direct IAP binding protein with low pI)	Smac/DIABLO is proapoptotic mitochondrial protein. It promotes caspase activation by binding to IAPs that subsequently leads to disruption in the interaction of IAPs with caspases.	Kroemer et al. (2007) Wong (2011)
Omi/HtrA2 (Omi stress-regulated endoprotease/ high temperature requirement protein A2)	Omi/HtrA2 is proapoptotic mitochondrial protein. It promotes caspase activation by binding to IAPs that subsequently leads to disruption in the interaction of IAPs with caspases.	Kroemer et al. (2007) Wong (2011)
CAD / ICAD (Caspase Activated DNase/ Inhibitor of Caspase Activated DNase)	CAD cleaves chromosomal DNA in a caspase-dependent manner during apoptosis. When apoptosis is activated ICAD is cleaved by executor caspases.	Nagata (2000) Omata et al. (2008)

Table 2. Some proteins involved in apoptosis.

cell arrest or/and apoptosis occur (Akiyama et al., 2002; Cong & Shay, 2008; Gao & Chen, 2007; Herbert et al., 1999; Lechel et al., 2005; Mattson et al., 2001; Mondello & Scovassi, 2004; Multani et al., 2000; Shay & Wright, 2006; Yuan & Mei, 2002; Zhang et al., 1999).

Signals leading to apoptosis in telomerase inhibited cells are still not fully understood. Upon loss of chromosome end protection function, uncapped telomeres are recognized by specialized DNA damage sensors. Uncapped telomeres activate signaling cascades involving the protein kinases member of PI3-kinase like (PIKK) family include Ataxia Telangiectasia Mutated (ATM), Ataxia Telangiectasia and Rad3 related protein (ATR), and DNA-PK. ATM and ATR are protein kinases which regulates cellular response to DNA breaks. ATM and ATR phosphorylate several proteins in response to DNA damage. These responses include the activation of cell cycle checkpoints, DNA repair and apoptosis. Two important phosphorylation substrates of ATM and ATR are cell cycle checkpoint kinase 1 (Chk1) and cell cycle checkpoint kinase 2 (Chk2). These proteins act by regulating cyclin dependent kinases (CDK) inhibitory effectors such as Cdc25a, Wee1 or p53. Chk1 and Chk2 are the central activators of p53 in response to DNA damage. The p53 transcription factor stops the cell cycle in case of an abnormal situation in the cell. PARP is connected to the broken DNA chain and adds poly (ADP-ribose) to nuclear proteins such as histone. Caspase 3 is connected to PARP in apoptosis and prevents repair of damaged DNA. Apoptosis, which is a highly-organized physiological mechanism, plays an essential role as a mechanism that is protective against carcinogenesis through elimination of genetically-damaged cells (Aggarwal & Shishodia, 2006; Ben-Porath & Weinberg, 2005; d'Adda di Fagagna, 2003; Ljungman, 2009; Lopez-Contreras & Fernandez-Capetillo, 2012; Mondello & Scovassi, 2004; Smith et al., 2003; Takai et al., 2003; Karlseder et al., 1999; Kurz& Lees-Miller, 2004; Roos & Kaina, 2006; von Zglinicki et al. 2005).

Various studies report that some compounds, in particular, natural compounds, inhibit telomerase activity and induce apoptosis. For this reason, it is of great importance for studies to focus on potentials of natural compounds to inhibit telomerase activation and induce apoptosis of tumour cells without giving harm to normal cells. The researches conducted generally emphasize on two beneficial effects of natural compounds. These beneficial effects of natural compounds are potential anti-carcinogenic effects and few or milder side effects in normal cells. Some researches showed that resveratrol, which is the most investigated among the compounds we will discuss in this chapter, does not induce apoptosis in normal cells. In vivo studies carried out with resveratrol clearly demonstrate that it is safe in pharmacological terms and it can be used in treatment of cancer. It was also revealed that similar to resveratrol, quercetin has minimized side effects on normal cells and therefore it is safe to be used in certain doses. On the other hand, the number of studies conducted with tannic acid is very limited. Through further studies to be conducted in the following years, behaviours of tannic acid on normal cells can be identified (Aalinkeel et al., 2008; Aggarwal et al., 2004; Fulda& Debatin, 2006; Granado-Serrano et al., 2006; Psahoulia et al., 2007; She et al., 2003; Shu et al., 2011).

Determination of a relation between telomerase enzyme/apoptosis and natural compounds is important as it suggests that undesired effects of the compounds used in the current treatment methods can be eliminated. In this review, an emphasis will be placed on telomerase regulation - which is quite important for formation of human cancers -and on mechanisms that result in apoptosis and impacts and inter-relations of resveratrol, quercetin and tannic acid. The molecular structure of these compounds is shown in **Figure 2.**

Resveratrol (3,5,4′ trihydroxystilbene)	Quercetin (3,5,7,3′,4′-pentahidroksiflavon)	Tannic Acid ([3,5-dihydroxy-4,6-bis[(3,4,5-trihydro xybenzoyl)oxy]oxan-2-yl]methyl3,4,5-trihydroxybenzoate)
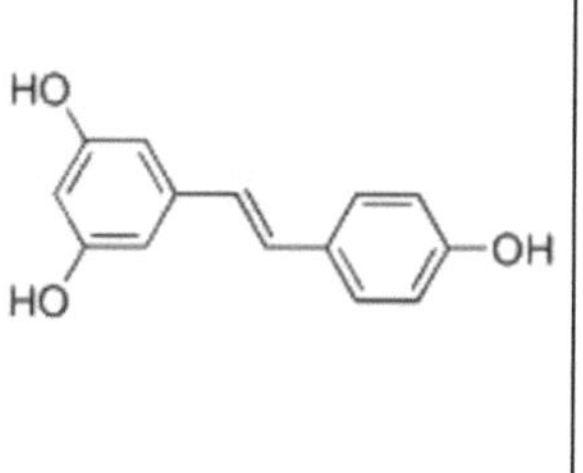	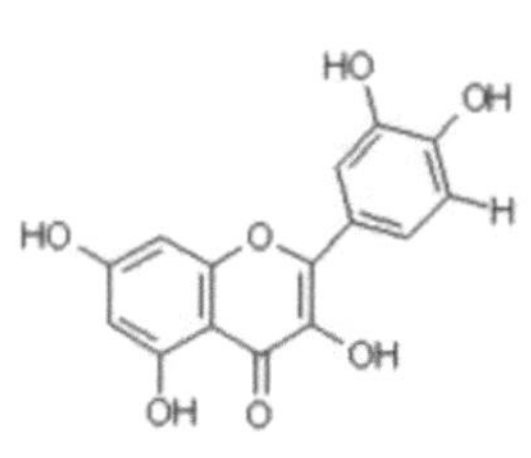	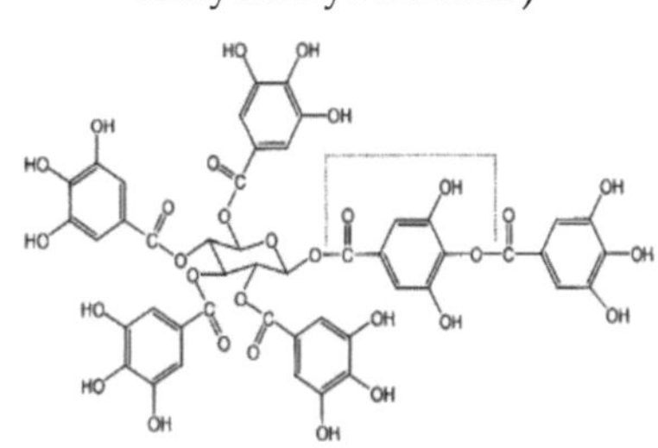

Fig. 2. Name of phenolic compounds and chemical formules.

2. Effects of polyphenols on telomerase activity and apoptosis in cancer cells

It is a known fact that cancer cells, which have the ability to reproduce infinitely, cannot resist some of the compounds in the food we consume daily. One of these compounds, polyphenols, bears anti-carcinogenic properties. These polyphenols are contained in fruits, vegetables, seeds and drinks and are classified as stilbenes, flavonoids, tannins, phenolic acids and their analogues, lignans and others depending on their chemical structures (Huang et al., 2010a; Ramos, 2008).

These polyphenolic compounds that taken by diet show their effects through similar or different molecules in the cells. As a result of these effects, they may lead to inhibition of telomerase activity while inducing apoptosis in cancer cells (Avci et al., 2011; Fuggetta et al., 2006; Lanzilli et al., 2006; Sadava et al., 2007; Turgut Cosan et al., 2011; Wang et al., 2007). The studies that underline the relationship between these two incidents are limited. In this chapter, we aim to draw attention to the effects of resveratrol, tannic acid and quercetin, which are among important polyphenols, on telomerase activity and apoptosis in multiple breast and colon cancer cases and their probable relationships. The effects on telomerase activity and apoptosis of these compounds are summarized in **Figure 3.**

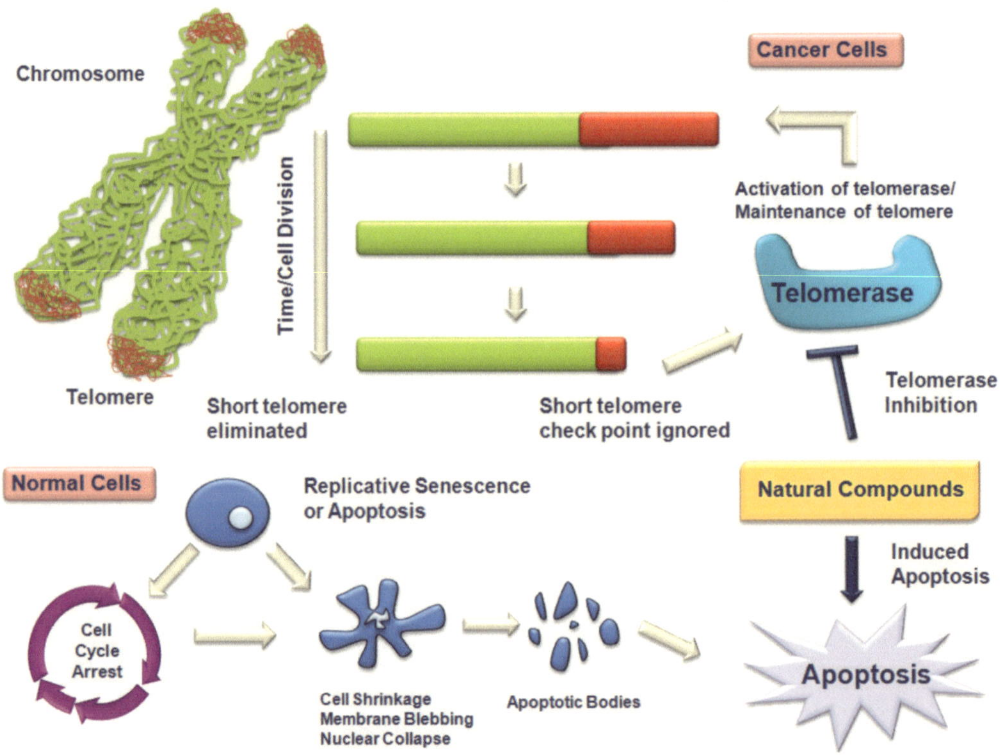

Fig. 3. Interaction of telomerase activity and apoptosis in cancer cells.

2.1 Resveratrol

Resveratrol (3,5,4′ trihydroxystilbene) is a phytoalexin phenolic compound. Resveratrol is contained in the root of *Polygonumcuspidatum* plant and peanut as well as small soft fruits such as grape, mulberry, strawberry, blackberry and drinks made of these. Resveratrol chelates copper, is neuroprotective, has oestrogen regulation activity, inhibits lipid peroxidation, causes alteration of eicosanoid, and inhibits platelet aggregation. It has anti-oxidant, anti-carcinogenic, anti-inflammatory, anti-mutagen, anti-proliferative, anti-viral, anti-bacterial activities, and cardioprotective and vasorelaxing activities (Aziz et al., 2003; Corre et al., 2005; Gusman et al., 2001; Ignatowicz &Baer-Dubowska, 2001; Pervaiz, 2003).

2.1.1 Resveratrol, telomerase and apoptosis

Studies have been carried out to investigate the effect of resveratrol on telomerase enzyme and apoptosis in cancer cells. In one of these researches, Del Bufalo et al. (2005) also stated that hTERT plays an important role in direct or indirect control of cell survival upon regulation of genes that function in apoptosis. hTERT appears to affect apoptosis by directly intervening in early phases of upstream of intrinsic apoptotic pathway.

Fuggetta et al. (2006) indicated that tumour growth and progression can be prevented through resveratrol. These authors examined the effect of resveratrol on telomerase activity and growth in human colon cancer cell lines HT-29 and WiDr. Resveratrol showed a dose-dependent inhibiting effect on cell proliferation in both cell lines. In addition, this compound down-regulated telomerase activity in higher concentrations. It was stated in this study that in various epithelial cancers including colon cancer, a close relationship existed between hTERT mRNA expression and high telomerase activity. hTERT inhibition results in telomere loss, which leads to apoptosis and limits tumour cells growth. In this case, telomeres of these cells reached a critically short length.

A study conducted by Lanzilli et al. (2006) investigated the potential role of resveratrol as chemoprevention/chemotherapy for breast cancer. They indicated that resveratrol showed direct inhibitive impact on cell proliferation. They demonstrated that resveratrol induced apoptosis in MCF-7 breast cancer cells depending on time and concentration. Furthermore, they indicated that it reduced telomerase activity, inhibited growth in connection with this and that it did so through induction of apoptosis and S-phase arrest. According to hypothesis of this study, resveratrol directly down-regulates telomerase activity and indirectly affects the signal pathways including apoptosis and cell cycle control.

Various studies demonstrate that the catalytic subunit hTERT can activate telomerase activity as a result of its post translational phosphorylation and nuclear translocation (Liu et al., 2001; Seimiya et al. 2000). In addition, in a research they conducted on colon cancers, Wang et al. (2010) reported that resveratrol reduced promoter activity of hTERT and, in this way, prevented proliferation of cancer cells by inhibiting hTERT expression.

In their studies, Turgut Cosan et al. (2011) examined the impacts of resveratrol on telomerase activity and apoptosis in MCF-7 human breast and CaCo-2 human colon cancer cell lines. They found that resveratrol was more effective in reducing cell viability of MCF-7 cells compared to CaCo-2 cells. Resveratrol also had a negative regulatory effect on telomerase activity. DNA fragmentation, which is seen at all times and concentrations, shows that apoptosis occurs in cells treated with resveratrol. These impacts do not entirely depend on time and concentration. The study supports this impact of resveratrol with the alterations in cell count and cell viability.

More studies are needed to further increase our knowledge of resveratrol induced telomerase-apoptosis interactions. In this way, whether resveratrol induces any link between telomerase and apoptosis and, if it does, which molecular mechanisms are utilized by it can be revealed clearly.

2.2 Tannic acid

Tannins are polyphenolic compounds with molecular weight of 500-3000 Dalton. Tannins are divided into two classes as hydrolyzed and condensed. Tannic acid, which is hydrolyzed tannin, is contained in tea, coffee, grapes, red wine, beans, and nuts such as hazelnut and most fruits and vegetables. Apart from their anti-angiogenic, anti-bacterial, anti-carcinogenic, anti-oxidant, anti-mutagenic, anti-microbial, anti-allergic and anti-proliferative activities, tannic acids have such biological activities as chemopreventive effects (Chen et al., 2003; Chung et al., 1998; Khan& Hadi, 1998; Khan et al., 2000; Naus et al., 2007; Taffetani et al., 2005).

2.2.1 Tannic acid, telomerase and apoptosis

Various studies are available in which cancer chemopreventive activity of tannic acid is presented (Chen et al., 2003; Chung et al., 1998; Gali-Muhtasib et al., 2000; Kazi et al., 2003; Khan & Hadi, 1998; Koide et al., 1999; Marienfeld et al., 2003; Nam et al., 2001a; Nepka et al., 1999a; Nepka et al., 1999b). Gali-Muhtasib et al., 2000, demonstrated that tannic acid can suppress promotion of skin tumour induced by ultraviolet-B radiation in an animal study. Nepka et al., 1999b, reported that dietary consumption of low-dose tannic acid strongly showed dose-dependent chemopreventative activity against spontaneous liver tumour development in C3H male rats. It was revealed by Koideet al., 1999 that tannic acid increased survival rate of Balb/c rats carrying syngeneic tumours. In other researches, it was demonstrated that ester bond-containing tea polyphenols of tannic acid inhibit potently and specifically chymotrypsin-like activity of proteasome in vitro and in vivo (Marienfeld et al., 2003; Nam et al., 2001a; Nam et al., 2001b). Nam et al., 2001a, and Kazi et al., 2003, reported that anti-cancer impact of tannic acid arose from induction of apoptosis as well as inhibition of proteasomal activity. Other researches executed also showed that tannic acid could induce apoptosis (Labieniec et al., 2006; Pan et al., 1999; Romero et al., 2002; Sakagami et al., 2000; Wang et al.; 2000; Yang et al., 2000).

However, the impacts of tannic acid on telomerase enzyme activity and apoptosis have not been addressed except in the research we executed (Turgut Cosan et al. 2011). We investigated the impact of tannic acid in breast and colon adenocarcinoma cells and found that cell viability and cell count dropped dramatically when cells were treated with tannic acid. Tannic acid reduced telomerase activity in all concentrations independent of time and dose. On the other hand, DNA fragmentation, which is seen at all times and concentrations, shows that tannic acid induces apoptosis in breast and colon cancer cells. Thus, it can be asserted that tannic acid has a suppression effect on telomerase activity and inducing effect on apoptosis. We also found that telomerase activity is lower in breast cancer cells than in colon cancer cells. In line with this conclusion, it can be mentioned that tannic acid has different effects in different cell lines.

In various studies, the impacts of (-) epigallocatechin-3-gallate (EGCG), a tea polyphenol like tannic acid, on telomerase enzyme activity and apoptosis in cancer cells were examined.

In 2007, Sadava et al. examined DNA fragmentation and telomerase activity in cancer cells treated with EGCG, similarly to studies by Turgut Cosan D et al. 2011. These studies were performed on drug resistant and drug sensitive lung cells (H69VP, H69). They reported that EGCG and green tea inhibit telomerase activity in cancer cells and these cells show molecular characteristics of apoptosis. These results imply that EGCG may have simultaneous impact on both apoptosis and telomerase activity in small cell lung carcinomas. There are some studies reporting that EGCG, abundant in green tea such as tannins, has growth inhibitory effect on cancer cells but not on normal cells (Bode& Dong, 2009; Chung et al., 2003).

Another study demonstrated that, following long term treatment of non-toxic low dose EGCG, carcinoma cells aged, telomere shortening was induced and telomerase inhibition occured in vitro (Naasani et al., 2003). In another study conducted on lung, oral cavity, thyroid and liver carcinoma cells, it was reported that low cytotoxic dose EGCG and (-) epigallocatechin (EGC) suppressed hTERT expression on reporter system and hTERT mRNA level (Lin et al., 2006). On the other hand, it was demonstrated in this study that tea polyphenols can materialize inhibition of cancer cells in many ways.

Understanding the effect of tea polyphenols like tannic acid on molecular mechanism of malignancies bears importance in order for these polyphenols, which seem to be advantageous for treatment and prevention, to become useable.

2.3 Quercetin

Quercetin (3,5,7,3′,4′-pentahidroksiflavon) is a flavonoid which is contained very commonly in fruits and vegetables including onion, tomato, broccoli, red wine, green tea, apples, grapes, berries, cherries, and citrus fruits. Apart from anti-cancer, anti-allergic, anti-inflammatory, anti-oxidant, anti-tumour, anti-viral and anti-microbial properties, quercetin has many beneficial impacts on human health such as inhibition of lipid peroxidation, anti-platelet, anti-hypertensive, anti-cataract and anti-neurodegenerative effects (Aherne &O'Brien, 2002; Bischoff, 2008; Middleton et al., 2000; Perez-Vizcaino, 2009).

2.3.1 Quercetin, telomerase and apoptosis

Biologically useful impacts of quercetin are revealed by many studies. One of the objectives of these studies is to be able to understand the molecular mechanisms of these useful impacts in cancer and the interactions among them. Various researches demonstrate that this polyphenol can play a role in cancer treatment and prevention by inhibiting telomerase activity and inducing apoptosis and cell cycle arrest.

In a 2000 study, Nakayama et al. stated that growth and telomerase activity was inhibited as a result of treatment with estrogen receptor beta ligands (such as quercetin and tamoxifen) in colon cancer cells. In another study, Naasani et al. (2003) also reported that quercetin has the ability to inhibit telomerase activity. On the other hand, Hu et al. (2004) indicated that quercetin administered to these cells did not inhibit hTERT mRNA in malignant melanoma cells. In literature, apart from studies reporting that quercetin has an effect on telomerase activity, information on its ineffectiveness is also available.

With respect to the researches on the impact of quercetin on apoptosis, Choi et al. (2001) reported that quercetin induces growth inhibition with at least two different mechanisms in

MCF-7 cell lines. One of these is the inhibition of cell cycle progression through a transient M phase accumulation and subsequent G2 arrest while the other one is induction of apoptosis. Kang & Liang (1997) administered quercetin to human promyelocytic leukemia cells (HL-60) and observed its anti-tumour activity. They emphasizes that one of the mechanisms used by quercetin is its inducing of apoptosis. Kuo et al. (2004) showed that quercetin induces apoptosis and cytotoxic effects in human lung cancer cell lines in a dose dependant manner. When quercetin is administered to the cells at higher doses, cell proliferation was almost completely inhibited. Lee et al. (2006) demonstrated that quercetin administered to human leukemic monocyte lymphoma cells increased DNA fragmentation in a dose dependent manner and induced apoptosis by caspase activation and G2/M phase arrest. In a different study, Kou (1996) observed that quercetin can induce apoptosis in colon cancer cells in a dose dependant manner. On the other hand, Gibellini et al. (2011) emphasized that in various types of cancer cells; quercetin can arrest the cells at different cycles and block their growth. Therefore, they exhibit pro-apoptotic feature. Furthermore, this article touches on quercetin showing anti-proliferative and pro-apoptotic effects as well as anti-carcinogenic properties. Therefore, it was pointed out that studies need be conducted on more complex and sophisticated animal models in order to understand mechanisms of chemopreventive and chemotherapeutic effects of quercetin. Tang et al. (2010) stated that quercetin shows many properties in cancer cells such as death receptor 5 (DR5) upregulation, p53 activation, cell cycle arrest and caspase-mediated apoptosis. It was underlined in this study that while quercetin down regulates expression of heat shock protein 90 (Hsp90) in prostate cancer cells and induces growth inhibition and apoptosis; it has no measurable effect on normal prostate epithelial cells. Unlike the unclear statements about the impact of quercetin on telomerase activity, the effect of quercetin on apoptosis is obvious. Almost all studies prove that quercetin induces apoptosis in cancer cells.

Although there are limited number of studies which examine both telomerase activity and apoptosis together, in a recent research conducted by Avci et al. in 2011, the impacts of quercetin on telomerase activity, apoptosis-mediated cell death, and cell reproduction in leukemic cells were addressed. In CCRF-CEM human T-cell acute lymphoblastic leukemia, HL-60 human acute promyelocytic leukemia, and K-562 human chronicmyeloid leukemia cells, quercetin suppresses telomerase activity and induces apoptosis. It was therefore stated that quercetin is a potential therapeutic agent for treatment of leukaemia. In 2007, Wang et al. demonstrated that quercetin inhibited growth in lung cancer cell line, induced apoptosis and down regulated hTERT expression in a dose dependant manner. Wei et al. (2007) reported that quercetin has a suppressing effect on growth in gastric cancer cells SGC-7901. They found that quercetin realized anti-cancer activity by suppressing telomerase activity and inducing apoptosis. Cheng et al. (1998) emphasized that treatment of nasophargeal carcinoma cells (NPC) with cisplatin or quercetin ensured activation of mitotic arrest and apoptotic pathways. They indicated that apoptosis of NPC cells can be induced through induction of mitotic arrest. Furthermore, it was emphasized that it has still not been clarified whether there is a correlation between apoptosis and telomerase activity. In another study conducted by Ak et al. (2011), it was reported that quercetin induce apoptosis in breast cancer cells but did not reduce telomerase activity. In a 2011 study, Turgut Cosan et al. stated that quercetin is effective on apoptosis in CaCo-2 human colon cancer cell lines. In this study, it was found that quercetin has no effect on cell viability and cell count, and that it has very little effect on telomerase activity. On the other hand, when the level of DNA fragmentation was examined, quercetin is reported as effective. In this case, a full correlation is not observed between apoptosis and telomerase activity. When all these studies are taken into consideration, it can be provided that quercetin is more effective on apoptosis and mainly shows its anti-carcinogenic effect via this mechanism.

After giving all the above information, we cannot proceed without mentioning the fact that natural compounds have separate impacts on cancer cells and they can have increased impact when combined. Zamin et al. (2009) found that quercetin and resveratrol combination forms a very strong synergy in inducing senescence-like growth arrest in glioblastoma cells. The same study revealed that apoptosis induction does not occur through combinations made at low concentrations but that higher concentration combinations are effective. Kuhar et al. (2007) administered curcumin and quercetin together with cisplatin to human laryngeal carcinoma (Hep-2) cells. It was concluded that both compounds induce apoptosis through mitochondrial pathway and their adverse effects can be minimized. Identification of therapeutic concentrations in anti-tumoural activity bears great importance in emergence of these effects.

It is beyond doubt that further research is needed where all important molecules in anti-cancer mechanisms are addressed together in order to understand better the mechanism of impacts of quercetin on telomerase enzyme activity and apoptosis.

3. Inhibition of telomerase and induction of apoptosis by other polyphenols

Dietary polyphenols are compounds contained in fruits, vegetables and seeds and classified according to their chemical and structural differences. The idea that these polyphenols, which approximately has 8,000 varieties, can play a role in preventing cancer has recently created the necessity to illuminate the mechanisms of their action in cancer cells (Han et al. 2007; Ramos, 2007; Saunders & Wallace, 2010).

In addition to some polyphenols focused on here, relationships of telomerase inhibition and apoptosis induction of other polyphenols with cancer are shown in **Table 3.**

Products	Cells	Mechanisms of action	Reference
Curcumin	MCF-10A Human mammary epithelial cells MCF-7 Human breast cancer cells	Inhibits telomerase activity by down-regulating hTERT expression.	Ramachandran et al. (2002)
	HL-60 Human acute myeloblastic leukemia cells	Induced apoptosis. Inhibition of telomerase activity in a dose dependent manner.	Mukherjee et al. (2007)
	K562 Human chronic myelogenous leukaemia cells	Induced apoptosis. Inhibits telomerase activity.	Chakraborty et al. (2006)
Ginsenoside Rk1	HepG2 Human hepatocellular liver carcinoma cells	Inhibited cell growth. Induce apoptosis. Inhibit telomerase activity.	Kim et al. (2008a)
Verbascoside	MKN45 Human gastric carcinoma cells	Inhibited telomerase activity. Reduced telomere length. Arrested tumor cell cycle in G2/M phase.	Zhang et al. (2002)

Products	**Cells**	**Mechanisms of action**	**Reference**
Allicin	SGC-7901 Human gastric cancer cells	Induce apoptosis. Inhibit telomerase activity.	Sun & Wang (2003).
Diterpenoids -Xerophilusin B -Macrocalin B -Eeriocalyxin B	K562 Human chronic myelogenous leukaemia cells HL-60 Human acute myeloblastic leukemia cells A549 Human lung carcinoma cells HCT Human colorectal carcinoma cells MKN Human gastric adenocarcinoma cells CA Human live carcinoma cells	Inhibit the proliferation and the telomerase activity.	Yang et al. (2009)
Salvicine	HL-60 Human acute myeloblastic leukemia cells	Induce apoptosis. Inhibit telomerase activity.	Liu et al. (2002)
(Z)-Stellettic acid	U937 Human leukemic cells	Dose-dependent growth inhibition. Induce apoptosis was associated with an increase in Bcl-2 family expression, activation of caspases and down regulation of IAPs family members. Down regulation of hTERT expression .	Park et al. (2007)
Methylenedioxy lignan	Hep-2 Human alveolar epithelial carcinoma cells MCF-7 Human breast cancer cells HeLa Human cervical cancer cells EL-1 Humanmonocyte cells	Induces apoptosis by Bcl-2 suppression and activation of caspases. Decrease in the activity of telomerase.	Giridharan et al. (2002)
Mistletoe Lectin (VCA)	SK-Hep-1 Human hepatocarcinoma cells (p53-positive) Hep 3B Human hepatocarcinoma cells (p53-negative)	Apoptosis by down regulation of Bcl-2 and by up regulation of Bax functioning upstream of caspase-3 in both cell lines. Down regulation of telomerase activity.	Lyu et al. (2002)
	A253 Human submandibular carcinoma cells	Induction of apoptotic cell death through activation of caspase. Inhibition of telomerase activity through	Choi et al. (2004)

Products	Cells	Mechanisms of action	Reference
		transcriptional down regulation of hTERT. Inhibition of telomerase activity and induction of apoptosis resulted from dephosphorylation of Akt in the survival signaling pathways.	
Daidzein	HeLa Human cervical cancer cells	Inhibited the cell growth and cell cycle. Induce apoptosis. Inhibit telomerase activity.	Guo et al. (2004)
Korean red ginseng	U937 Human leukemic cells	Induction of apoptosis. Inhibit telomerase activity. Cell growth inhibition.	Park et al. (2009a)
Cordyceps militaris (WECM)	A549 Human lung carcinoma cells NSCLC Human non-small cell lung cancer cells	Cell growth inhibition. Apoptosis induction (associated with the induction of Fas, catalytic activation of caspase-8, and Bid cleavage). Dose-dependent inhibition of telomerase activity via down regulation of human telomerase reverse transcriptase (hTERT), c-myc and Sp1 expression	Park et al. (2009b)
Wogonin	HL-60 Human acute myeloblastic leukemia cells	Growth inhibition. Induction of Bax/Bcl-2 apoptosis. Telomerase inhibition through suppression of c-myc.	Huang et al. (2010b)
Platycodin D	U937 Human leukemic cells THP-1 Human acute monocytic leukemia cells K562 Human chronic myelogenous leukaemia cells	Induces apoptosis. Represses telomerase activity.	Kim et al. (2008b)

Table 3. Mechanisms of action of natural products.

4. Conclusion

In this chapter, recent research results of the impacts of natural compounds on telomerase inhibition and apoptosis induction in cancer cells are summarized. Researches suggest that polyphenols alter telomerase activity and induce apoptosis by affecting proteins that function in various signal pathways. We showed that the possible relationship between the impacts of natural compounds on telomerase inhibition and apoptosis induction. Some studies suggest that telomerase activity is connected to regulation of apoptosis in physiological and pathological terms. However, it is also a fact that every compound cannot directly affect both of the mechanisms simultaneously. More detailed knowledge about polyphenols and the mechanism responsible for telomerase inhibition and apoptosis induction and the true effectiveness of polyphenols would help to determine whether polyphenols is a potential chemopreventive and chemotherapeutic reagent for treatment of cancer.

5. References

Aalinkeel,R.; Bindukumar, B.; Reynolds, J.L.; Sykes, D.E.; Mahajan, S.D.; Chadha, K.C. & Schwartz, S. A. (2008). The Dietary Bioflavonoid, Quercetin, Selectively Induces Apoptosis of Prostate Cancer Cells by Down-Regulating the Expression of Heat Shock Protein 90. *Prostate.* Vol.68, No.16, pp. 1773-1789.

Aggarwal, B.B. & Shishodia, S. (2006). Molecular targets of dietary agents for prevention and therapy of cancer.*Biochem Pharmacol.* Vol.71, No.10, pp. 1397-421.

Aggarwal, B.B.; Bhardwaj, A.; Aggarwal, R.S.; Seeram, N.P.; Shishodia, S. & Takada, Y. (2004). Role of resveratrol in prevention and therapy of cancer: preclinical and clinical studies. *Anticancer Res.* Vol.24, No.5A, pp. 2783-840.

Aherne, S.A. & O'Brien, N.M. (2002). Dietary flavonols: chemistry, food content, and metabolism.*Nutrition.* Vol. 18, pp. 75–81.

Ak, A.; Basaran, A.; Dikmen, M.; Turgut Cosan, D.; Degirmenci, I. & Gunes, H.V. (2011). Evaluation of Effects of Quercetin (3, 3', 4', 5, 7-pentohidroxyfl avon) on Apoptosis and Telomerase Enzyme Activity in MCF-7 and NIH-3T3 Cell Lines Compared with Tamoxifen.*Balkan Med J.* Vol. 28, No.3, 293-299.

Akiyama, M.; Hideshima, T.; Hayashi, T.; Tai, Y.T.; Mitsiades, C.S.; Mitsiades, N.; Chauhan, D.; Richardson, P.; Munshi, N.C. &Anderson, K.C. (2002). Cytokines modulate telomerase activity in a human multiple myeloma cell line. *Cancer Res.* Vol. 62, No.13, pp. 3876-82.

Andres Joaquin Lopez-Contreras and Oscar Fernandez-Capetillo (2012). Signalling DNA Damage, Protein Phosphorylation in Human Health, Cai Huang (Ed.), ISBN: 978-953-51-0737-8, InTech, Available from: http://www.intechopen.com/books/protein-phosphorylation-in-human-health/signalling-dna-damage

Avci, C.B.; Yilmaz, S.; Dogan, Z.O.; Saydam, G.; Dodurga, Y.; Ekiz, H.A.; Kartal, M.; Sahin, F.; Baran, Y. & Gunduz, C. (2011). Quercetin-induced apoptosis involves increased hTERT enzyme activity of leukemic cells. *Hematology*, Vol.16, No.5, pp. 303-307.

Aziz, M.H.; Kumar, R. &Ahmad, N. (2003). Cancer chemoprevention by resveratrol:In vitro and in vivo studies and the underlying mechanisms. *International Journal of Oncology,*Vol. 23, pp. 17-28.

Bae, N.S. & Baumann, P. (2007). A RAP1/TRF2 complex inhibits nonhomologous end-joining at human telomeric DNA ends. *Mol Cell.,* Vol. 26, No: 3, pp. 323-34.

Bailey, S.M.; Conforth, M.N.; Kurimasa, A.; Chen, D.J. &Goodwin, E.H. (2001). Strand-specific postreplicative processing of mammalian telomeres. *Science,* Vol. 293, pp. 2462–2465.

Baumann, P. & Cech, T.R. (2001). Pot1, the Putative Telomere End-Binding Protein in Fission Yeast and Humans. *Science*, Vol. 292, pp. 1171-1175

Ben-Porath, I. & Weinberg, R.A. (2005). The signals and pathways activating cellular senescence. *Int J Biochem Cell Biol.* Vol. 37, No. 5, pp. 961-76.

Bischoff, S.C. (2008). Quercetin: potentials in the prevention and therapy of disease. *Current Opinion in Clinical Nutrition and Metabolic Care*.Vol.11, No.6, pp. 733–740.

Blackburn, E. H. (2001). Switching and signaling at the telomere. *Cell,* Vol.106, pp. 661–673.

Blackburn, E.H. (2000). Telomere states and cell fates. *Nature*, Vol. 408, pp. 53-56.

Bode, A.M. & Dong, Z. (2009). Epigallocatechin 3-gallate and green tea catechins: United they work, divided they fail. *Cancer Prev Res (Phila).* Vol. 2, No. 6, pp. 514-7.

Bradshaw, R. & Edward Dennis, E. (2003). Apoptosis signaling: a means to an End. *Handbook of Cell Signaling,* Vol.3, No.331, pp. 431-439.

Bryan, T.M. & Cech, T.R. (1999). Telomerase and the maintenance of chromosome ends. *Current Opinion in Genetics & Development*, Vol.11, pp. 318-324.

Cain, K.; Bratton, S.B. & Cohen, G.M. (2002). The Apaf-1 apoptosome: a large caspase-activating complex. *Biochimie.* Vol. 84, pp. 203-14.

Celli, G.B. & de Lange, T.(2005). DNA processing is not required for ATM mediated telomere damage response after TRF2 deletion. *Nat. Cell Biol.*,Vol. 7, pp. 712–718.

Chakraborty, S.; Ghosh, U.; Bhattacharyya, N.P.; Bhattacharya, R.K. & Roy, M.(2006).Inhibition of telomerase activity and induction of apoptosis by curcumin in K-562 cells.*Mutation Research,* Vol. 596, pp. 81–90.

Chan, S. W-L. & Blackburn, E. H. (2002). New ways not to make ends meet: telomerase, DNA damage proteins and heterochromatin. *Oncogene,* Vol.21, pp. 553–563.

Chatziantoniou, V.D. (2001). Telomerase: Biological function and potential role in cancer management. *Pathology Oncology Research,* Vol. 7, No.3, pp. 161-170.

Chen, X.; Beutler, J.A;, McCloud, T.G.; Loehfelm, A.; Yang, L.; et al. (2003). Tannic acid is an inhibitor of CXCL12 (SDF-1α)/CXCR4 with antiangiogenic activity. Clinical Cancer Research.Vol. 9, pp. 3115-3123.

Cheng, R.Y.S.; Yuen, P.W.; Nicholls, J.M.; et al. (1998).Telomerase activation in nasopharyngeal carcinoma.*Brit J Cancer,* Vol.77, pp. 456–460.

Choi, J.A.; Kim, J.Y.; Lee, J.Y.; Kang, C.M.; Kwon, H.J. & Yoo, Y.D. (2001).Induction of Cell Cycle Arrest and Apoptosis in Human Breast Cancer Cells by Quercetin.*Int. J. Oncol.,* Vol.19, pp. 837-844.

Choi, S.H.; Lyu, S.Y. & Park, W.B. (2004).Mistletoe Lectin Induces Apoptosis and Telomerase Inhibition in Human A253 Cancer Cells through Dephosphorylation of Akt. *Arch Pharm Res,* Vol.27, No.1, pp. 68-76.

Chung, J.H.; Han, J.H.; Hwang, E.J.; Seo, J.Y.; Cho, K.H.; Kim, K.H.; Youn, J.I. & Eun HC. (2003). Dual mechanisms of green tea extract (EGCG)-induced cell survival in human epidermalkeratinocytes. *Faseb J.* Vol. 17, No.13, pp. 1913-5.

Chung, K.T.; Wong, T.Y.; Wei, C.I.; Huang, Y.W. & Lin, Y. (1998). Tannins and human health: a review. *Crit Rev Food Sci Nutr.* Vol. 38, No. 6, pp. 421-64.

Collins, K. (2006). The biogenesis and regulation of telomerase holoenzymes. *Nature reviews Mol Cell Biol.,* Vol.7, pp. 484-494.

Cong, Y.& Shay, J.W. (2008). Actions of human telomerase beyond telomeres. *Cell Research.* Vol. 18, pp. 725-732.

Cong, Y.S.; Wright, W.E. & Shay, J.W. (2002). Human telomerase and its regulation. *Microbiol Mol Biol Rev.,* Vol.66, pp. 407-425.

Corre, L.L.; Chalabi, N.; Delort, L.; Bingon, Y.J.; Bernard-Gallon, D.J. (2005). Resveratrol and breast cancer chemoprevention: Molecular mechanisms, *Mol. Nutr. Food Res.* Vol. 49, pp. 462-471.

Cory, S. & Adams, J.M. (2002). The Bcl2 family: regulators of the cellular life-or-death switch. *Nature Reviews Cancer*. Vol.2, pp. 647-656.

D'Adda di Fagagna, F.; Reaper, P.M.; Clay-Farrace, L.; Fiegler, H.; Carr, P.; von Zglinicki, T.; Saretzki, G.; Carter, N.P. & Jackson, S.P. (2003).A DNA damage checkpoint response in telomere-initiated senescence. *Nature,* Vol. 426, pp. 194-198.

Dantzer, F.; Giraud-Panis, M.J.; Jaco, I.; Ame, J.C.; Schultz, I.; Blasco, M.; Koering, C.E.; Gilson, E.; Menissier-de Murcia, J.; Murcia, G. & Schreiber, V. (2004). Functional interaction between poly(ADP-ribose) polymerase 2 (PARP-2) and TRF2: PARP activity negatively regulates TRF2. *Mol Cell Biol,* Vol.24, pp. 1595–1607.

De Lange, T. (2002). Protection of mammalian telomeres.*Oncogene,* Vol. 21, pp. 532–540.

De Lange, T. (2009). How telomeres solve the end-protection problem. *Science,* Vol. 326, pp. 948–952.

Debatin, K.M. (2004). Apoptosis pathways in cancer and cancer therapy. *Cancer Immunol Immunother,* Vol.53, pp. 153–159.

Del Bufalo, D.; Rizzo, A.; Trisciuoglio, D.; Cardinali, G.; Torrisi, M.R.; Zangemeister-Wittke, U.; Zupi, G. & Biroccio, A. (2005). Involvement of hTERT in apoptosis induced by interference with Bcl-2 expression and function.*Cell Death Differ* Vol. 12, pp. 1429-1438.

Diotti, R. & Loayza, D. (2011). Shelterin complex and associated factors at human telomeres.*Nucleus,* Vol.2, No. 2, pp.119-35.

Espejel, S.; Franco, S.; Rodriguez-Perales, S.; Bouffler, D.S.; Cigudosa, J.C. &Blasco, M.A. (2002).Mammalian Ku86 mediates chromosomal fusions and apoptosis caused by critically short telomeres. *EMBO J.,* Vol. 21, pp. 2207–2219.

Feng, J.; Funk, W.D.; Wang, S.S.; Weinrich, S.L.; Avilion, A.A.; Chiu, C.P.; Adams, R.R.; Chang, E.; Allsopp, R.C.; Yu, J., et al. (1995). The RNA component of human telomerase. *Science,* Vol.269, pp. 1236–1241.

Fuggetta, M.P.; Lanzilli, G.; Tricarico, M.; Cottarelli, A.; Falchetti, R.; Ravagnan, G. & Bonmassar E. (2006). Effect of resveratrol on proliferation and telomerase activity of human colon cancer cells in vitro. *J Exp Clin Cancer Res.* Vol.25, No.2, pp. 189-93.

Fulda, S. & Debatin, K.M. (2006). Resveratrol modulation of signal transduction in apoptosis and cell survival: a mini-review. *Cancer Detect Prev.* Vol.30, No.3, pp. 217-23.

Gali-Muhtasib, H.U.; Yamout, S.Z. & Sidani, M.M. (2000). Tannins protect against skin tumor promotion induced by ultraviolet-B radiation in hairless mice. *Nutr Cancer,* Vol.37, pp. 73-77.

Gao, X.D. & Chen, Y.R. (2007). Inhibition of telomerase with hTERT antisense enhances TNF-alpha-induced apoptosis in prostate cancer cells PC3.[Article in Chinese] *Zhonghua Nan Ke Xue.* Vol.13, No.8, pp. 723-6.

Gibellini, L.; Pinti, M.; Nasi, M.; Montagna, J.P.; Biasi, S.D.; Roat, E.; Bertoncelli, L.; Cooper, E.L. & Cossarizza, A. (2011). Quercetin and Cancer Chemoprevention.*Evidence-Based Complementary and Alternative Medicine,* Vol.2011, Article ID 591356, 15.

Giridharan, P.; Somasundaram, S.T.; Perumal, K.; Vishwakarma, R.A.; Karthikeyan, N.P.; Velmurugan, R. & Balakrishnan, A. (2002). Novel substituted methylenedioxy lignan suppresses proliferation of cancer cells by inhibiting telomerase and activation of c-myc and caspases leading to apoptosis. *British Journal of Cancer* , Vol.87, pp. 98–105.

Granado-Serrano, A.B.; Martín, M.A.; Bravo, L.; Goya, L&, Ramos, S. (2006). Quercetin induces apoptosis via caspase activation, regulation of Bcl-2, and inhibition of PI-3-kinase/Akt and ERK pathways in a human hepatoma cell line (HepG2). *J Nutr.*, Vol. 136, No.11, pp. 2715-21.

Green, D. & Kroemer, G. (1998). The central executioners of apoptosis: caspases or mitochondria? *Trends Cell Biol.*, Vol.8, No.7, pp. 267-71.

Greider, C.W. &Blackburn, E.H. (1989). A telomeric sequence in the RNA of Tetrahymena telomerase required for telomere repeat synthesis. *Nature*, Vol. 337, pp. 331–337.

Griffith, J.D.; Comeau, L.; Rosenfield, S.; Stansel, R.M.; Bianchi, A.; Moss, H. & de Lange, T.(1999). Mammalian telomeres end in a large duplex loop. *Cell*, Vol. 97, pp. 503–514.

Guo, J.M.;.Kang, G.Z.; Xiao, B.X.; Li, D.H. & Zhang. S. (2004). Effect of daidzein on cell growth, cell cycle, and telomerase activity of human cervical cancer in vitro.*Int J Gynecol Cancer*, Vol.14, pp. 882-888.

Gusman, J.; Malonne, H. & Atassi, G. (2001). A reappraisal of the potential chemopreventive and chemotherapeutic properties of resveratrol, *Carcinogenesis*,Vol. 22, No. 8, pp. 1111-1117.

Han, X.; Shen, T. & Lou, H. (2007).Dietary Polyphenols and Their Biological Significance. *International Journal of Molecular Sciences*. Vol. 8, No. 9, pp. 950-988.

Herbert, B.; Pitts, A.E.; Baker, S.I.; Hamilton, S.E.; Wright, W.E.; Shay, J.W. & Corey, D.R. (1999). Inhibition of human telomerase in immortal human cells leads to progressivetelomere shortening andcelldeath. *Proc Natl Acad Sci U S A*. Vol. 96, No.25, pp. 14276-81.

Hiyama, E. & Hiyama, K. (2002). Clinical utility of telomerase in cancer. *Oncogene*. Vol. 21, No. 4, pp. 643-649.

Holdenrieder, S. & Stieber P. (2004). Apoptotic markers in cancer. *Clinical Biochemistry*, Vol.37, No.7, pp. 605-617.

Hu, S.; Liao, S.K.; Pang, J.H.S.; Chen, M.C.; Chen, C.H. & Hong, H.S. (2004). Screening of Inhibitors of Human Telomerase Reverse Transcriptase in a Cultured Malignant Melanoma Cell Lines. *British Journal of Dermatology*, Vol.150, pp. 367–399.

Huang, S.T.; Wang, C.Y.; Yang, R.C.; Chu, C.J.; Wu, H.T. & Pang, J.H.S. (2010b) Wogonin, an active compound in Scutellaria baicalensis, induces apoptosis and reduces telomerase activity in the HL-60 leukemia cells. *Phytomedicine* , Vol.17, pp. 47–54.

Huang, W.U.; Cai, Z.Y. & Zhang, J. (2010a). Natural phenolic compounds from medicinal herbs and dietary plants: potential use for cancer prevention. *Nutr Cancer*.Vol.62, No.1, pp. 1-20.

Ignatowicz, E. &Baer-Dubowska, W. (2001).Resveratrol, a natural chemopreventive agent against degenerative diseases.*Pol. J. Pharmacol.*, Vol. 53, pp. 557-569.

Kaminker, P.G.; Kim, S.H.; Taylor, R.D.; Zebarjadian, Y.; Funk, W.D.; et al. (2001). TANK2, a new TRF1-associated PARP, causes rapid induction of cell death upon overexpression. *J. Biol. Chem.*, Vol. 276, pp. 35891–99.

Kang, T.B. & Liang, M. (1997). Studies on the Inhibitory Effects of Quercetin on the Growth of HL460 Leukemia Cells.*Biochemical Pharmacology*, Vol.54, pp. 1013-1018.

Karlseder, J.; Broccoli, D.; Dai, Y.; Hardy, S. & DeLange, T. (1999). p53- and ATM-dependent apoptosis induced by telomeres lacking TRF2. *Science*. Vol. 283, pp. 1321–1325.

Kaufmann, S.H. & Earnshaw, W.C. (2000). Induction of apoptosis by cancer chemotherapy. *Exp. Cell Res.*, Vol. 256, pp. 42–49.

Kazi, A.; Urbizu, D.A.; Kuhn, D.J.; Acebo, A.L.; Jackson, E.R.; Greenfelder, G.P.; Kumar, N.B. & Dou, Q.P. (2003) A natural musaceas plant extract inhibits proteasome activity and induces apoptosis selectively in human tumor and transformed, but not normal and non-transformed, cells. *Int J Mol Med.* Vol.12, No.6, pp. 879-87.

Kerr, J. F. ; Wyllie, A. H. & Currie, A. R. (1972). Apoptosis: A basic biologic phenomenon with wide-ranging implications in tissue-kinetics. *Br J Cancer,* Vol.26, pp. 239-57.

Khan, N.S.& Hadi, S.M. (1998). Structural features of tannic acid important for DNA degradation in the presence of Cu(II). *Mutagenesis.* Vol. 13, No. 3, pp. 271-4.

Khan, N.S.; Ahmad, A. & Hadi,S.M. (2000). Anti-oxidant, pro-oxidant properties of tannic acid and its binding to DNA. *Chemico-Biological Interactions.*Vol. 125, pp. 177–189.

Kim, M.O.; Moon, D.O.; Choi, Y.H.; Shin, D.Y.; Kang, H.S.; Choi, B.T.; Lee, J.D.; Li, W. & Kim, G.Y. (2008b). Platycodin D induces apoptosis and decreases telomerase activity in human leukemia cells. *Cancer Letters,* Vol.261, pp. 98–107.

Kim, N.W. (1997). Clinical implications of telomerase in cancer. *Eur. J. Cancer,* Vol. 33, pp. 781-786.

Kim, S.H.; Beausejour, C.; Davalos, A.R.; Kaminker, P.; Heo, S.J. & Campisi, J. (2004). TIN2 mediates functions of TRF2 at human telomeres. *J. Biol. Chem.*, Vol. 279, pp. 43799-43804.

Kim, Y.J.; Kwon, H.C.; Ko, H.; Park, J.H.; Kim, H.Y.; Yoo, J.H. & Yang, H.O. (2008a). Anti-tumor activity of the ginsenoside Rk1 in human hepatocellular carcinoma cells through inhibition of telomerase activity and induction of apoptosis. *Biol Pharm Bull,* Vol.31, pp. 826-830.

Koide, T.; Kamei, H.; Hashimoto, Y., Kojima, T. & Hasegawa, M. (1999). Tannic acid raises survival rate of mice bearing syngeneic tumors. *Cancer Biother Radiopharm,* Vol.14, pp. 231-234.

Kou, S.M. (1996). Antiproliferative Potency of Structurally Distinct Dietary Flavonoids on Human Colon Cancer Cells.*Cancer Letters (Ireland), Vol.*110, No.1-2, pp. 41-48.

Kroemer, G.; Galluzzi, L.& Brenner C. (2007). Mitochondrial membrane permeabilisation in cell death. *Physiol Rev.* Vol.87, No.1, pp. 99-163.

Kuhar, M.; Imran, S. & Singh, N. (2007). Curcumin and Quercetin Combined with Cisplatin to Induce Apoptosis in Human Laryngeal Carcinoma Hep-2 Cells through the Mitochondrial Pathway. *Journal of Cancer Molecules,* Vol.3, No.4, pp. 121-128.

Kuo, P.C.; Liu, H.F. & Chao, J.I. (2004). Survivin and p53 Modulate Quercetin- induced Cell Growth Inhibition and Apoptosis in Human Lung Carcinoma Cells. *The Journal of Biological Chemistry,* Vol.279, pp. 55875-55885.

Kurz, E.U. & Lees-Miller, S.P. (2004). DNA damage-induced activation of ATM and ATM-dependent signaling pathways. *DNA Repair (Amst).* Vol.3, pp.889-900.

Labieniec, M. & Gabryelak, T. (2006). Oxidatively modified proteins and DNA in digestive gland cells of the fresh-water mussel Unio tumidus in the presence of tannic acid and its derivatives. *Mutation Research,* Vol.603, pp. 48-55.

Lanzilli, G.; Fuggetta, M.P.; Tricarico, M.; Cottarelli, A.; Serafino, A.; Falchetti, R.; Ravagnan, G.; Turriziani, M.; Adamo, R.; Franzese, O. &Bonmassar, E. (2006). Resveratrol down- regulates the growth and telomerase activity of breast cancer cells in vitro. *Int J Oncol.* Vol. 28, No.3, pp. 641-8.

Lechel, A.; Satyanarayana, A.; Ju, Z.; Plentz, R.R.; Schaetzlein, S.; Rudolph, C.; Wilkens, L.; Wiemann, S.U.; Saretzki, G.; Malek, N.P.; Manns, M.P.; Buer, J. & Rudolph, K.L. (2005). The cellular level of telomere dysfunction determines induction of senescence or apoptosis in vivo. *EMBO Rep.* Vol.6, No.3, pp.275–281.

Lee, T.J.; Kim, O.H.; Kim, Y.H.; Kim, S.; Park, J.W. & Kwon, T.K. (2006). Quercetin arrests G2/M phase and induces caspase-dependent cell death in U937 cells. *Cancer Lett.*, Vol.240, pp. 234-242.

Lenain, C.;Bauwens, S.; Amiard, S.; Brunori, M.; Giraud-Panis, M.J. &Gilson, E. (2006). The Apollo 5' exonuclease functions together with TRF2 to protect telomeres from DNA repair. *Curr Biol*, Vol.16, No.13, pp. 1303-10.

Letai, A.G. (2008). Diagnosing and exploiting cancer's addiction to blocks in apoptosis. *Nat. Rev. Cancer*, Vol. 8, pp. 121–132.

Li, B. & de Lange, T. (2003). Rap1 affects the length and heterogeneity of human telomeres. *Mol. Biol. Cell*, Vol. 14, pp. 5060–68.

Li, B., Oestreich, S. & de Lange, T. (2000). Identification of human Rap1: implications for telomere evolution. *Cell*, Vol. 101, pp. 471–83.

Lichtsteiner, S.P.; Lebkowski, J.S. & Vasserot, A.P. (1999).Telomerase. A target for anticancer therapy. *Ann N Y Acad Sci.*, Vol. 886, pp. 1-11.

Lin, S.C.; Li, W.C.; Shih. J.W.; Hong, K.F.; Pan, Y.R.; Lin, J.J. (2006). The tea polyphenols EGCG and EGC repress mRNA expression of human telomerasereverse transcriptase (hTERT) in carcinoma cells. *Cancer Lett.* Vol.236, No.1, pp. 80-8.

Liu, D.; Safari, A.; O'Connor, M.S.; Chan, D.W.; Laegeler, A.; et al. (2004). PTOP interacts with POT1 and regulates its localization to telomeres. *Nat.Cell Biol.*Vol. 6, pp. 673–80.

Liu, K.; Hodes, R.J. & Weng, N.P. (2001) Cutting edge: telomerase activation in human T lymphocytes does not require increase in telomerase reverse transcriptase (hTERT) protein but is associated with hTERT phosphorylation and nuclear translocation. *J. Immunol.* Vol.166, pp.4826–4830.

Liu, W.J.; Jiang, J.F.; Xiao, D. & Ding, J. (2002). Down-regulation of telomerase activity via protein phosphatase 2A activation in salvicine-induced human leukemia HL-60 cell apoptosis.*Biochemical Pharmacology*, Vol.64, No.12, pp. 1677-1687.

Ljungman, M. (2009).Targeting the DNA Damage Response in Cancer. *Chem. Rev.* Vol.109, pp. 2929–2950.

Loayza, D. & de Lange,T. (2003). POT1 as a terminal transducer of TRF1 telomere length control. *Nature*, Vol. 423, pp. 1013-1018.

Lyu, S.Y.; Choi, S.H. & Park, W.B. (2002).Korean Mistletoe Lectin-induced Apoptosis in Hepatocarcinoma Cells is Associated with Inhibition of Telomerase *via* Mitochondrial Controlled Pathway Independent of p53. *Arch Pharm Res.* Vol.25, No.1, pp. 93-101.

Marienfeld, C.; Tadlock, L.; Yamagiwa, Y. & Patel, T. (2003).Inhibition of cholangiocarcinoma growth by tannic acid.*Hepatology*, Vol.37, pp. 1097-1104.

Martínez, P. &Blasco, M.A. (2010). Role of shelterin in cancer and aging. *Aging Cell*, Vol. 9, No.5, pp.653-66.

Martinez, P.; Thanasoula, M.; Carlos, A.R.; Gomez-Lopez, G.; Tejera, A.M.; Schoeftner, S.; et al. (2010). Mammalian Rap1 controls telomere function and gene expression through binding to telomeric and extratelomeric sites. *Nat Cell Biol*, Vol.12, pp.768–780.

Mattson, M.P.; Fu, W. & Zhang, P. (2001). Emerging roles for telomerase in regulating cell differentiation and survival: a neuroscientist's perspective. *Mech Ageing Dev.* Vol. 122, No.7, pp. 659-71.

Middleton, E.; Kandaswamı, C. &Theoharıdes, T.C. (2000). The effects of plant flavonoids on mammalian cells: implications for inflammation, heart disease, and cancer.*Pharmacol Rev.* Vol. 52, pp. 673–751.

Mondello, C. & Scovassi, A.I. (2004). Telomeres, Telomerase, and Apoptosis.*Biochemistry and Cell Biology*; Vol.82, No.4, pp. 498-507.

Morin, G.B. (1997).Telomere Control of Replicative Lifespan. *Exp Gerontol*, Vol.32, pp. 375-82.

Moyzis, R.K.; Buckingham, J.M.; Scott Crams, L.; Dani, M.; Deavent, L.L.; Jones, M.D.; Meyne, J.; Ratliff, R.L. & Wu, J.-R. (1988). A highly conserved repetitive DNA sequence (TTAGGG)n, present at the telomeres of human chromosomes. *Proc. Natl Acad. Sci.* Vol. 85, pp. 6622–6626.

Mukherjee Nee Chakraborty, S.; Ghosh, U.; Bhattacharyya, N.P.; Bhattacharya, R.K.; Dey, S. & Roy, M. (2007). Curcumin-induced apoptosis in human leukemia cell HL-60 is associated with inhibition of telomerase activity. *Molecular and Cellular Biochemistry*, Vol.297, pp. 31–39.

Multani,A.S.; Ozen,M.;Narayan,S.; Kumar,V.; Chandra,J.; McConkey,D.J.; Newman, R.A. &Pathak, S.(2000). Caspase-Dependent Apoptosis Induced by Telomere Cleavage and TRF2 Loss. *Neoplasia*.Vol.2, No.4, pp. 339–345.

Naasani, I.; Oh-Hashi, F.; Oh-Hara, T.; Feng, W.Y.; Johnston, J.; Chan, K.& Tsuruo T. (2003). Blocking telomerase by dietary polyphenols is a major mechanism for limiting the growth of human cancer cells in vitro and in vivo. *Cancer Res.* Vol.63, No.4, pp. 824-30.

Nagata, S. (2000). Apoptotic DNA fragmentation. *Exp Cell Res.* Vol. 256, No.1, pp.12-8.

Nakayama, Y.; Sakamoto, H.; Satoh, K. & Yamamoto, T. (2000). Tamoxifen and Gonadal Steroids Inhibit Colon Cancer Growth in Association with Inhibition of Thymidylate Synthase, Survivin and Telomerase Expression Through Estrogen Receptor Beta Mediated System. *Cancer Letters, Vol.* 161, pp. 63-71.

Nam, S.; Smith, D.M. & Dou, Q.P. (2001a). Tannic acid potently inhibits tumor cell proteasome activity, increases p27 and Bax expression, and induces G1 arrest and apoptosis. *Cancer Epidemiology, Biomarkers & Prevention*,Vol.10, pp. 1083-1088.

Nam, S.; Smith, D.M. & Dou, Q.P. (2001b). Ester bond-containing tea polyphenols potently inhibit proteasome activity *in vitro* and *in vivo*. *J Biol Chem*, Vol.276, pp. 13322-13330.

Naus, P.J.; Henson, R.; Bleeker, G.; Wehbe, H.; Meng, F. & Patel, T. (2007). Tannic acid synergizes the cytotoxicity of chemotherapeutic drugs in human cholangiocarcinoma by modulating drug efflux pathways. Journal of Hepatology. Vol. 46, pp. 222-229.

Nepka, C.; Asprodini, E. & Kouretas, D. (1999a).Tannins, xenobiotic metabolism and cancer chemoprevention in experimental animals.*Eur J Drug Metab Pharmacokinet*, Vol.24, pp.183-189.

Nepka, C.; Sivridis, E.; Antonoglou, O.; Kortsaris, A.; Georgellis, A.; Taitzoglou, I.; Hytiroglou, P.; Papadimitriou, C.; Zintzaras, I. & Kouretas, D. (1999b). Chemopreventive activity of very low dose dietary tannic acid administration in hepatoma bearing C3H male mice.*Cancer Lett*, Vol.141, pp. 57-62.

Nuñez, G.; Benedict, M.A.; Hu, Y. & Inohara N. (1998). Caspases: the proteases of the apoptotic pathway. *Oncogene.* , Vol. 17, No.25, pp. 3237-45.

O'Connor, M.S.; Safari, A.; Liu, D.; Qin, J. & Songyang, Z. (2004). The human Rap1 protein complex and modulation of telomere length. *J Biol Chem,*Vol. 279, No. 27, pp. 28585-91.

Omata, K.; Suzuki, R.; Masaki, T.; Miyamura, T.; Satoh, T. & Suzuki, T. (2008). Identification and characterization of the human inhibitor of caspase-activated DNase gene promoter. *Apoptosis.* Vol.13, No.7, pp.929-37.

Palm, W. & de Lange, T. (2008). How shelterin protects mammalian telomeres. *Annu Rev Genet,* Vol. 42, pp. 301–34.

Pan, M.H.; Lin, J.H.; Lin-Shiau, S.Y. & Lin, J.K. (1999). Induction of apoptosis by penta-O-galloyl--D-glucose through activation of caspase-3 in human leukemia HL-60 cells. *Eur. J. Pharmacol.,* Vol.381, pp. 171–183.

Park, C.; Kim, G.Y.; Kim, W.I.; Hong, S.H.; Park, D.I.; Kim, N.D.; Bae, S.J.; Jung, J.H. & Choi, Y.H. (2007). Induction of Apoptosis by (Z) -Stellettic Acid C, an Acetylenic Acid from the Sponge Stelletta sp., Is Associated with Inhibition of Telomerase Activity in Human Leukemic U937 Cells. *Chemotherapy,* Vol.53, pp. 160–168.

Park, S.E.; Park, C.; Kim, S.H.; Hossain, M.A.; Kim, M.Y.; Chung, H.Y.; Son, W.S.; Kim, G.Y.; Choi, Y.H.; Kim, N.D. (2009a). Korean red ginseng extract induces apoptosis and decreases telomerase activity in human leukemia cells. *Journal of Ethnopharmacology,* Vol.121, pp. 304–312.

Park, S.E.; Yoo, H.S.; Jin, C.Y.; Hong, S.H.; Lee, Y.W.; Kim, B.W.; Lee, S.H.; Kim,W.J.; Cho, C.K. & Choi, Y.H. (2009b). Induction of apoptosis and inhibition of telomerase activity in human lung carcinoma cells by the water extract of Cordyceps militaris. *Food and Chemical Toxicology,* Vol.47, pp. 1667–1675.

Parone, P.A.; James, D. & Martinou, J.C. (2002). Mitochondria: regulating the inevitable. *Biochimie.* Vol. 84, pp. 105-11.

Perez-Vizcaino, F.; Duarte, J.; Jimenez, R.; Santos-Buelga, C. & Osuna, A. (2009).Antihypertensive effects of the flavonoid quercetin. Pharmacological Reports. Vol. 61, pp. 67–75.

Pervaiz, S. (2003). Resveratrol: from grapevines to mammalian biology, *The FASEB Journal,*Vol. 17, pp. 1975-1985.

Pfingsten, J.S.; Goodrich, K.J.; Taabazuing, C.; Ouenzar, F.; Chartrand, P. & Cech, T.R. (2012). Mutually exclusive binding of telomerase RNA and DNA by Ku alters telomerase recruitment model. *Cell,* Vol.148, No.5, pp. 922-32.

Psahoulia, F.H.; Drosopoulos, K.G.; Doubravska, L.; Andera, L. & Pintzas, A. (2007). Quercetin enhances TRAIL-mediated apoptosis in colon cancer cells by inducing the accumulation of death receptors in lipid rafts. *Mol Cancer Ther.* Vol. 6, No.9, pp. 2591-9.

Ramachandran, C.; Fonseca, H.B.; Jhabvala, P.; Escalon, E.A. & Melnick S.J. (2002). Curcumin inhibits telomerase activity through human telomerase reverse transcritpase in MCF-7 breast cancer cell line. *Cancer Letters.* Vol.184, pp. 1–6.

Ramos, S. (2007). Effects of dietary flavonoids on apoptotic pathways related to cancer chemoprevention.*The Journal of Nutritional Biochemistry* Vol.18, No. 7, pp. 427-442.

Ramos, S. (2008). Cancer chemoprevention and chemotherapy: Dietary polyphenols and signalling pathways. *Mol. Nutr. Food Res.*Vol. 52, pp. 507-526.

Romero, I.; Paez, A.; Ferruelo, A.; Lujan, M. & Berenguer, A. (2002). Polyphenols in red wine inhibit the proliferation and induce apoptosis of LNCaP cells. *BJU International*, Vol.89, pp. 950-954.

Roos, W.P. & Kaina, B. (2006).DNA damage-induced cell death by apoptosis. *Trends Mol Med.* Vol.12, No.9, pp.440-50.

Sadava, D.; Whitlock, E. & Kane, S.E. (2007). The green tea polyphenol, epigallocatechin-3-gallate inhibits telomerase and induce apoptosis in drug-resitant lung cancer cells. *Biochemical and Biophysical Research Communications,* Vol.360, pp. 233-237.

Sakagami, H.; Jiang, Y.; Kusama, K.; Atsumi, T.; Ueha, T.; Toguchi, M.; Iwakura, I.; Satoh, K.; Ito, H.; Hatano, T. & Yoshida, T. (2000). Cytotoxic activity of hydrolyzable tannins against human oral tumor cell lines—a possible mechanism. *Phytomedicine*, Vol.7, pp. 39–47.

Sarthy, J.; Bae, N.S.; Scrafford. J. & Baumann, P. (2009). Human RAP1 inhibits non-homologous end joining at telomeres. *EMBO J*,Vol. 28, No. 21, pp. 3390-9.

Saunders, F.R. & Wallace H.M. (2010).On the natural chemoprevention of cancer.*Plant Physiol Biochem.* Vol. 48 No. 7, pp. 621-6.

Seimiya, H.; Sawada, H.; Muramatsu, Y.; Shimizu, M.; Ohko, K.; Yamane, K. &Tsuruo, T. (2000). Involvement of 14-3-3 proteins in nuclear localization of telomerase. *EMBO J.* Vol.19, pp.2652–2661.

Sfeir, A.; Kabir, S.; van Overbeek, M.; Celli, G.B. & de Lange T. (2010). Loss of Rap1 induces telomere recombination in the absence of NHEJ or a DNA damage signal. *Science,* Vol. 327, pp.1657–1661.

Sfeir, A.; Kosiyatrakul, S.T.; Hockemeyer, D.; Macrae, S.L.; Karlseder, J.; Schildkraut, C.L.; & De Lange, T. (2009). Mammalian telomeres resemble fragile sites and require TRF1 for efficient replication. *Cell*, Vol. 138, pp. 90–103.

Shay, J.W. & Bacchetti, S. (1997). A survey of telomerase activity in human cancer. *Eur. J. Cancer*, Vol. 33, pp. 787-791.

Shay, J.W. & Wright, W.E. (2005). Senescence and immortalization: role of telomeres and telomerase. *Carcinogenesis,* Vol.26, pp. 867-874.

Shay, J.W. & Wright, W.E. (2006). Telomerase therapeutics for cancer: challenges and new directions. *Nat Rev Drug Discov.* Vol. 7, pp. 577-584.

Shay, J.W. & Wright, W.E. (2011). Role of telomeres and telomerase in cancer. *Seminars in Cancer Biology.*, Vol. 21, pp. 349-353.

She, Q.B.; Ma, W.Y.; Wang, M.; Kaji, A.; Ho, C.T. & Dong, Z. (2003). Inhibition of cell transformation by resveratrol and its derivatives: differential effects and mechanisms involved. *Oncogene.* Vol.22, No.14, pp. 2143-50.

Shu, X.H.; Li, H.; Sun, X.X.; Wang, Q.; Sun, Z.; et al. (2011) Metabolic Patterns and Biotransformation Activities of Resveratrol in Human Glioblastoma Cells: Relevance with Therapeutic Efficacies. *PLoS ONE,* Vol.6, No.11, e27484. doi:10.1371/journal.pone.0027484

Smith, L.L.; Coller, H.A. & Roberts, J.M. (2003). Telomerase modulates expression of growth-controlling genes and enhances cell proliferation. *Nature Cell Biology*, Vol.5, pp. 474 - 479.

Smith, S., Giriat, I., Schmitt, A., & de Lange, T. (1998). Tankyrase, a poly(ADP-Ribose) polymerase at human telomeres. *Science*, Vol. 282, pp. 1484–1487.

Smogorzewska, A.; Bianchi, A.; Oelmann, S.; Schaefer, M.R.; Schnapp, G. &De Lange, T.(2000). Control of human telomere length by TRF1 and TRF2.*Mol. Cell. Biol.*, Vol. 20, pp. 1659–1668.

Sun, L. & Wang, X. (2003).Effects of allicin on both telomerase activity and apoptosis in gastric cancer SGC-7901 cells. *World J Gastroenterol*, Vol.9, No.9, pp. 1930-1934.

Taffetani, S.; Ueno, Y.; Meng, F., Venter, J.; Francis, H.; et al. (2005). Tannic acid inhibits cholangiocyte proliferation after bile duct ligation via a cyclic adenosine 5′,3′-monophosphate-dependent pathway. American Journal of Pathology.Vol. 166 No. 6, pp. 1671-1679.

Takai, H.; Smogorzewska, A. & de Lange, T. (2003). DNA damage foci at dysfunctional telomeres. *Curr Biol.* Vol.13, No.17, pp. 1549-56.

Takai, K.K.; Kibe, T.; Donigian, J.R.; Frescas, D. & de Lange, T. (2011). Telomere protection by TPP1/POT1 requires tethering to TIN2. *Mol Cell*, Vol. 44, No.4, pp. 647-59.

Tang, S.N.; Singh, C.; Nall, D.; Meeker, D.; Shankar, S. & Srivastava, R.K. (2010). The dietary bioflavonoid quercetin synergizes with epigallocathechin gallate (EGCG) to inhibit prostate cancer stem cell characteristics, invasion, migration and epithelial-mesenchymal transition. *Journal of Molecular Signaling*, Vol.18, pp. 5-14.

Turgut Cosan, D. & Soyocak, A. Induction of Apoptosis by Polyphenolic Compounds in Cancer Cells. In: Diederich, Marc; Noworyta, Karoline (eds.) Natural compounds as inducers of cell death. Springer; 2012. pp 185-214.

Turgut Cosan, D.; Soyocak, A.; Basaran, A.; Degirmenci, I.; Gunes, H.V. & Mutlu Sahin, F. (2011). Effects of various agents on DNA fragmentation and telomerase enzyme activities in adenocarcinoma cell lines. *Mol. Biol. Rep.*Vol. 38, pp. 2463–2469.

van Overbeek, M. &de Lange T. (2006). Apollo, an Artemis-related nuclease, interacts with TRF2 and protects human telomeres in S phase. *Curr. Biol.* Vol:16, pp. 1295–302.

van Steensel, B. & de Lange, T.(1997). Control of telomere length by the human telomeric protein TRF1.*Nature*, Vol. 385, pp. 740–743.

van Steensel, B.; Smogorzewska, A. & de Lange, T. (1998). TRF2 protects human telomeres from end-to end fusions. *Cell*, Vol. 92, pp. 401–413.

von Zglinicki, T.; Saretzki, G.; Ladhoff, J.; d'Adda di Fagagna, F. & Jackson, S.P. (2005). Human cell senescence as a DNA damage response. *Mech Ageing Dev.* Vol. 126, No. 1, pp. 111-7.

Wang, C.C.; Chen, L.G. & Yang, L.L. (2000). Cuphiin D1, the macrocyclic hydrolyzable tannin induced apoptosis in HL- 60 cell line. *Cancer Lett.*, Vol.149, 77–83.

Wang, J.; Zhang, P.H. & Tu, Z.G. (2007).Effects of quercetin on proliferation of lung cancer cell line A549 by down-regulating hTERT gene expression. *Journal of Third Military Medical University*,Vol.29, No.19, pp. 1852-1854.

Wang, X.Y.; Fan, Y.; Zhang, Y.L. & Zhong, X.M. (2010).Effect of resveratrol on promoter and human telomerase reverse transcriptase (hTERT) expression of human colorectal carcinoma cell.*Journal of Jiangsu University (Medicine Edition)* Vol. 23 pp. 3-23

Wang, F. & Lei, M. (2011). Human telomere POT1-TPP1 complex and its role in telomerase activity regulation. *Methods Mol Biol*, Vol. 735, pp. 173-87.

Wei, J.W.; Fan, Y.; Zhang, Y.L. & Wu, Y. (2007).Effects of Quercetin on telomerase activity and apoptosis in gastric cancer cells.*Shandong Medical Journal*, Vol.35

Wong, L.S.M.; van der Harst, P.; de Boer, R.A.; Huzen, J.; van Gilst, W.H.& van Veldhuisen, D.J. (2010). Aging, telomeres and heart failure. *Heart Fail Rev.*, Vol.15, No:5, pp. 479-486.

Wong, R.S.Y. (2011). Apoptosis in cancer: from pathogenesis to treatment. *J Exp Clin Cancer Res.* Vol.30, pp. 87-91.

Wu, P.; Takai, H. & de Lange, T. (2012). Telomeric 3' overhangs derive from resection by Exo1 and Apollo and fill-in by POT1b-associated CST. *Cell,* Vol.150, No.1, pp. 39-52.

Wu,Y.; Mitchell, T.R.H. & Zhu, X.D. (2008). Human XPF controls TRF2 and telomere length maintenance through distinctive mechanisms. *Mech. Ageing Dev.,* Vol: 129, No: 10, pp. 602–610.

Wyllie, A. H. (1992). Apoptosis & regulation of cell numbers in normal & neoplastic tissues: an overview. *Cancer Metast Rev.* Vol. 11, pp. 95-103.

Yang, L.L.; Lee, C.Y. & Yen, K.Y. (2000).Induction of apoptosis by hydrolyzable tannins from Eugenia jambos L. on human leukemia cells.*Cancer Lett.*, Vol.157, pp. 65–75.

Yang, Y.; Sun, H.; Zhou, Y.; Ji, S. & Li, M. (2009). Effects of three diterpenoids on tumour cell proliferation and telomerase activity. *Natural Product Research,* Vol. 23, No. 11, pp. 1007–1012.

Ye, J.Z.; Donigian, J.R.; van Overbeek, M.; Loayza, D.; Luo, Y.; Krutchinsky, A.N.; Chait, B.T. & de Lange, T. (2004a). TIN2 binds TRF1 and TRF2 simultaneously and stabilizes the TRF2 complex on telomeres. *J. Biol. Chem.,* Vol. 279, pp. 47264-47271.

Ye, J.Z.; Hockemeyer, D.; Krutchinsky, A.N.; Loayza, D.; Hooper, S.M.; et al. (2004b). POT1-interacting protein PIP1: a telomere length regulator that recruits POT1 to the TIN2/TRF1 complex. *Genes Dev.* Vol. 18, pp. 1649–54.

Yuan, Z. & Mei, H.D. (2002). Inhibition of telomerase activity with hTERT antisense increases the effect of CDDP-induced apoptosis in myeloid leukemia. *Hematol J.* Vol.3, No.4, pp. 201-5.

Zakian, V.A. (1995).Telomeres: Beginning to understand the end. *Science,* Vol. 270, pp. 1601-6.

Zamin, L.L.; Filippi-Chiela, E.C.; Dillenburg-Pilla, P; Horn, F.; Salbego, C. & Lenz, G. (2009). Resveratrol and quercetin cooperate to induce senescence-like growth arrest in C6 rat glioma cells. *Cancer Sci,* Vol.100, pp. 1655–1662.

Zhang, F.; Jia, Z.; Deng, Z.; Wie, Y.; Zheng, R. & Yu, L. (2002). In vitro modulation of telomerase activity, telomere length and cell cycle in MKN45 cells by verbascoside. *Planta Med.,* Vol.68, pp. 115-118.

Zhang, X.; Mar, V.; Zhou, W.; Harrington, L. & Robinson, M.O. (1999). Telomere shortening and apoptosis in telomerase-inhibited human tumor cells. *Genes Dev.* Vol.13, No.18, pp. 2388-99.

Zhong, F.L.; Batista, L.F.; Freund, A.; Pech, M.F.; Venteicher, A.S. & Artandi, S.E. (2012).TPP1 OB-Fold Domain Controls Telomere Maintenance by Recruiting Telomerase to Chromosome Ends. *Cell,* Vol. 150, No.3, pp. 481-94.

Zhou, X.Z. & Lu, K.P. (2001). The Pin2/TRF1-interacting protein PinX1 is a potent telomerase inhibitor. *Cell,*Vol. 107, pp. 347-359.

Zhu, X.D.; Kuster, B.; Mann, M.; Petrini, J.H. &de Lange, T. (2000). Cell-cycle-regulated association of RAD50/MRE11/NBS1 with TRF2 and human telomeres. *Nat Genet,* Vol. 25, pp. 347-352.

Zhu, X.D.; Niedernhofer, L.; Kuster, B.; Mann, M.; Hoeijmakers, J.H. &de Lange, T. (2003). ERCC1/XPF Removes the 3′ overhang from uncapped telomeres and represses formation of telomeric DNA-containing double minute chromosomes. *Mol. Cell,* Vol. 12, pp. 1489–98.

6

Telomeres and Reproductive Aging

Sena Aydos
Department of Medical Biology University of Ankara,
Faculty of Medicine, Ankara
Turkey

1. Introduction

Telomeres are special deoxyribonucleic acid (DNA) structures that "cap" the ends of eukaryote chromosomes. The term telomere derives from the Greek words telos, meaning "end", and meros meaning "part". The existence of these end-parts of chromosomes was first suggested in 1938 by Muller (Muller, 1938). Telomere length is involved in biological aging and disease processes. Telomere length is affected by several factors, such as aging, aging related diseases, gender, genetic and environmental factors. Telomere length, which is a highly variable and heritable trait (Jeanclos et al., 2000; Slagboom et al., 1994; Nawrot et al., 2004; Vasa-Nicotera et al., 2005; Andrew et al., 2006; Biscoff et al., 2005), is greater in women than men (Jeanclos et al., 2000, Nawrot et al., 2004; Vasa-Nicotera et al., 2005; Biscoff et al., 2005, Benetos et al., 2001; Mayer et al., 2006; Fitzpatrick et al., 2007). As well as genetic factors environmental factors are also influential on leukocyte telomere dynamics. Environmental factors, including smoking (Nawrot et al., 2004; Valdes et al., 2005), obesity (Fitzpatrick et al., 2007; Valdes et al., 2005; Gardner et al., 2005), psychological stress (Epel et al., 2005) and low socio-economic status (Cherkas et al., 2006) are associated with shortened leukocyte telomere length. Leukocyte telomere length can be determined relatively easily and the processing of leukocytes is rather simple. Leukocyte telomere length has been studied extensively in humans in relation to both the aging process and several pathologies. There are many correlative studies demonstrating a link between telomere length and aging (Slagboom et al, 1994, Wu et al, 2003).

Aging has been defined as a normal biological process, which involves the cumulative deposition of damaged and defective cellular components, loss of cell or organ physiological functions and inability to perform physical activity. Cellular senescence and aging have been reported to be related to shortening telomere length (Aubert & Lansdorp, 2008). Multiple surveys conducted in human populations have demonstrated the shortening of telomere length in various tissues during the aging process. Many theories have been proposed for aging, yet still, no single theory is able to account for all the different views. Among the most widely accepted theories on aging are the Hayflic limit theory and telomere theory (Gavrilov & Gavrilova, 2003). Shortened leukocyte telomere length is observed in individuals with aging-related diseases, including hypertension (Jeanclos et al., 2000; Benetos et al., 2001), insulin resistance (Gardner et al., 2005; Demissie et al., 2006; Aviv et al., 2006), atherosclerosis (Brouilette et al., 2003; Benetos et al., 2004), myocardial infarction (Brouilette et al., 2003, 2007; Cawthon et al., 2003), stroke (Fitzpatrick et al., 2007) and dementia (von Zglinicki et al., 2000; Panossian et al., 2003). Furthermore, it is suggested that the relationship between leukocyte telomere length and some of these variables could be modified by the aging process itself (Aviv et al., 2006). Unlike other systems, first signs of reproductive aging begin at mid 30 in normal condition. Telomere may be one of the responsible factors in also reproductive aging especially in women.

2. Telomere biology

The nucleoprotein complexes, referred to as telomeres, are specialized structures located at both ends of linear eukaryote chromosomes. Human telomeres are composed of a short repetitive DNA sequence (TTAGGG) and bound by a six-protein complex known as shelterin. TTAGGG repeat-binding factors (TRF) 1 and 2, bind to the TTAGGG sequences in double-stranded DNA, and one subunit, proteins for the protection of telomeres (POT1), bind to these sequences in single stranded form (de Lange, 2005; Pan et al., 2011). They are linked by three additional shelterin proteins, TIN2, TPP1, and Rap1, composing a complex called shelterin that enables cells to distinguish telomeres from sites of DNA damage (Fig.1). Three shelterin subunits, TRF1, TRF2, and POT1 directly recognize TTAGGG repeats. TRF1 and TIN2 regulate telomere length, TRF2 prevents end to end fusion and activation of DNA damage response. It has been reported that, additional proteins capable of interacting with telomeric proteins which are involved in DNA damage response and double-strand break repair also have implications for telomere length regulation and chromosome end protection (De Boeck et al., 2009; Gilson and Geli, 2007; Palm and de Lange, 2008).

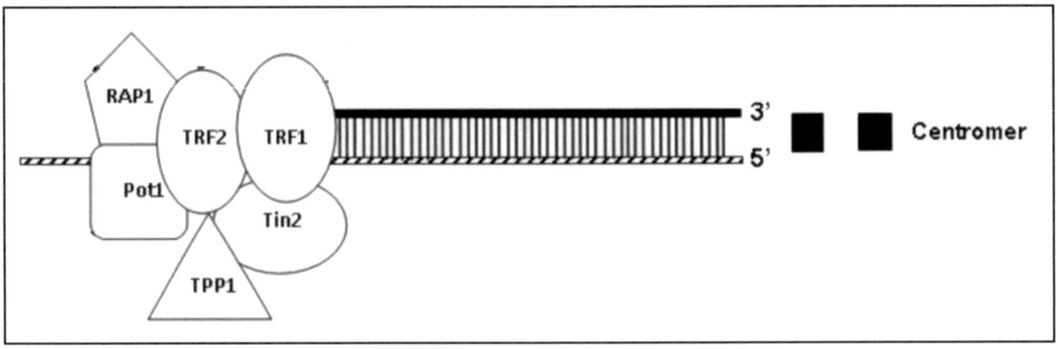

Fig. 1. **Schematic representation of chromosome termini. In mammals** telomeric sequences are enclosed by a complex which is composed of 6 different proteins **(TRF1, TRF2, POT1, TIN2, TPP1 AND RAP1)** that have specificity for either the single or double stranded DNA, **called shelterin.**

Telomeres act as the cap of the chromosome and maintain genomic integrity by preventing end-to-end fusions. (Murnane & Sabatier, 2004). Telomeres shorten with age through at least two mechanisms: (*1*) replicative senescence in dividing cells (*2*) and a damage response to reactive oxygen in non-dividing cells (Passos & von Zglinicki, 2005).

The shortening of telomeres occurs in each round of cell division consequential to the inability of conventional DNA polymerases to replicate the ends of linear chromosomes, in other words, as a result of the so-called 'end replication problem'. DNA replication involves the simultaneous copying of antiparallel DNA strands, such that replication proceeds in opposite directions, along a "leading" strand and a "lagging" strand. Daughter strand DNA synthesis takes place progressively on the leading template in the 5' to 3' direction, whilst on the lagging strand template, although seemingly backward in the form of Okazaki fragments, DNA synthesis also proceeds in the 5' to 3' direction. The leading daughter strand is almost completely synthesized, by the time the DNA polymerase reaches the 5' end of the leading template. However, a primer is required to start replication. If the RNA primer occupying the 5' end of the daughter strand is removed, it is not possible for the overlapping single strand to be replicated. The localization of this primer is the beginning of the leading strand and the end of the lagging strand. Consequently, the 5' end of each of the antiparallel daughter strands becomes one primer-length shorter. Chromosomes grow shorter with each consecutive replication (Fig 2).

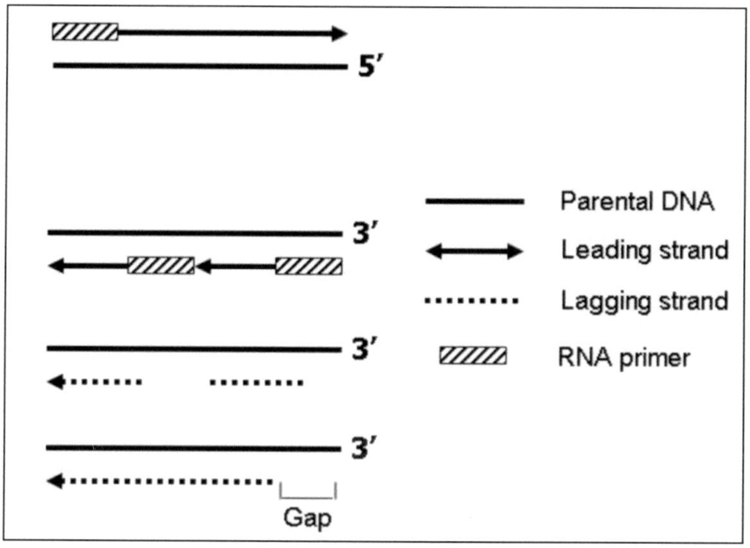

Fig. 2. In a linear chromosome, the leading strand can be synthesized by DNA polymerase until the end of the chromosome. On the other hand, in the lagging strand, synthesis by DNA polymerase is based on a series of fragments, referred to as Okazaki fragments, each of which requires an RNA primer. When the RNA primer occupying the 5' end of the daughter strand is removed, it is not possible for the overlapping single strand to be replicated. The localization of this primer is the beginning of the leading strand and the end of the lagging strand. Consequently, the 5' end of each of the antiparallel daughter strands becomes one primer-length shorter. Chromosomes grow shorter with each consecutive replication.

Due to the end replication problem, it is estimated that, in most human cells, a loss of less than 10 base pairs occurs per division. In fact, most often, the rate of loss is much higher, calculated as 50–200 base pairs per division in humans (Takai et al., 2003). The underlying reason of this difference has aroused great interest, but remains poorly understood (Lansdorp, 2005). Oxidative stress is thought to be one of the main factors involved (Houben et al., 2008). Exonuclease activity degrading the 5′ end is another major factor. The degradation of the primer on the lagging strand and the action of a putative 5' to 3' exonuclease lead to shortening of the 5' end of the telomere and the formation of a 3'-end overhang structure (Wai, 2004). Both, the nuclease-dependent resection of telomeres create single-stranded G-rich-strand overhangs and the inability of DNA polymerase to copy through the ends in lagging-strand during DNA replication cause to loss of telomeric repeats in each replication (Shay & Wright, 2000). Telomeric DNA is much more susceptible to oxidative damage than nontelomeric DNA, at least partly due to its high guanine content. While most studies investigating the effects of oxidative stress on telomere loss have been conducted in vitro (Richter & von Zglinicki, 2007), correlative and experimental studies have begun to demonstrate the link between oxidative stress and the rate of telomere loss in vivo (Houben et al., 2008; Cattan et al., 2008). Telomeres shorten throughout the lifespan of human cells. When telomeres shorten to a critical length, the cell ceases mitotic division, thus, replicative senescence occurs. This phenomenon, which is referred to as the Hayflick limit (Hayflick & Moorhead, 1961), demonstrates that telomere length acts as a major determinant of replicative capacity. Therefore, it is indicated that, telomere length, in a way, serves as a mitotic clock and constitutes a marker of biological aging, representative of the aging process other than chronological aging (the measure of time elapsed since a person' birth). In his research dating back to 1961, Hayflick showed that a cell culture population of normal human fetal cells divided between 40 and 60 times. Accordingly, he suggested that cells were capable of undergoing only a limited number of cell divisions before entering a senescence phase (Hayflick & Moorhead, 1961). Because of limited telomerase activity in normal somatic cells, it is presumed that, at the Hayflick limit (Ml), one or more telomeres lose TTAGGG beyond a crtical threshold activating a checkpoint mechanism that arrest cell growth. If partially transformed cells that skip this checkpoint without telomerase being activated, they continuously lose telomeres until "crisis" (M2). Cells capable of activating telomerase, most probably by mutation, as seen in most of cancer cells could survive the crisis. Only then can telomeres be maintained at stable length (Fig 3).

Senescent cells may produce protein aggregates different than those pertaining to quiescent but non-senescent adjacent cells. The homeostasis of tissues characterized by the senescence of cells, which emerges and is recognized as aging, could be changed (Shay & Wright, 2007). The shortening of telomeres is encountered in rapidly proliferating cells of the skin, gastrointestinal system and blood.

An oxidation-trigerred DNA damage response that excises the oxidized sequence leads to telomere attrition also exist in non-dividing cells (Passos & von Zglinicki, 2005). ROS-induced telomere shortening may result from direct injury to guanine repeat telomere DNA by ROS. A large number of independent studies have shown that (von Zglinicki, 2002; Serra et al., 2003) telomere shortening increased significantly under mild oxidative stress, in comparison to that observed under normal conditions. In somatic cells, the rate of telomere shortening can be suppressed by the addition of an antioxidant. Furumoto et al showed that the telomere shortening rate slowed after enrichment with ascorbic acid, which is a strong antioxidant (Furumoto et al., 1998). In most cases, the contribution of oxidative damage to telomere loss is much greater than that of the end-replication problem alone. Telomeres, as triple-G-containing structures, are highly sensitive to damage by oxidative stress (Henle et al., 1999), alkylation (Petersen et al., 1998) or ultraviolet (UV) irradiation (Oikawa et al., 200)]. Thus, stresses of high intensity may lead to telomere shortening without DNA replication, as a result of the induction of telomeric double-strand breaks at high frequency (Bar-Or et al., 2001; Oikawa et al., 2001).

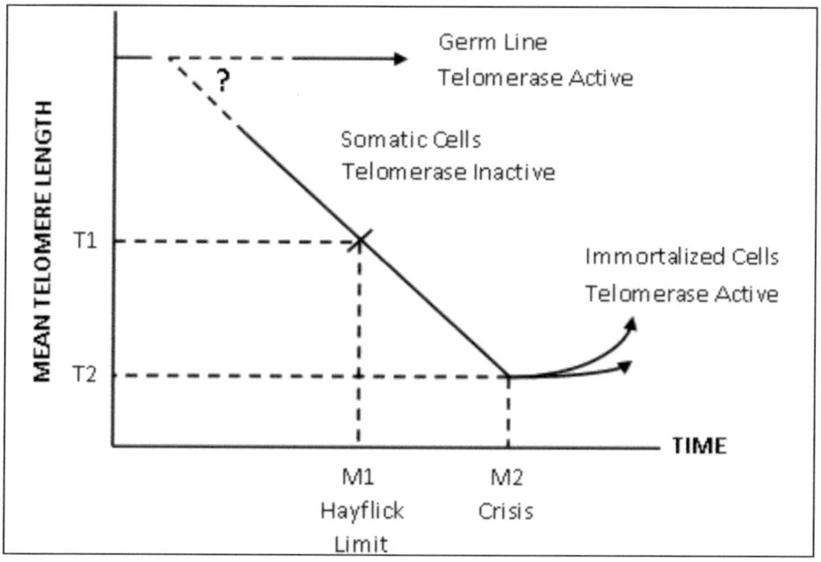

Fig. 3. **Schematic representation of the telomere hypothesis of cell aging and immortalization.** Alterations observed in telomere length over time (in cell divisions) are shown for germ line, normal somatic and transformed cells. Events in the early embryonic stage, at the beginning of the time axis, remain unknown (dotted lines). As telomere length is maintained in germ-line cells, it is thought that telomerase is activated at some point in gametogenesis, yet it is unclear whether telomerase activity is present in the early embryo prior to germ-line development. On the contrary, the decrease observed in telomere length and the lack of telomerase activity in normal somatic cells, suggest that telomerase is repressed in these cells. It is presumed that, at the Hayflick limit (Ml), one or more telomeres lose a threshold amount of TTAGGG, pointing out to a checkpoint in cell growth. The mean telomere length at this point is shown as T1. Partially transformed cells that skip this checkpoint without telomerase being activated, continuously lose telomeres until "crisis" (M2), at the point where most cells have critically short telomeres on many chromosomes (mean telomere length = T2). Cells capable of activating telomerase, most probably by mutation, could survive the crisis. Only then can telomeres be maintained at stable length.

The telomere end replication problem is solved by the use of a cellular enzyme called telomerase. Telomerase is a ribonucleoprotein complex composed of a catalytic subunit of component telomerase reverse transcriptase (TERT) responsible for the synthesis of new telomeric DNA repeats, and a telomerase RNA component (TERC) that functions as a template (Aubert & Lansdorp, 2008). This enzyme is capable of compensating for progressive telomere attrition through the de novo addition of TTAGGG repeats to chromosome ends (Greider & Blackburn, 1985) as well as of preventing telomere shortening in some cells, including male germ, stem and cancer cells (Keefe & Liu, 2009). The accelerated aging phenotype occurs in both TERC and TERT gene knockout mice (Greer & Brunet, 2008). As well as various pathologies, telomere dysfunction in late generations also leads to decline in fertility in female mice, eventually resulting in sterility (Lee et al., 1998; Herrera et al., 1999). Recent studies have revealed that telomerase function is regulated by an epigenetic mechanism involving histone methylation and deacetylation as well as CpG methylation. Strikingly extended telomeres were detected in mouse embryonic stem cells with deficient DNA methyltransferase (DNMT)1, or both DNMT3a and DNMT3b (Gonzalo et al., 2006). Increased telomere length is observed in histone methyltransferase-deficient MEFs. Elimination of acetylated histone H4 lysine 12 (H4K12) at telomeric heterochromatin resulted in reduction of telomere replication and recombination (Zhou et al., 2011).

Meiocytes may display telomerase independent mechanisms for telomere elongation that are based on homologous recombination between telomeres of different chromosomes. In other words, these cells may present with an alternative pathway for the lengthening of telomeres (ALT) (Chin et al., 1999). A high degree of heterogeneity of telomeres, including among others elongated and shortened telomeres, is generated by the ALT pathway in somatic cells with ALT activity (Nittis et al., 2008). However, to date, the presence of this mechanism in germ cells has not been proven.

Leukocyte telomere length varies greatly among individuals and shortens with aging. Significant variations are observed, in particular, during the first few years of life (Rufer et al., 1999). Telomere length remains relatively stable throughout childhood, preadolescence and adolescence. Eventually, telomere length attrition reaches its peak at very old age, beyond 100.

3. Reproductive aging

3.1 In males

Spermatogenesis and male reproductive functions gradually decline with aging. Semen quality and pregnancy outcomes appear to decline. Dunson et al showed that semen parameters begin to decline after 35 years of age. As a result, male fertility also decreases substantially in the late 30s and continues to decrease after the age of 40 (Dunson et al., 2004).

In a study on couples undergoing intracytoplasmic sperm injection (ICSI), it was found that increased age in men with oligozoospermia resulted in decreased implantation and pregnancy rates. In these couples, pregnancy rates decreased 5% for each year of paternal age, however, this effect was not observed in normozoospermic men (Ferreira et al., 2010). Levels of ROS that bind to the DNA that may cause DNA fragmentation have been found to be significantly higher in seminal ejaculates of healthy fertile men older than 40 years. Protective antioxidant scavenging enzyme concentrations are low in spermatozoa, which may reduce the chances of pregnancy, as men become progressively less fertile with age (Desai et al., 2010; Cocuzza et al., 2008). Based on findings detected in infertile men, it has been shown that aging affects the chromatin integrity of spermatozoa (Vagnini et al., 2007; Plastira et al., 2007). Numerical (such as disomy of chromosome 3, higher incidence of extra group C chromosomes including X chromosome, and group G chromosome or by extra group D and F chromosome) (Sartorelli et al., 2001) and structural aberrations in sperm chromosome also increase with paternal age. When a female baby is born, mitotic divisions of primordial germ cells have already been completed and meiosis has been arrested at prophase I. Therefore, a female baby is born with all the eggs she will have throughout her life, whilst mitotic spermatogenesis is an ongoing process throughout most of the male's life. The number of germ-line divisions is much higher in males than females. Consequently, more replications enhance the chance for spontaneous germ-line mutations that arise during the mitotic phase of spermatogenesis (Crow, 2000; Glaser & Jabs, 2004; Tarin et al. 1998; Kuhnert & Nieschlag, 2004). Transmitted to their offspring by older fathers, these germline mutations might cause an increased rate of clinical disorders such as autism, schizophrenia, and autosomal dominant disorders including achrondroplasia, osteogenesis imperfecta, and Marfan syndrome. As well as numerical and structural aberrations in sperm chromosome, some clinical manifestations such as cryptorchidism, hypospadias, and testicular cancer also increase with paternal age (Stewart & Kim, 2011). Fisch et al found that a paternal effect on the increased risk of Down syndrome was an important factor when both parents were over 35, but not when the female partner was younger than 35 years of age. In this study, the incidence of Down syndrome seemed to be related to paternal age at an approximate rate of 50% when the male was older than 35 and the female was older than 40 (Fisch et al., 2003).

Two previous studies conducted in 125 (Unryn et al., 2005) and 2,433 (De Meyer et al., 2007) participants demonstrated that leukocyte telomere length in adult offspring and paternal age were positively correlated with each other. This could be explained by the presence of a subset of sperm with longer telomeres in older men. It is possible that numerous replications of the male germ-line that occur with advancing age exert a powerful selection pressure that produces stem cells resistant against the effects of aging (Wallenfang et al., 2006). Sperm with greater telomere length might emerge from a subset of germ-line stem cells less resistant to aging-related oxidative stress, either due to increased resistance to its action—or having undergone fewer replications before meiosis. Epigenetic processes that occur in germ-line stem cells with advancing age in men may result in the elongation of telomeres (Blasco, 2007). Through the inheritance of the particular genetic constitution of such sperm (with or without DNA mutations) across generations, some offspring with longer leukocyte telomere length would emerge.

Although available data stress the important impact of male aging on telomere status, further studies are needed to clarify such correlation.

3.2 In females

During the aging process, in addition to several physiological changes in other systems, age-related changes, including the decline of ovarian functions resulting from reductions in the quantity and quality of the oocyte/follicle pool, also occur. Two important changes are observed in human ovaries with aging: 1) decline in oocyte genomic stability leading to aneuploidy (Hassold & Hunt, 2001) and 2) depletion of ovarian follicles (Faddy et al., 1992; Faddy, 2000).

Women display a marked increase in infertility, chromosomal nondisjunction associated miscarriage, and birth defects, as a result of reproductive aging characterized by a markedly increased duration of meiotic dysfunction. In women, fertility begins to decline starting from the mid-30s. Furthermore, as women grow older, the rate of miscarriage and/or aneuploid offspring increases dramatically. In clinically diagnosed pregnancies, trisomy incidence tends to be low (2-3%) in women in their 20's, yet rises to about 35% in women in their 40's (Hassold & Hunt, 2001). Previously conducted studies on *in vitro* fertilization (IVF) have proven that female age constitutes the most significant factor influential on clinical outcome (Wright et al., 2006). Based on studies investigating the effects of aging on oocytes, it has been concluded that maternal age has negative effect on the expression of oocyte genes responsible for major cellular activities such as cell cycle regulation, energy pathways and mitochondrial functions, and oxidative stress (Hamatani et al., 2004, Steuerwald et al., 2007).

3.2.1 Decline in oocyte genomic stability leading to aneuploidy

Most human aneuploidies occurring in embryos originate from the egg and not sperm (May et al., 1990; Hassold et al., 1987, 1991; Takaesu et al., 1990; Martin & Rademaker, 1987). Indirect proof suggests that, in addition to the reduction of oocyte quantity, impaired oocyte quality also contributes significantly to the age-related decline of fertility in women (Ottolenghi et al., 2004). As women age, their oocytes increasingly show abnormalities in chromosome segretion and spindle morphology. Keefe and co workers proposed a telomere theory of reproductive aging in women (Keefe et al., 2006). According to this theory, telomere dysfunction in oocytes is responsible for several reproductive changes including meiotic dysfunction, increased aneuploidy resulting in miscarriage, decreased fertility rate and birth defects. In older women, the prolonged exit of oocytes from the production line and their chronic exposure to reactive oxygen results in the shortening of telomeres. In return, the shortening of telomeres brings about a reduction in chiasmata, the presence of abnormal meiotic spindles in oocytes, as well as cell cycle arrest, apoptosis and cytogenetic abnormalities in resulting embryos (Keefe et al., 2006).

3.2.1.1 Oocyte senescence

In females, meiosis begins during fetal development, becomes arrested at prophase I before birth, and remains in this stage until prior to ovulation in adulthood, up to 50 years later in humans, by means of the synthesis of several RNAs and proteins. At that time, oocytes with a diameter of 15–20 μm develop to become fully grown oocytes of 70–150 μm (Bacharova, 1985). Based on observations in the mouse model, it has been suggested that aging impairs the accumulation of maternal RNAs either required for oocyte-specific processes and metabolism, or presumably stored for later use during early embryonic development prior to activation of the embryonic genome (Hamatani et al., 2004). The long interval between meiotic prophase I arrest in the fetus and each ovulation cycle in aged women increases the incidence of aneuploidy.

3.2.1.1.1 Meiotic chromosome and telomere

The aging oocyte is responsible for problems associated with maternal age (Sauer, 1998; Stolwijk et al., 1997). As they are involved in the tethering of chromosomes and the facilitation of their alignment, pairing and synapsis, as well as the formation of chiasmata during early meiosis, telomeres play a major role in meiotic reproduction (Scherthan et al., 1996; Scherthan, 2006; Roig et al., 2004; Bass et al., 1997). The mechanisms of meiotic telomere maintenance and dynamics, including attachment to the nuclear envelope, are only partially understood (Adelfalk et al., 2009). In the early stage of meiosis, in order to facilitate the homologue alignment required for the formation of chiasmata, telomeres aggregate around the nuclear envelope, forming 'bouquets' with a stalklike attachment to the nuclear envelope. This structure aids in the formation of the meiotic spindle and is therefore critical to chromosomal division. In oocytes, the main cause of telomere shortening is reactive oxygen species (Liu et al., 2002a), which increase with maternal aging. Experimental telomere shortening by several generations in the telomerase-null state (Liu et al., 2002b), or exposure to pharmacologically induced reactive oxygen in mice, results in impaired chiasmata and synapsis, and even abnormal spindles and chromosome misalignment (Liu et al, 2002b; Liu et al., 2004). Furthermore, females present with chromosome misalignment, lack of efficient metaphase checkpoint control during meiosis, progression from the MI stage to the MII stage (LeMaire-Adkins et al., 1997; Roeder, 1997). Structural abnormalities in the meiotic spindle, including asymmetry of the spindle poles and failure of chromosomes to align on the metaphase plate, are present in almost 80% of eggs aspirated from women over the age of 40, compared to only 17% of eggs from younger controls (Keefe et al., 2007). The mechanisms underlying chromosome misalignment and disruption of meiotic spindles caused by telomere dysfunction are not well understood. In a study conducted by Wood et al, female Mlh 1 mutant mice, which lacked normal recombination, also exhibited abnormal spindle assembly (Woods et al., 1999), and this may have caused improper homologous chromosome pairing and recombination during early meiosis. But still there is no clear information on whether telomeres play a role in spindle organization and chromosome segregetion in meiosis (Liu et al., 2002a). Experimental studies in adult mice have demonstrated that checkpoints for meiotic chromosome behaviour during the metaphase-to-anaphase transition are more efficient in males compared to females (Hunt et al., 1995; Le-Maire Adkins et al., 1997)]. Making use of telomerase null mice, it was investigated whether telomerase deficiency and/or telomere shortening could influence meiotic progression. The meiotic resumption and division (maturation) of germinal vesicle oocytes from fourth-generation telomerase null mice and first-generation telomerase null mice, as well as wild-type controls were compared. Chromosome misalignment and disruption of meiotic spindles at the metaphase stage appeared frequently in oocytes from fourth-generation telomerase null mice with very short telomeres, while meiotic progression, chromosome behavior, and spindle morphology in first-generation telomerase null mouse oocytes were comparable to those of wild-type mouse oocytes (Liu et al., 2002b).

In mammalian oogenesis, the sister chromatid cohesion is mediated by the multi-subunit protein complex called cohesin, which is composed of the meiosis-specific subunits REC8, STAGE3, SMC1β, and SMC3 (Garcia-Cruz et al., 2010; Prieto et al., 2004; Revenkova & Jessberger, 2005). It has been proposed that chromosome missegregation and aneuploidy in aged oocytes could result from loss of sister chromatid cohesion (SCC) through slow deterioration of cohesin (Hassold & Hunt, 2001; Hunt & Hassold 2008; Hodges et al., 2005). The cohesin component SMC1β prevents oocyte telomere shortening in mice (Adelfalk et al., 2009). It was observed that, in the oocytes of aged senescence-accelerated mice (SAM), meiotic cohesin proteins including REC8 (recombinant 8), STAG3 (stromal antigen 3) and

SMC1β that are located between sister chromatids were significantly reduced. In the study of Adelfalk et al., it was reported that, cohesion SMC1β which was reduced significantly in aging, is necessary to prevent telomere shortening, and SMC3, present in all known cohesion complexes, properly localizes to telomeres only if SMC1β is present (Adelfalk et al., 2009). Therefore it is one of the responsible factors, aging related telomere shortening in oocyte and meiotic-dysfunction in female. Furthermore, cohesion degradation was more pronounced in SAM compared to hybrid F1 mice with age, which may explain the vulnerability of SAM to aneuploidy. This ageing mouse model revealed that defective cohesin is associated with increased incidence of chromosome misalignment and precocious segregation (Liu & Keefe, 2008). In a study conducted by Hodges et al, the aging of female SMC1β-/- mice was associated with a dramatic loss of chiasmata. In parallel with the aging of SMC1β-/- oocytes, the loss of sister chromatid cohesion in metaphase I oocytes increases significantly (Hodges et al., 2005). This supports the increasingly distal localization of chiasmata on metaphase chromosomes, indicative of the inability of chiasmata being prevented from moving and slipping off chromosomes without SMC1β mediated sister chromatid cohesion (SCC). The expression of SMC1β cohesin takes place during prophase I prior to the primordial follicle stage with an aim of ensuring SCC in mice with advancing age. Slow degradation of SMC1β-mediated cohesion has a major role in age-dependent increase of aneuploidy (Revenkova et al, 2010). Telomeres shortened by several generations in the telomerase-null state (Liu et al., 2002b), or exposure to pharmacologically induced reactive oxygen in mice (Liu et al., 2003), produce similar abnormalities in meiotic spindles, with asymmetry and congression failure (Battaglia et al., 1996).

Oocytes contain a maternally transmitted pool of mitochondria throughout the reproductive process, including the initiation and progression of preimplantation embryo development. This pool may be involved in oocyte development, and may be required for the modulation of sperm-triggered calcium oscillations (Dumollard et al., 2007). Denham Harman was the first to hypothesize that the dysfunction of mitochondria, which constitute the main cellular site of ROS production, could be responsible for aging, due to progressive accumulation of oxidative damage (Harman, 1956, 1972). Though sufficient evidence is lacking to show a causal connection between mitochondrial DNA damage, ROS production, and aging, the free radical theory remains one of the best explanations for aging. Thouas and co workers (Thouas et al., 2005) studied the developmental ability of both young and aged oocytes, in the event of mitochondrial injury, with an aim to determine the impact of mitochondrial dysfunctions on oocyte alterations observed in aging females. The researchers ascertained a decline in blastocyst development in both groups with this trend being sudden in aged embryos. Therefore, they proposed that, due to their greater sensitivity to mitochondrial damage, aged oocytes should be protected against the potential damage of IVF procedures. Despite the possibility of being abrogated by the transfer of injured germinal vesicles (GV) into healthy ooplasts, compromised developmental potential as a result of induced mitochondrial damage in young oocytes at GV stage (Takeuchi et al., 2005) further supports the involvement of mitochondria in the reduced developmental potential of aged oocytes.

As confirmed by the observations referred to above, age-related ooplasmic dysfunction can be corrected by germinal vesicle transplantation, or micro-aspiration and transfer of ooplasm from younger eggs to older eggs. Preliminary studies suggest that novel IVF-based methods, including the transfer of mitochondria, have some clinical efficacy in rejuvenating fertility in older women (Malter & Cohen., 2002). However, the development of these highly invasive methods in ART requires a better understanding of processes that involve mitochondrial DNA replication and transcription, since asynchrony between mitochondrial and nuclear genomes could lead to problems in mitochondrial function, localization, and biogenesis (Harvey et al., 2007). Oocyte aging being a result of oxidative stress, in other words, a consequence of accumulated damage caused by increased levels of reactive oxygen species (ROS), is the most widely accepted proposal related to reproductive aging (Harman 1956; Tarin, 1995). It has been demonstrated that the expression of genes, including oxidative stress genes, differs between aged and younger oocytes (Hamatani et al., 2004, Steuerwald et al., 2007). Oxidative stress genes downregulated in aged oocytes belong to the family of thioredoxins, which are ATP-binding proteins that act as antioxidants against oxidative stress-induced apoptosis. The hypothesis that aging is related to decreased antioxidant defenses is supported by findings in mice. It has been observed that mature oocytes from aged mice display decreased activity levels of glutathione (GSH) and GSH-transferase (Tarin et al., 2004), which are factors that play an important role in cellular defense against ROS. In addition to endogenous ROS, oocytes may also be damaged by those produced in the follicular microenvironment during their prolonged stay in the ovary and/or as a consequence of a compromised oxygen supply (van Blerkom, 2000). Available data on how ROS production and mitochondrial function contribute to replicative senescence remains limited (Passos & von Zglinicki, 2005). Research has demonstrated that accelerated telomere shortening is observed under increased oxidative stress, and that this could be reversed by antioxidants (Xu et al., 2000, Bar-Or et al., 2001). Damage-induced telomere shortening cannot be attributed solely to the induction of double-strand breaks, yet, unrepaired nucleotide or base damage of telomeres increases the proportion of unreplicated ends. Furthermore, it has been confirmed by Honda and colleagues that telomere single-strand-break frequency and shortening rate are positively correlated with each other (Honda et al., 2001a, 2001b). It remains unclear how the existence of single-strand breaks accelerates telomere shortening and why single-strand break repair is less efficient in telomeres compared to the interstitial noncoding regions of the genome (von Zglinicki, 2002). The prolonged interval between the birth of oocytes and ovulation (up to 45 years in some women) would also render oocytes susceptible to telomere independent replicating shortening, as guanine rich sequence and location in the nuclear membrane make telomeres susceptible to reactive oxygen species (ROS). Keefe and co workers suggested that telomeres provide a cytogenetic mechanism to explain the "two hits" of aging on the female reproductive system, one active during fetal life and the other during adult life (Keefe et al., 2006). Increased mitochondrial DNA (mtDNA) mutations from chronic exposure to ROS during the prolonged interval between the birth of oocytes and ovulation shorten telomeres in oocytes from older women. Short telomeres cause a reduced number of chiasmata, as well as abnormal meiotic spindles in oocytes, cell cycle arrest and apoptosis, and clinically, result in infertility, miscarriage, birth defects and cytogenetic abnormalities in embryos.

3.2.2 Depletion of ovarian follicles

Age-related changes in the human ovary involve not only oocyte aging with decline in oocyte genomic stability that leads to aneuploidy, but also the depletion of ovarian follicles (Faddy et al., 1992; Faddy, 2000; Hassold & Hunt, 2001). During fetal life the ovaries have a stock of follicles, which should serve throughout the woman's reproductive lifespan. Besides the possible presence of germ stem cells in the postnatal ovary (Johnson et al., 2004; Liu et al., 2007), the number of follicles reduces exponentially, with a marked increase in the rate of disappearance from age 37–38 years onwards. When the supply drops below a thousand follicles, a number insufficient to sustain the cyclic hormonal process necessary for menstruation, menopause occurs at a mean age of 51 years (Faddy et al., 1992).

The timing of the menopause-related consequence of depletion of oocyte reserves, which occurs any time between 40-60 years of age (Kato et al., 1998; te Velde & Pearson, 2002; Toner et al., 1991; Baker, 1963), displays a large amount of inter-individual variability. The risk of conceiving a trisomic pregnancy, similarly, displays inter-individual variability (Warburton et al., 2004; Nicolaides et al., 2005). This natural variation in reproductive aging may be the result of environmental and genetic factors that affect individual rates of cellular aging. Although several environmental factors have been proposed as risk factors for the early onset of menopause (Brambilla & McKinlay 1989; Cramer et al., 1995; Kline et al., 2000; Pines et al., 2002), factors influencing the timing of menopause are not well understood (Snieder et al., 1998). Some genetic factors have recently been proposed to be determinants of the age at which menopause occurs. This idea is strongly supported by the following studies; the twin study which showed that the onset of menopause is genetically determined, yielding a heritability for age at menopause of 63% (Whelan et al., 1990); the study on the correlation between the menopausal age of mother and daughter (Torgerson et al., 1997); and another study which ascertained family history as a predictor of early menopause (Cramer et al., 1995). Based on animal model research and epidemiological studies in human populations, it has been proposed that longevity is associated with prolonged reproductive lifespan. It has been reported that women living till a minimum age of 100 years are greater than four times more likely to have given birth while in their 40s, compared to women living to the age of 73 (Perls et al., 1997). Several alternative mechanisms have been proposed for the relationship between longevity and age at menopause: (i) positive effect of prolonged estrogen exposure in association with later menopause on life expectancy (Perls et al., 1997), (ii) direct effect of effective ovarian age on longevity (Hsin & Kenyon, 1999; Cargill et al., 2003) or (iii) positive selection for women with slower rates of cellular aging by the use of selective pressures for maximizing female reproductive years by slow reproductive aging (Perls & Fretts, 2001; Perls et al., 2002). As their length declines with each cell division, telomeres are accepted as a marker for cellular aging. Telomere length varies among individuals (Hastie et al., 1990) and it is suggested that it may have a role in the variability observed in reproductive aging. The variability of telomere length may arise from differences in telomere length at conception, telomerase activity during early development, rate of cell division and rate of telomere loss per cell division.

Telomeres shorten by at least two mechanisms, including replicative senescence and response to damage from reactive oxygen (Passos & von Zglinicki 2005). As oocytes do not divide in adults, replicative senescence does not seem agreeable for them. However, female primordial germ cells divide during fetal life before entering meiosis. Inter-individual variations of telomere length in primordial germ cells may result from different sizes of follicular pools, and shorter telomeres may limit mitotic capacity during fetal development, reducing the size of the follicular pool (Keefe et al., 2006, Aydos et al., 2005). Previous studies have shown that telomere length is a strong predictor of the developmental potential of sister oocytes from women undergoing in vitro fertilization procedures (Keefe et al., 2007) and is also correlated with reproductive lifespan in women (Aydos et al., 2005). Research conducted by Keefe and co workers on sister eggs, aspirated during clinical in vitro fertilization procedures, demonstrated that, compared to patient age and other clinical parameters, telomere length is a more reliable indicator of pregnancy outcome following in vitro fertilization procedures, even in cases where telomere length is measured in only spare eggs. It was determined that, telomere length in chromosomes from spare eggs was strongly correlated with that in their associated first polar bodies (R2 = 0.98). Therefore, it was considered that the telomere length of the actual embryo transferred could be estimated with greater accuracy in the future, compared to estimations based on the measurement of telomere length in a spare, sister oocyte (Keefe et al, 2004). Data obtained in a study carried out by Aydos et al revealed that telomere lengths of women at the same age were correlated with their reproductive life span. Dorland et al. (Dorland et al., 1998) studied general aging, ovarian aging and telomere length. In this study, women older than 34 years of age, who presented with unexplained infertility and had less than five oocytes following an induced cycle, were investigated. The women's reproductive lifes were accepted to cease soon. The researchers expected that if there was a relation between general aging and ovarian aging, women who were accepted to have aged ovaries would have shorter telomeres than the fertile women included in the control group. The contradictory results obtained were surprising. These results showed that, in the case of infertile women, cell divisions in all cells were less than that observed in the control (fertile) group. This was attributed to growth hormone deficiency. This study also showed that reproductive life span and telomere length were correlated with each other. Results were interpreted such that, in the presence of factors with negative impact on reproductivity and cell division, the mitotic capacity of cells would decrease. Accordingly, cells, in general, including leukocytes and primordial germ cells, divided less, and thus less primordial follicles were formed. For this reason, these women had less ovarian follicles, aged ovaries and also long leukocyte telomeres. Increased telomere length in premature ovarian failure (POF) reported in the study of Hanna et al, similar to the study conducted by Dorland et al, was explained by longer telomeres in blood, reflecting fewer mitotic divisions in the initial germ cell pool, which could also explain a smaller follicular pool and early menopause in POF patients (Hanna et al., 2009).

4. Conclusion

Aging, a normal biological process, which involves the cumulative deposition of damaged and defective cellular components, loss of cell or organ physiological functions and inability to perform physical activity also includes telomere shortening. Although aging affects female reproductive function more evidently then male, declining in fertility and conception rate, meiotic dysfunction, birth defects, increase failure rate of implantation, fertilization and resulting unsuccess outcome of pregnancy that are performed assisted reproduction techniques are seen both in men and women as a result of reproductive aging. In men spermatogenesis and reproductive functions gradually decline with aging. It was shown that semen parameters begin to decline after 35 years of age. Numerical and structural aberrations, DNA fragmentation in sperm chromosome also increases with paternal age (Vagnini et al., 2007; Plastira et al., 2007; Dunson et al., 2004). As a result, male fertility also decreases substantially in the late 30s and continues to decrease after the age of 40 (Dunson et al., 2004). Though telomere theory of reproductive aging proposed by Keefe and co workwers does not explain the aging of reproductive function in male, as telomere length is maintained by telomerase activity and telomere attrition of germ cells is not evident in men, this theory is appropriate for female reproductive aging. According to this theory, telomere dysfunction in oocytes is responsible for several reproductive changes including meiotic dysfunction, increased aneuploidy resulting in miscarriage, decreased fertility rate and birth defects. In older women, the prolonged exit of oocytes from the production line and their chronic exposure to reactive oxygen results in the shortening of telomeres. In return, the shortening of telomeres brings about a reduction in chiasmata, the presence of abnormal meiotic spindles in oocytes, as well as cell cycle arrest, apoptosis and cytogenetic abnormalities in resulting embryos (Keefe et al., 2006). Age-related changes in the human ovary involve not only oocyte aging with decline in oocyte genomic stability that leads to aneuploidy, but also the depletion of ovarian follicles (Faddy et al., 1992; Faddy, 2000; Hassold & Hunt, 2001). During fetal life the ovaries have a stock of follicles, which should serve throughout the woman's reproductive lifespan. Besides the possible presence of germ stem cells in the postnatal ovary (Johnson et al., 2004; Liu et al., 2007), the number of follicles reduces exponentially, with a marked increase in the rate of disappearance from age 37–38 years onwards. When the supply drops below a thousand follicles, a number insufficient to sustain the cyclic hormonal process necessary for menstruation, menopause occurs at a mean age of 51 years (Faddy et al., 1992). The timing of the menopause-related consequence of depletion of oocyte reserves, which occurs any time between 40-60 years of age (Kato et al., 1998; te Velde & Pearson, 2002; Toner et al., 1991; Baker, 1963), displays a large amount of inter-individual variability. This may be also explained by telomere length. Female primordial germ cells divide during fetal life before entering meiosis. Inter-individual variations of telomere length in primordial germ cells may result from different sizes of follicular pools, and shorter telomeres may limit mitotic capacity during fetal development, reducing the size of the follicular pool (Keefe et al, 2006, Aydos et al 2003). Previous studies have shown that telomere length is a strong predictor of the developmental potential of sister oocytes from women undergoing in vitro fertilization procedures (Keefe et al., 2007) and is also correlated with reproductive lifespan in women (Aydos et al., 2005). Therefore, telomeres most likely play a crucial role in female reproductive aging. However, the molecular mechanisms of telomere regulation in early and late meiosis need to be clarified not only for a better understanding of normal development but also of human diseases associated with female reproductive aging as well.

5. References

Adelfalk, C.; Janschek, J.; Revenkova, E.; Blei, C.; Liebe, B.; Gob, E.; Alsheimer, M.; Benavente, R., de Boer, E.; Novak, I.; Hoog, C.; Scherthan, H. & Jessberger, R. (2009). Cohesin SMC1beta protects telomeres in meiocytes. *J Cell Biol*, Vol.187, No.2, (October 2009), pp.185–199, ISSN 0021-9525

Andrew, T.; Aviv, A.; Falchi, M.; Surdulescu, G.L.; Gardner, J.P.; Lu, X.; Kimura, M.; Kato, B.S.; Valdes, A.M. & Spector, T.D. (2006). Mapping genetic loci that determine leukocyte telomere length in a large sample of unselected, female sibling pairs. *Am J Hum Genet*, Vol.78, No.3, (March 2006), pp.480–486, ISSN 0002-9297

Aubert, G. & Lansdorp, P. M. (2008). Telomeres and aging. *Physiol Rev*, Vol.88, No.2, (April 2008), pp.557–579, ISSN 0031- 9333

Aviv, A.; Valdes, A.M. & Spector, T.D. (2006). Human telomere biology: pitfalls of moving from the laboratory to epidemiology. *Int J Epidemiol*, Vol.35, No.6, (December 2006), pp.1424–1429, ISSN 0300-5771

Aydos, S.E.; Elhan, A.H. & Tukun, A. (2005). Is telomere length one of the determinants of reproductive life span? *Arch Gynecol Obstet*, vol.272, No.2, (July 2005), pp. 113-116, ISSN 09320067. ISBN 09320067

Aviv, A.; Valdes, A.; Gardner, J.P.; Swaminathan, R.; Kimura, M. & Spector, T.D. (2006). Menopause modifies the association of leukocyte telomere length with insulin resistance and inflammation. *J Clin Endocrinol Metab*, Vol.91, No.2, (February 2006), pp.635–640, ISSN 0021-972X

Bacharova, R. (1985). Gene expression during oogenesis and oocyte development in mammals. *Dev Biol*, Vol.1, pp.453–524

Baker, T.G. A quantitative and cytological study of germ cells in human ovaries. *Proc R Soc Lond B Biol Sci*, Vol.158, (October 1963), pp.417–433, ISSN 0080-4649

Bar-Or, D.; Thomas, G.W.; Rael, L.T.; Lau, E.P. & Winkler, J.V. (2001). Asp-Ala-His-Lys (DAHK) inhibits copper-induced oxidative DNA double strand breaks and telomere shortening. *Biochem. Biophys Res Commun*, Vol.282, No.1, (March 2001), pp.356–360, ISSN 0006-291X

Bass, H.W.; Marshall, W.F.; Sedat, J.W.; Agard, D.A. & Cande, W.Z. (1997) Telomeres cluster de novo before the initiation of synapsis: a three-dimensional spatial analysis of telomere positions before and during meiotic prophase. *J. Cell Biol*, Vol.137, No.1, (April 1997), pp.5–18, ISSN 0021-9525

Battaglia, D.E.; Goodwin, P.; Klein, N.A. & Soules, M.R. (1996). Influence of maternal age on meiotic spindle assembly in oocytes from naturally cycling women. *Hum Reprod, Vol.11, No.10, (October* 1996), pp.2217–2222, ISSN 0268-1161

Benetos, A.; Okuda, K.; Lajemi, M.; Kimura, M.; Thomas, F.; Skurnick, J.; Labat, C.; Bean, K. & Aviv, A. (2001). Telomere length as an indicator of biological ageing: the gender effect and relation with pulse pressure and pulse wave velocity. *Hypertension*, Vol.37, No.2, (February 2001), pp.381–385, ISSN 0194-911X

Benetos, A.; Gardner, J.P.; Zureik, M.; Labat, C.; Xiaobin, L.; Adamopoulos, C.; Temmar, M.; Bean, K.E.; Thomas, F.; Aviv, A. (2004). Short telomeres are associated with increased carotid atherosclerosis in hypertensive subjects. *Hypertension*, Vol.43, No.2, (February 2004), pp.182–185, ISSN 0194-911X

Bischoff, C.; Graakjaer, J.; Petersen, H.C.; Hjelmborg, J.B.; Vaupel, J.W.; Bohr, V.; Koelvraa, S. & Christensen, K. (2005). The heritability of telomere length among the elderly and oldest-old. *Twin Res Hum Genet*, Vol.8, No.5, (october 2005), pp.433–439, ISSN 1832-4274

Blasco, M.A. (2007). The epigenetic regulation of mammalian telomeres. *Nat Rev Genet*, Vol.8, No.4, (April 2007), pp.299–309, ISSN 1471-0056

Brouilette, S.; Singh, R.K.; Thompson, J.R.; Goodall, A.H. & Samani, N.J. (2003). White cell telomere length and risk of premature myocardial infarction. *Arterioscler Thromb Vasc Biol*, Vol.23, No.5, (May 2003), pp.842–846, ISSN 1079-5642

Brouilette, S.W.; Moore, J.S.; McMahon, A.D.; Thompson, J.R.; Ford, I.; Shepherd, J.; Packard, C.J.; Samani, N.J. & West of Scotland Coronary Prevention Study Group. (2007).

Telomere length, risk of coronary heart disease, and statin treatment in the West of Scotland Primary Prevention Study: a nested case-control study. *Lancet*, Vol.369, No.9556, pp.107–114, ISSN 0140-6736

Brambilla, D.J. & McKinlay, S.M. (1989). A prospective study of factors affecting age at menopause. *J Clin Epidemiol*, Vol.42, No.11, (March 1989), pp.1031–1039, ISSN 0895-4356

Cargill, S.L; Carey, J.R; Muller, H.G. & Anderson, G. (2003). Age of ovary determines remaining life expectancy in old ovariectomized mice. *Aging Cell*, Vol.2, No.3, (June 2003), pp.185–190, ISSN 1474-9718

Cattan, V.; Mercier, N.;, Gardner, J.P.; Regnault, V.; Labat, C.; Mäki-Jouppila, J.; Nzietchueng. R.; Benetos, A.; Kimura, M.; Aviv, A. & Lacolley, P. (2008). Chronic oxidative stress induces a tissue-specific reduction in telomere length in CAST/Ei mice. *Free Radical Biol Med*, Vol.44, No.8, (April 2008), pp.1592–1598, ISSN 0891-5849

Cawthon, R.M.; Smith, K.R.; O'Brien, E.; Silvatchenko, A. & Kerber, R.A. (2003). Association between telomere length in blood and mortality in people aged 60 years or older. *Lancet*, Vol.361, No.9355, (February 2003), pp.393–395, ISSN 0140-6736

Cherkas, L.F.; Aviv, A.; Valdes, A.M.; Hunkin, J.L.; Gardner, J.P.; Surdulescu, G.L.; Kimura, M. & Spector, T.D. (2006). The effects of social status on biological ageing as measured by white-blood-cell telomere length. *Aging Cell*, Vol.5, No.5, (October 2006), pp.361–365, ISSN 1474-9718

Chin, L.; Artandi, S.E.; Shen Q.; Tam, A.; Lee, S.L.; Gottlieb, G.J.; Greider, C.W. & DePinho R.A. (1999). p53 deficiency rescues the adverse effects of telomere loss and cooperates with telomere dysfunction to accelerate carcinogenesis. *Cell*, Vol.97, No.4, (May 1999), pp.527–538, ISSN 0092-8674

Cocuzza, M.; Athayde, K.S.; Agarwal, A.; Sharma, R.; Pagani, R.; Lucon, A.M.; Srougi, M. & Hallak, J. (2008). Age-related increase of reactive oxygen species in neat semen in healthy fertile men. *Urology*, Vol.71, No.3, (March 2008), pp.490-494, ISSN 0090-4295

Cramer, D.W.; Xu, H. & Harlow, B.L. (1995). Family history as a predictor of early menopause. *Fertil Steril*, Vol.64, No.4, (October 1995), pp.740–745, ISSN 0015-0282

Crow, J.F. (2000). The origins, patterns and implications of human spontaneous mutations. *Nat Rev Genet*, Vol.1, No.1, (October 2000), pp.40-47, ISSN 1471-0056

De Boeck, G.; Forsyth, R.G.; Praet, M. & Hogendoorn, P.C. (2009). Telomere-associated proteins: cross-talk between telomere maintenance and telomere-lengthening mechanisms. *J Pathol*, Vol.217, No.3, (February 2009), pp.327-344, ISSN 0022-3417

de Lange, T. (2005). Shelterin: the protein complex that shapes and safeguards human telomeres. *Genes Dev*, Vol.19, No.18, (September 2005), pp.2100–2110, ISSN 0890-9369

De Meyer, T.; Rietzschel, E.R.; De Buyzere, M.L.; De Bacquer, D.; Van Criekinge, W.; De Backer, G.G.; Gillebert, T.C.; Van Oostveldt, P.; Bekaert, S. & Asklepios investigators. (2007). Paternal age at birth is an important determinant of offspring telomere length. *Hum Mol Genet*, Vol.16, No.24, (December 2007), pp.3097-3102, ISSN 0964-6906

Demissie, S.; Levy, D.; Benjamin, E.J.; Cupples, L.A.; Gardner, J.P.; Herbert, A.; Kimura, M.; Larson, M.G.; Meigs, J.B.; Keaney, J.F. & Aviv, A. (2006). Insulin resistance, oxidative stress, hypertension, and leukocyte telomere length in men from the

Framingham Heart Study. *Aging Cell*, Vol.5, No.4, (August 2006), pp.325–330, ISSN 1474-9718

Desai, N.; Sabanegh, E. Jr.; Kim, T. & Agarwal, A. (2010). Free radical theory of aging: implications in male infertility. *Urology*, Vol.75, No.1, (January 2010), pp.14-19, ISSN 0090-4295

Dorland, M.; Van Kooij, R.J. & te Velde, E.R. (1998). General ageing and ovarian ageing. *Maturitas*, Vol.30, No.2, (October 1998), pp.113–118, ISSN 0378-5122

Dumollard, R.; Duchen, M. & Carroll, J. (2007). The role of mitochondrial function in the oocyte and embryo. *Curr Top Dev Biol*, Vol.77, pp.21–49, ISSN 0070-2153

Duncan, F.E.; Chiang, T.; Schultz, R.M. & Lampson, M.A. (2009). Evidence that a defective spindle assembly checkpoint is not the primary cause of maternal age-associated aneuploidy in mouse eggs. *Biol Reprod, Vol.81, No.4, (October* 2009), pp.768–776, ISSN 0006-3363

Dunson, D.B.; Baird, D.D. & Colombo, B. (2004). Increased infertility with age in men and women. *Obstet Gynecol*, Vol.103, No.1, (January 2004), pp.51-56, ISSN 0029-7844

Epel, E.S.; Blackburn, E.H.; Lin, J.; Dhabhar, F.S.; Adler, N.E.; Morrow, J.D. & Cawthon, RM. (2004). Accelerated telomere shortening in response to life stress. *Proc Natl Acad Sci U S A*, Vol.101, No.49, (December 2004), pp.17312–17315, ISSN 0027-8424

Faddy, M.J.; Gosden, R.G.; Gougeon, A.; Richardson, S.J. & Nelson, J.F. (1992). Accelerated disappearance of ovarian follicles in mid-life: implications for forecasting menopause. *Hum Reprod*, Vol.7, No.10, (November 1992), pp.1342–1346, ISSN 0268-1161

Faddy, M.J. (2000). Follicle dynamics during ovarian ageing. *Mol Cell Endocrinol*, Vol.163, No1-2, (May 2000), pp.43–48, ISSN 0303-7207

Ferreira, R.C.; Braga, D.P.; Bonetti, T.C.; Pasqualotto, F.F.; Iaconelli, A. Jr. & Borges, E. Jr. (2010). Negative influence of paternal age on clinical intracytoplasmic sperm injection cycle outcomes in oligozoospermic patients. *Fertil Steril*, Vol.93, No.6, (April 2010), pp.1870-1874, ISSN 0015-0282

Fisch, H.; Hyun, G.; Golden, R.; Hensle, T.W.; Olsson, C.A. & Liberson, G.L. (2003). The influence of paternal age on Down syndrome. *J Urol*, Vol.169, No.6, (June 2003), pp.2275-2278, ISSN 0022-5347

Fitzpatrick, A.L.; Kronmal, R.A.; Gardner, J.P.; Psaty, B.M.; Jenny, N.S.; Tracy, R.P.; Walston, J.; Kimura, M. & Aviv, A. (2007). Leukocyte telomere length and cardiovascular disease in the cardiovascular health study. *Am J Epidemiol*, Vol.165, No.1, (January 2007), pp.14–21, ISSN 0002-9262

Furumoto, K.; Inoue, E.; Nagao, N.; Hiyama, E. & Miwa, N. (1998). Age-dependent telomere shortening is slowed down by enrichment of intracellular vitamin C via suppression of oxidative stress. *Life Sci*, Vol.63, No.11, (August 1998), pp.935-948, ISSN 0024-3205

Garcia-Cruz, R.; Brieno, M.A.; Roig, I.; Grossmann, M.; Velilla, E.; Pujol, A.; Cabero, L.; Pessarrodona, A.; Barbero, J.L.; Garcia Caldes, M. (2010). Dynamics of cohesin proteins REC8, STAG3, SMC1 beta and SMC3 are consistent with a role in sister chromatid cohesion during meiosis in human oocytes. *Hum Reprod*, Vol.25, No.9, (September 2010), pp.2316–2327, 0268-1161

Gardner, J.P.; Li, S.; Srinivasan, S.R.; Chen, W.; Kimura, M.; Lu, X.; Berenson, G.S. & Aviv, A. (2005). Rise in insulin resistance is associated with escalated telomere attrition. *Circulation*, Vol.111, No.17, (May 2005), pp.2171–2177, ISSN 0009-7322

Gavrilov, L. A. & Gavrilova, N. S. (2003). The quest for a general theory of aging and longevity. *Sci Aging Knowledge Environ,* Vol.28, (July 2003), RE5, ISSN 1539-6150

Gilson, E. & Géli, V. (2007). How telomeres are replicated. *Nat Rev Mol Cell Biol,* Vol.8, No.10, (October 2007), pp.825-838, ISSN 1471-0072

Ginsburg, J. (1991). What determines the age at the menopause? The number of ovarian follicles seems the most important factor. *BrMedJ* Vol.302, No.6788, (June 2001), pp.1288–1289, ISSN 09598138. ISBN 09598138

Glaser, R.L. & Jabs, E.W. (2004) Dear old dad. *Sci Aging Knowledge Environ,* Vol.21, No.3, (January 2004), pp.re1, ISSN 1539-6150

Gonzalo, S.; Jaco, I.; Fraga, M.F.; Chen, T.; Li, E.; Etseller, M. & Blasco, M.A. (2006). DNA methyltransferases control telomere length and telomere recombination in mammalian cells. *Nat Cell Biol,* Vol.8, No.4, (April 2006), pp. 416–424, ISSN 1465-7392

Greer, E.L. & Brunet, A. (2008). Signaling networks in aging. *J Cell Sci,* Vol.121, No.4, (February 2008), pp.407-412, ISSN 0021-9533

Greider, C.W. & Blackburn, E.H. (1985). Identification of a specific telomere terminal transferase activity in Tetrahymena extracts. *Cell,* Vol.43, No.2, (December 1985), pp.405-413, ISSN 0092-8674

Hamatani, T.; Falco, G.; Carter, M.G.; Akutsu, H.; Stagg, C.A.; Sharov, A.A.; Dudekula, D.B.; VanBuren, V. & Ko, M.S. (2004). Ageassociated alteration of gene expression patterns in mouse oocytes. *Hum Mol Genet,* Vol.13, No.19, (October 2004), pp.2263–2278, ISSN 0964-6906

Hanna, C.W.; Bretherick, K.L.; Gair, J.L.; Fluker, M.R.; Stephenson, M.D. & Robinson, W.P. (2009). Telomere length and reproductive aging. *Hum Reprod,* Vol.24, No.5, (May 2009), pp.1206-11, ISSN 0268-1161

Harman, D. (1956). Aging: a theory based on free radical and radiation chemistry. *J Gerontol,* Vol.11, No.3, (July 1956), pp.298–300, ISSN 0022-1422

Harman, D. (1972). The biologic clock: the mitochondria? *J Am Geriatr Soc,* Vol.20, No.4, (April 1972), pp.145–147, ISSN 0002-8614

Harvey, A.J; Gibson, T.C.; Quebedeaux, T.M. & Brenner, C.A. (2007). Impact of assisted reproductive technologies: a mitochondrial perspective of cytoplasmic transplantation. *Curr Top Dev Biol,* Vol.77, pp.229–249, ISSN 0070-2153

Hassold, T. & Chiu, D. (1985). Maternal age-specific rates of numerical chromosome abnormalities with special reference to trisomy. *Hum Genet, Vol.70, No.1, pp.*11–17, ISSN 0340-6717

Hassold, T.; Jacobs, P.A.; Leppert, M. & Sheldon, M. (1987). Cytogenetic and molecular studies of trisomy 13. *J Med Genet,* Vol.24, No.2, (December 1987), pp.725-732, ISSN 0022-2593

Hassold, T.J.; Pettay, D.; Freeman, S.B.; Grantham, M. & Takaesu, N. (1991). Molecular studies of nondisjunction in trisomy 16. *J Med Genet,* Vol.28, No.3, (March 1991), pp.159-162, ISSN 0022-2593

Hassold, T. & Hunt, P. (2001). To err (meiotically) is human: the genesis of human aneuploidy. *Nat Rev Genet,* Vol.2, No.4, (April 2001), pp.280–291, ISSN 14710056. ISBN 1471-0056

Hastie, N.D; Dempster, M.; Dunlop, M.G.; Thompson, A.M.; Green, D.K. & Allshire, R.C. (1990). Telomere reduction in human colorectal carcinoma and with ageing. *Nature,* Vol.346, No.6287, (August 1990), pp.866–868, ISSN 0028-0836

Hayflick, L. & Moorhead, P.S. (1961). The serial cultivation of human diploid cell strains. *Exp Cell Res,* Vol.25, (December 1961), pp.585–621, ISSN 0014-4827

Henderson, S.A. & Edwards, R.G. (1968). Chiasma frequency and maternal age in mammals. *Nature, Vol.218, No.5136, (April 1968), pp.22-28, ISSN 0028-0836*

Henle, E.S.; Han, Z.; Tang, N.; Rai, P.; Luo, Y. & Linn, S. (1999). Sequence-specific DNA cleavage by Fe2+-mediated Fenton reactions has possible biological implications. *J Biol Chem,* Vol.274, No.2, (January 1999), pp.962–971, ISSN 0021-9258

Herrera, E.; Samper, E.; Martín-Caballero, J.; Flores, J.M.; Lee, H.W &, Blasco, M.A. (1999). Disease states associated with telomerase deficiency appear earlier in mice with short telomeres. *EMBO J,* Vol.18, No.11, (June 1999), pp.2950-2960, ISSN 0261-4189

Hodges, C.A.; Revenkova, E.; Jessberger, R.; Hassold, T.J. & Hunt, P.A. (2005). SMC1beta-deficient female mice provide evidence that cohesins are a missing link in age-related nondisjunction. *Nat Genet.* Vol.37, No.12, December 2005), pp.1351–1355, ISSN 1061-4036

Honda, S.; Hjelmeland, L.M. & Handa, J.T. (2001a). Oxidative stress-induced single strand breaks in chromosomal telomeres of human retinal pigment epithelial cells in vitro. *Invest Ophthalmol Vis Sci,* Vol.42, No.9, (August 2001), pp.2139–2144, ISSN 0146-0404

Honda, S.; Weigel, A.; Hjelmeland, L.M. & Handa, J.T. (2001b). Induction of telomere shortening and replicative senescence by cryopreservation. *Biochem Biophys Res Commun,* Vol.282, No.2, (March 2001), pp.493–498, ISSN 0006-291X

Houben, J.M.; Moonen, H.J.; van Schooten, F.J. & Hageman G.J. (2008). Telomere length assessment: biomarker of chronic oxidative stress? *Free Radic Biol Med,* Vol.44, No.3, (February 2008), pp.235–246, ISSN 0891-5849

Hsin, H. & Kenyon, C. Signals from the reproductive system regulate the lifespan of C. elegans. *Nature,* Vol.399, No.6734, (May 1999), pp.362–366, ISSN 0028-0836

Hunt, P.; LeMaire, R.; Embury, P.; Sheean, L. & Mroz, K. (2007). Analysis of chromosome behavior in intact mammalian oocytes: monitoring the segregation of a univalent chromosome during female meiosis. *Hum Mol Genet,* Vol.4, No.11, (November 1995), pp.2007-2012, ISSN 0964-6906

Hunt, P.A. & Hassold, T.J. (2008). Human female meiosis: What makes a good egg go bad? *Trends Genet, Vol.24, No.2, (February 2008), pp.*86–93, ISSN 0168-9525

Jeanclos, E.; Schork, N.J.; Kyvik, K.O.; Kimura, M.; Skurnick, J.H. & Aviv, A. (2000). Telomere length inversely correlates with pulse pressure and is highly familial. *Hypertension,* Vol.36, No.2, (August 2000), pp.195–200, ISSN 0194-911X

Johnson, J.; Canning, J.; Kaneko, T.; Pru, J.K. & Tilly, J.L. (2004). Germline stem cells and follicular renewal in the postnatal mammalian ovary. *Nature,* Vol.428, No.6979, (March 2004), pp.145–150, ISSN 0028-0836

Kato, I.; Toniolo, P.; Akhmedkhanov, A.; Koenig, K.L.; Shore, R. & Zeleniuch-Jacquotte, A. (1998). Prospective study of factors influencing the onset of natural menopause. *J Clin Epidemiol,* Vol.51, No.12, (December 1998), pp.1271- 1276, ISSN 0895-4356

Keefe, D. L.; Franco, S.; Liu, L.; Cho, B.; Weitzen, S. & Blasco, M.A. (2004). Telomere length and reproductive outcome in women. *Am J Obstet Gynecol,* Vol.192, No.4, (April 2005), pp.1256-1260, ISSN 0002-9378

Keefe, D.L; Marquard, K. & Liu, L. (2006). The telomere theory of reproductive senescence in women. *Curr Opin Obstet Gynecol,* Vol.18, No.3, (June 2006), pp.280-285, ISSN 1040-872X

Keefe, D.L.; Liu, L. & Marquard, K. (2007). Telomeres and aging-related meiotic dysfunction in women. *Cell Mol Life Sci,* Vol.64, No.2, (January 2007), pp.139–143, ISSN 1420-682X

Keefe, D.L. & Liu, L. (2009). Telomeres and reproductive aging. *Reprod Fertil Dev,* Vol.21, No.1, pp.10-14, ISSN 1031-3613

Kline, K.; Kinney, A.; Levin, B. & Warburton, D. (2000). Trisomic pregnancy and early age at menopause. *Am J Hum Genet,* Vol.67, No.2, (August 2000), pp.395–404, ISSN 0002-9297

Kruk, P.A.; Rampino, N.J. & Bohr, V.A. (1995). DNA damage and repair in telomeres: relation to aging. *Proc Natl Acad Sci USA,* Vol.92, No.1, (January 1995), pp.258–262, ISSN 0027-8424

Kuhnert, B. & Nieschlag, E. (2004). Reproductive functions of the ageing male. *Hum Reprod Update,* Vol.10, No.4, (July-August 2004), pp.327–339, ISSN 1355-4786

Lansdorp, P.M. (2005). Major cutbacks at chromosome ends. *Trends Biochem Sci,* Vol.30, No.7, (July 2005), pp.388–395, ISSN 0968-0004

Lee, H.W.; Blasco, M.A.; Gottlieb, G.J.; Horner, J.W. 2nd, Greider, C.W. & DePinho, R.A. (1998). Essential role of mouse telomerase in highly proliferative organs. *Nature,* Vol.392, No.6676, (April 1998), pp.569-74, ISSN 0028-0836

LeMaire-Adkins, R.; Radke, K. & Hunt, P. A. (1997) Lack of checkpoint control at the metaphase/anaphase transition: a mechanism of meiotic nondisjunction in mammalian females. *J Cell Biol,* Vol.139, No.7, (December 1997), pp. 1611–1619, ISSN 0021-9525

Liu, L.; Trimarchi, J.R.; Smith, P.J. & Keefe, D.L. (2002a). Mitochondrial dysfunction leads to telomere attrition and genomic instability. *Aging Cell,* Vol.1, No.1, (October 2002), pp.40–46, ISSN 1474-9718

Liu, L.; Blasco, M. & Kefe, D.L. (2002b) Requirement of functional telomeres for metaphase chromosome alignments and integrity of meiotic spindles. *EMBO Rep,* Vol.3, No.3, (March 2002), pp.230–234, ISSN 1469-221X

Liu L, Trimarchi JR, Navarro P, Blasco MA, Keefe DL. (2003). Oxidative stress contributes to arsenic-induced telomere attrition, chromosome instability, and apoptosis. *J Biol Chem,* Vol. 278, No.34, (May 2003), pp.1998-2004, ISSN 0021-9258

Liu, L.; Franco, S.; Spyropoulos, B.; Moens, P.B.; Blasco, M.A. & Kefe, D.L. (2004). Irregular telomeres impair meiotic synapsis and recombination in mice. *Proc Natl Acad Sci USA,* Vol.101, No.17, (April 2004), pp.6496–6501, ISSN 0027-8424

Liu, Y.;Wu, C.; Lyu, Q. & Yang, D. (2007). Albertini DF, Keefe DL, Liu L. Germline stem cells and neo-oogenesis in the adult human ovary. *Dev Biol,* Vol.306, No.1, (June 2007), pp.112–120, ISSN 0012-1606

Liu, L. & Keefe, D.L. (2008). Defective cohesin is associated with age-dependent misaligned chromosomes in oocytes. *Reprod Biomed Online,* Vol.16, No.1, (January 2008), pp.103-112, ISSN 1472-6483

Malter, H.E. & Cohen, J. (2002). Ooplasmic transfer: animal models assist human studies. *Reprod Biomed Online,* Vol.5, No.1, (July-August 2002), pp.26–35, ISSN 14726483

Martin, R.H. & Rademaker, A.W. (1987) The effect of age on the frequency of sperm chromosomal abnormalities in normal men. *Am J Hum Genet,* Vol.41, No.3, (September 1987), pp.484-492, ISSN 0002-9297

Matthews, T.J. & Hamilton, B.E. (2009). Delayed childbearing: More women are having their first child later in life. *NCHS Data Brief, Vol.21, (August* 2009), pp.1–8, ISSN 1941-4935

May, K.M.; Jacobs, P.A.; Lee, M.; Ratcliffe, S.; Robinson, A.; Nielsen, J. & Hassold, T.J. (1990). The parental origin of the extra X chromosome in 47,XXX females. *Am J Hum Genet,* Vol.46, No.4, (April 1990), pp.754-761, ISSN 0002-9297

Mayer, S.; Bruderlein, S.; Perner, S.; Waibel, I.; Holdenried, A.; Ciloglu, N.; Hasel, C.; Mattfeldt, T.; Nielsen, K.V. & Möller, P. (2006) Sex-specific telomere length profiles and age-dependent erosion dynamics of individual chromosome arms in humans. *Cytogenet Genome Res,* Vol.112, No.3-4, (July 2005), pp.194–201, ISSN 1424-8581

Muller, H.J. (1938) The remaking of chromosomes. Collecting Net 13:15

Murnane, J.P. & Sabatier, L. (2004). Chromosome rearrangements resulting from telomere dysfunction and their role in cancer. *Bioessays,* Vol.26, No.11, (November 2004), pp.1164-1174, ISSN 0265-9247

Nawrot, T.S.; Staessen, J.A.; Gardner, J.P. & Aviv, A. (2004). Telomere length and possible link to X chromosome. *Lancet,* Vol.363, No.9408, (February 2004), pp.507–510, ISSN 0140-6736

Nicolaides, K.H.; Spencer, K.; Avgidou, K.; Faiola, S. & Falcon, O. (2005). Multicenter study of first-trimester screening for trisomy 21 in 75821 pregnancies: results and estimation of the potential impact of individual risk-orientated two-stage first-trimester screening. *Ultrasound Obstet Gynecol,* Vol.25, No.3, (March 2005), pp.221–226, ISSN 0960-7692

Nittis, T., Guittat, L. & Stewart, S.A. (2008). Alternative lengthening of telomeres (ALT) and chromatin: is there a connection? *Biochimie,* Vol.90, No.1, (January 2008), pp.5–12, ISSN 0300-9084

Oikawa, S.; Tada-Oikawa, S. & Kawanishi, S. (2001). Site-specific DNA damage at the GGG sequence by UVA involves acceleration of telomere shortening. *Biochemistry,* Vol.40, No.15, (April 2001), pp.4763–4768, ISSN 0006-2960

Ottolenghi, C.; Uda, M.; Hamatani, T.; Crisponi, L.; Garcia, J.E.; Ko, M.; Pilia, G.; Sforza, C.; Schlessinger, D. & Forabosco, A. (2004). Aging of oocyte, ovary, and human reproduction. *Ann N Y Acad Sci,* Vol.1034, (December 2004), pp.117–131, ISSN 0077-8923

Palm, W.& de Lange, T. (2008). How shelterin protects mammalian telomeres. *Annu Rev Genet,* Vol.42, (December 2008), pp.301-334, ISSN 0066-4197

Pan, H.; Ma, P.; Zhu, W. & Schultz, R.M. (2008). Age-associated increase in aneuploidy and changes in gene expression in mouse eggs. *Dev Biol, Vol.*316, No.2, (April 2008), pp.397–407, ISSN 0012-1606

Pan, M.H.; Lai, C.S.; Tsai, M.L.; Wu, J.C. & Ho, C.T. (2011). Molecular mechanisms for anti-aging by natural dietary compounds. *Mol Nutr Food Res*, Vol.(November 2011), doi: 10.1002/mnfr.201100509. [Epub ahead of print] ISSN 1613-4125

Panossian, L.A.; Porter, V.R.; Valenzuela, H.F.; Zhu, X.; Reback, E.; Masterman, D.; Cummings, J.L. & Effros, R.B. (2003). Telomere shortening in T cells correlate with Alzheimer's disease status. *Neurobiol Aging*, Vol.24, No.1, (January-February 2003), pp.77–84, ISSN 0197-4580

Passos, J. F., & von Zglinicki, T. (2005). Mitochondria, telomeres and cell senescence. *Exp Geronto,* Vol.40, No.6, (June 2005), pp.466–472, ISSN 0531-5565

Passos, J.F.; Saretzki, G. & von Zglinicki, T. (2007). DNA damage in telomeres and mitochondria during cellular senescence: is there a connection? *Nucleic Acids Res*, Vol.35, No.22, pp.7505-7513, ISSN 0305-1048

Petersen, S.; Saretzki, G. & von Zglinicki, T. (1998). Preferential accumulation of single-stranded regions in telomeres of human fibroblasts. *Exp Cell Res*, Vol.239, No.1, (February 1998), pp.152–160, ISSN 0014-4827

Perls, T.T.; Alpert, L. & Fretts, R.C. (1997). Middle-aged mothers live longer. *Nature* Vol.389, No.6647, (September 1997), pp.133, ISSN 0028-0836

Perls T, Levenson R, Regan M, Puca A. (2002). What does it take to live to 100? *Mech Ageing Dev*, Vol.123, No.2-3, (January 2002), pp.231–242, ISSN 0047-6374

Perls, T.T. & Fretts, R.C. (2001). The evolution of menopause and human life span. *Ann Hum Biol*, Vol.28, No.3, (May-June 2001), pp.237–245, ISSN 0301-4460

Petersen, S.; Saretzki, G. & von Zglinicki, T. (1998). Preferential accumulation of single-stranded regions in telomeres of human fibroblasts. *Exp Cell Res,* Vol.239, No.1, (February 1998), pp.152–160, ISSN 0014-4827

Pines, A.; Shapira, I.; Mijatovic, V.; Margalioth, E.J. & Frenkel, Y. (2002). The impact of hormonal therapy for infertility on age at menopause. *Maturitas,* Vol.41, No.4, (April 2002), pp.283–287, ISSN 0378-5122

Plastira, K.; Msaouel, P.; Angelopoulou, R.; Zanioti, K.; Plastiras, A.; Pothos, A.; Bolaris, S.; Paparisteidis, N. & Mantas, D. (2007). The effects of age on DNA fragmentation, chromatin packaging and conventional semen parameters in spermatozoa of oligoasthenoteratozoospermic patients. *J Assist Reprod Genet,* Vol.24, No.10, (October 2007), pp.437-443, ISSN 1058-0468

Prieto, I.; Tease, C.; Pezzi, N.; Buesa, J.M,.; Ortega, S.; Kremer, L.; Martinez, A.; Martinez, A.C.; Hulten, M.A. & Barbero, J.L. (2004). Cohesin component dynamics during meiotic prophase I in mammalian oocytes. *Chromosome Res,* Vol.12, No.3, pp.197–213, ISSN 0967-3849

Revenkova, E. & Jessberger, R. (2005). Keeping sister chromatids together: cohesins in meiosis. *Reproduction*, Vol.130, No.6, (December 2005), pp.783–790, ISSN 1470-1626

Revenkova, E.; Herrmann, K; Adelfalk, C. & Jessberger, R. (2010). Oocyte cohesin expression restricted to predictyate stages provides full fertility and prevents aneuploidy. *Curr Biol*, Vol.20, No.17, (September 2010), pp.1529-1533, ISSN 0960-9822

Richter, T. & von Zglinicki, T. (2007). A continuous correlation between oxidative stress and telomere shortening in fibroblasts. *Exp Gerontol*, Vol.42, No.11, (November 2007), pp.1039–1042, ISSN 0531-5565

Roeder, G.S. (1997). Meiotic chromosomes:it takes two to tango. *Genes Dev*, Vol.11, No.20, (October 1997), pp.2600-2621, ISSN 0890-9369

Roig, I.; Liebe, B.; Egozcue, J.; Cabero, L.; Garcia, M. & Scherthan, H. (2004). Female-specific features of recombinatorial double-stranded DNA repair in relation to synapsis and telomere dynamics in human oocytes. *Chromosoma*, Vol.113, No.1, (August 2004), pp.22–23, ISSN 0009-5915

Rufer, N.; Brummendorf, T.H.; Kolvraa, S.; Bischoff, C.; Christensen, K.; Wadsworth, L.; Schulzer, M. & Lansdorp, P.M. (1999). Telomere fluorescence measurements in granulocytes and T lymphocyte subsets point to a high turnover of hematopoietic stem cells and memory T cells in early childhood. *J Exp Med*, Vol.190, No.2, (July 1999), pp.157–167, ISSN 0022-1007

Saretzki, G.; Sitte, N.; Merkel, U.; Wurm, R.E. & von Zglinicki, T. (1999). Telomere shortening triggers a p53-dependent cell cycle arrest via accumulation of G-rich single stranded DNA fragments. *Oncogene*, Vol.18, No.37, (September 1999), pp.5148–5158, ISSN 0950-9232

Sartorelli, E.M.P.; Mazuccatto, L.F & de Pina-Neto J.M. (2001). Effect of paternal age on human sperm chromosomes. *Fertil Steril*, Vol.76, No.6, (December 2001), pp.1119-1123, ISSN 0015-0282

Sauer, M.V. (1998). The impact of age on reproductive potential: lessons learned from oocyte donation. *Maturitas*, Vol. 30, No.2, (October 1998), pp.221-225, ISSN 0378-5122

Scherthan, H.; Weich, S.; Schwegler, H.; Heyting, C.; Harle, M. & Cremer, T. (1996). Centromere and telomere movements during early meiotic prophase of mouse and man are associated with the onset of chromosome pairing. *J. Cell Biol*, Vol.134, No.5, (September 1996), pp.1109–1125, ISSN 0021-9525

Scherthan, H. (2006). Factors directing telomere dynamics in synaptic meiosis. *Biochem Soc Trans*, Vol.34, No.4, (August 2006), pp.550–553, ISSN 0300-5127

Serra, V.; von Zglinicki, T.; Lorenz, M. & Saretzki, G. (2003). Extracellular superoxide dismutase is a major antioxidant in human fibroblasts and slows telomere shortening. *J Biol Chem*, Vol.278, No.9, (February 2003), pp.6824-6830, ISSN 0021-9258

Shay, J.W. & Wright, W.E. (2000). Hayflick, his limit, and cellular ageing. *Nat Rev Mol Cell Biol*, Vol.1, No.1, (October, 2000), pp.72-76, ISSN:1471-0072.

Shay, J.W. & Wright, W.E. (2007). Hallmarks of telomeres in ageing research. *J Pathol*, Vol.211, No.2, (January 2007), pp. 114–123, ISSN 0022-3417

Sitte, N.; Saretzki, G. & von Zglinicki, T. (1998). Accelerated telomere shortening in fibroblasts after extended periods of confluency. *Free Radic Biol Med*, Vol.24, No.6, (April 1998), pp.885–893, ISSN 0891-5849

Slagboom, P.E.; Droog, S. & Boomsma, D.I. (1994). Genetic determination of telomere size in humans: a twin study of three age groups. *Am J Hum Genet*, Vol.55, No.5, (November 1994), pp.876–882, ISSN 0002-9297

Snieder, H.; MacGregor, A.J. & Spector, T.D. (1998). Genes control the cessation of a woman's reproductive life: a twin study of hysterectomy and age at menopause. *J Clin Endocrinol Metab*, Vol.83, No.6, (June 1998), pp.1875–1880, ISSN 0021-972X

Steuerwald, N.M; Bermudez, M.G.; Wells, D.; Munne, S. & Cohen, J. Maternal age-related differential global expression profiles observed in human oocytes. *Reprod Biomed Online*, Vol.14, No.6, (June 2007), pp.700–708, ISSN 14726483

Stewart, A.F. & Kim, E.D. (2011). Fertility Concerns for the Aging Male. *Urology*, Vol.78, No.3, (September 2011), pp.496-499, ISSN 0090-4295

Stolwijk, A.M.; Zielhuis, G.A.; Sauer, M.V.; Hamilton, C.J. & Paulson, R.J. (1997). The impact of the woman's age on the success of standard and donor in vitro fertilization. *Fertil Steril*, Vol.67, No.4, (April 1997), pp.702-710, ISSN 0015-0282

Takaesu, N.; Jacobs, P.A.; Cockwell, A.; Blackston, R.D.; Freeman, S.; Nuccio, J.; Kurnit, D.M.; Uchida, I.; Freeman, V. & Hassold, T. Nondisjunction of chromosome 21. (1990). *Am J Med Genet Suppl*, Vol.7, pp.175-181, ISSN 1040-3787

Takeuchi, T.; Neri, Q.V.; Katagiri, Y.; Rosenwaks, Z. & Palermo, G.D. (2005). Effect of treating induced mitochondrial damage on embryonic development and epigenesis. *Biol Reprod,* Vol.72, No.3, (March 2005), pp.584–592, ISSN 0006-3363

Takai, H.; Smogorzewska, A. & de Lange, T. (2003). DNA damage foci at dysfunctional telomeres. *Curr Biol,* Vol.13, No.17, (September 2003), pp.1549–1556, ISSN 0960-9822

Tarin, J.J. (1995). Aetiology of age-associated aneuploidy: a mechanism based on the 'free radical theory of ageing'. *Hum Reprod,* Vol.10, No.6, (June 1995), pp.1563–1565, ISSN 0268-1161

Tarin, J.J.; Brines, J. & Cano, A. (1998). Long-term effects of delayed parenthood. *Hum Reprod,* Vol.13, No.9, (September 1998), pp.2371–2376, ISSN 0268-1161

Tarin, J.J.; Gomez-Piquer, V.; Pertusa, J.F.; Hermenegildo, C. & Cano, A. (2004). Association of female aging with decreased parthenogenetic activation, raised MPF, and MAPKs activities and reduced levels of glutathione S-transferases activity and thiols in mouse oocytes. *Mol Reprod Dev,* Vol.69, No.4, (December 2004), pp.402–410, ISSN 1040-452X

Tarín, J.J.; Pérez-Albalá, S. & Cano, A. (2001). Cellular and morphological traits of oocytes retrieved from aging mice after exogenous ovarian stimulation. *Biol Reprod, Vol.65, No.1, (July* 2001), pp.141–150, ISSN 0006-3363

Terry, D.F.; Nolan, V.G.; Andersen, S.L.; Perls, T.T. & Cawthon, R. (2008). Association of longer telomeres with better health in centenarians. *J Gerontol A Biol Sci Med Sci,* Vol.63, No.8, (August 2008), pp.809-812, ISSN 1079-5006

te Velde ER, Pearson PL. The variability of female reproductive ageing. (2002). *Hum Reprod Update,* Vol.8, No.2, (March-April 2002), pp.141-154, ISSN 1355-4786

Thouas, G.A.; Trounson, A.O. & Jones, G.M. (2005). Effect of female age on mouse oocyte developmental competence following mitochondrial injury. *Biol Reprod,* Vol.73, No.2, (August 2005), pp.366–373, ISSN 0006-3363

Toner, J.P.; Philput, C.B.; Jones, G.S. & Muasher, S.J. (1991). Basal follicle-stimulating hormone level is a better predictor of in vitro fertilization performance than age. *Fertil Steril,* Vol.55, No.4, (April 1991), pp.784–791, ISSN 0015-0282

Torgerson, D.J.; Thomas, R.E. & Reid, D.M. (1997). Mothers and daughters menopausal ages: is there a link? *Eur J Obstet Gynecol Reprod Biol,* Vol.74, No.1, (July 1997), pp.63–66, ISSN 0301-2115

Unryn, B.M.; Cook, L.S. & Riabowol, K.T. (2005). Paternal age is positively linked to telomere length of children. *Aging Cell,* Vol.4, No.2, (April 2005), pp.97–101, ISSN 1474-9718

Vagnini, L.; Baruffi, R.L.; Mauri, A.L.; Petersen, C.G.; Massaro, F.C.; Pontes, A.; Oliveira, J.B. & Franco, J.G. Jr. (2007). The effects of male age on sperm DNA damage in an infertile population. *Reprod Biomed Online,* Vol.15, No.5, (November 2007), pp.514-519, ISSN 1472-6483

Valdes, A.M.; Andrew, T.; Gardner, J.P.; Kimura, M.; Oelsner, E.; Cherkas, L.F.; Aviv, A. & Spector, T.D. (2005) Obesity, cigarette smoking, and telomere length in women. Lancet, Vol.366, No.9486, (August 2005), pp.662-664, ISSN 0140-6736

Van Blerkom, J. (2000). Intrafollicular influences on human oocyte developmental competence: perifollicular vascularity, oocyte metabolism and mitochondrial function. *Hum Reprod*, Vol.15, No.Suppl 2, (July 2000), pp.173–188, ISSN 0268-1161

Vasa-Nicotera, M.; Brouilette, S.; Mangino, M.; Thompson, J.R.; Braund, P.; Clemitson, J.R.; Mason, A.; Bodycote, C.L.; Raleigh, S.M.; Louis, E. & Samani, N.J. (2005) Mapping of a major locus that determines telomere length in humans. *Am J Hum Genet*, Vol.76, No.1, (January 2005), pp.147–151, ISSN 0002-9297

Ventura, S.J. (1989). Trends and variations in first births to older women, United States, 1970-86. *Vital Health Stat 21, Vol.47, (June* 1989), pp.1–27, ISSN 1057-7629

von Zglinicki, T.; Saretzki, G.; Döcke, W. & Lotze, C. (1995). Mild hyperoxia shortens telomeres and inhibits proliferation of fibroblasts: a model for senescence? *Exp Cell Res*, Vol.220, No.1, (September 1995), pp.186–193, ISSN 0014-4827

von Zglinicki, T.; Pilger, R. & Sitte, N. (2000). Accumulation of single-strand breaks is the major cause of telomere shortening in human fibroblasts. *Free Radic Biol Med*, Vol.28, No.1, (January 2000), pp.64–74, ISSN 0891-5849

Von Zglinicki, T. (2002). Oxidative stress shortens telomeres. *TRENDS in Biochemical Sciences*, Vol.27, No.7, (July 2002), pp. 339-344, ISSN 0968-0004

von Zglinicki, T.; Serra, V.; Lorenz, M.; Saretzki, G.; Lenzen-Grossimlighaus, R.; Gessner, R.; Risch, A. & Steinhagen-Thiessen, E. (2000). Short telomeres in patients with vascular dementia: an indicator of low antioxidative capacity and possible risk factors? *Lab Invest*, Vol.80, No.11, (November 2010), pp.1739–1747, ISSN 0023-6837

Wai, L.K. (2004). Telomeres, Telomerase, and Tumorigenesis: Telomeres, the Chromosome-End Protectors. *MedGenMed*, Vol.6, No.3, (July, 2004), pp.19, ISSN:1531-0132

Wallenfang, M.R.; Nayak, R. & DiNardo, S. (2006). Dynamics of the male germline stem cell population during aging of Drosophila melanogaster. *Aging Cell*, Vol.5, No.4, (August 2006), pp.297–304, ISSN 1474-9718

Warburton, D.; Dallaire, L.; Thangavelu, M.; Ross, L.; Levin, B. & Kline, J. (2004). Trisomy recurrence: a reconsideration based on North American data. *Am J Hum Genet*, Vol.75, No.3, (September 2004), pp.376–385, ISSN 0002-9297

Whelan, E.A.; Sandler, D.P.; McConnaughey, D.R. & Weinberg C.R. (1990). Menstrual and reproductive characteristics and age at natural menopause. *Am J Epidemiol*, Vol.131, No.4, (April 1990), pp.625–632, ISSN 0002-9262

Wright, V.C.; Chang, J.; Jeng, G. & Macaluso, M. (2006). Assisted reproductive technology surveillance - United States, 2003. *MMWR Surveill Summ*, Vol.55, No.4, (May, 2006), pp.1–22, ISSN 1546-0738

Wu, X.; Amos, C.I.; Zhu, Y.; Zhao, H.; Grossman, B.H.; Shay, J.W.; Luo, S.; Hong, W.K. & Spitz, M.R. (2003). Telomere dysfunction: a potential cancer predisposition factor. *J Natl Cancer Inst*, Vol.95, No.6, (August 2003), pp.1211–1218, ISSN 0027-8874

Xu, D.; Neville, R. & Finkel, T. (2000). Homocysteine accelerates endothelial cell senescence. *FEBS Lett*, Vol.470, No.1, (March 2000), pp.20–24, ISSN 0014-5793

Zhou, B.O.; Wang, S.S.; Zhang, Y.; Fu, X.H.; Dang, W.; Lenzmeier, B.A. & Zhou, J.Q. (2011). Histone H4 lysine 12 acetylation regulates telomeric heterochromatin plasticity in Saccharomyces cerevisiae. *PloS Genet,* Vol.7, No.1, (January 2011), pp.1-8, ISSN 1553-7390

Telomeres and Lifestyle Choices

Cigir Biray Avci
Ege University
Turkey

1. Introduction

Telomeres, the specific DNA-protein structures found at both ends of each chromosome, protect genome from nucleolytic degradation, unnecessary recombination, repair, and interchromosomal fusion. Telomeres therefore play a vital role in preserving the information in our genome. As a normal cellular process, a small portion of telomeric DNA is lost with each cell division. Telomeres shorten with age. When telomere length reaches a critical limit, the cell undergoes senescence and/or apoptosis. Shorter telomeres have also been implicated in genomic instability and oncogenesis. People older than 60 with short telomeres have three and eight times increased risk to die from heart and infectious diseases, respectively [Starr et al., 2007.] Rate of telomere shortening is therefore critical to an individual's health and pace of aging. Telomere length may therefore serve as a biological clock to determine the lifespan of a cell. The telomere length limits a cell proliferative ability in cultured human primary cells. Telomere shortens in the absence of telomerase in non-ALT cells. Certain agents associated with specific lifestyles may expedite telomere shortening by inducing damage to DNA in general or more specifically at telomeres and may therefore affect health and lifespan of an individual.

Smoking [McGrath et al., 2007; Morla ´ M et al., 2006; Song et al., 2010; Valdes et al., 2005], exposure to pollution [Hoxha et al., 2009; Pavanello et al., 2010.], lack of physical activity [Cherkas et al., 2008; Werner et al., 2009], obesity [Valdes et al., 2005], stress [Von et al., 2002], and an unhealthy diet [Jennings et al., 1999; Jennings et al., 2000.] increase oxidative burden and the rate of telomere shortening. To preserve telomeres and reduce cancer risk and pace of aging, we may consider to eat less; include antioxidants, fiber, soy protein and healthy fats (derived from avocados, fish, and nuts) in our diet; and stay lean, active, healthy, and stress-free through regular exercise and meditation. Foods such as tuna, salmon, herring, mackerel, halibut, anchovies, catfish, grouper, flounder, flax seeds, chia seeds, sesame seeds, kiwi, black raspberries, lingonberry, green tea, broccoli, sprouts, red grapes, tomatoes, olive fruit, and other vitamin C-rich and E-rich foods are a good source of antioxidants. These combined with a Mediterranean type of diet containing fruits, and whole grains would help protect telomeres.

2. Structure and function of telomeres

Telomeres, the DNA-protein complexes at chromosome ends, protect genome from degradation and interchromosomal fusion. Telomeric DNA is associated with telomere-binding proteins and a loop structure mediated by TRF2, which protects the ends of human chromosomes against exonucleolytic degradation [Van Steensel et al., 1998], and may also prime telomeric DNA synthesis by a mechanism similar to 'gap filling' in homologous recombination [Griffith et al., 1999]. Telomere shortening occurs at each DNA replication, and if telomere length reaches below a critical limit, this leads to chromosomal degradation and cell death [Shin et al, 2006]. Telomerase activity, the ability to extend telomeres, is present in germline and certain hematopoietic cells, whereas somatic cells have low or undetectable levels of this activity and their telomeres undergo a progressive shortening with cell proliferation [Kim et al., 1994; Wright et al., 1996.]. Telomerases are reactivated in most cancers and immortalized cells. However, a subset of cancer/ immortalized cells lack telomerase activity and maintain telomere length by alternative mechanisms, probably involving genetic (homologous) recombination [Dunham et al., 2000], which is elevated in most immortal/cancer cell lines [Shammas et al., 2009].

3. Telomere shortening, cancer, and aging

Telomeres shorten with age and rate of telomere shortening may indicate the pace of aging [Epel et al., 2004; Irie et al., 2003; Patel et al., 2002; Von et al., 2002.].

3.1 Telomere length decreases with age and may predict lifespan

Normal human somatic cells lose telomeres with each cell division and therefore have a limited lifespan in culture. Telomeres protect chromosome ends from being recognized as DNA damage and chromosomal rearrangements. Conventional replication leads to telomere shortening, but telomere length is maintained by the enzyme telomerase that synthesizes telomere sequences de novo onto chromosome ends. Telomerase is specialized reverse transcriptase, requiring both a catalytic protein and an essential RNA component. In the absence of telomerase, telomeres shorten progressively as cells divide, and telomere function is lost. For this reason, telomerase is required for cells that undergo many rounds of divisions, especially tumor cells and some stem cells. [de Lange et al., 1990; Harley et al., 1990.]. Human liver tissues have been reported to lose 55 base pairs of telomeric DNA per year [Takubo et al., 2000]. The expression of stathmin and EF-1a, the biomarkers for telomeric dysfunction and DNA damage in a cell, increases with age and age-related diseases in humans [Jiang et al., 2008; Song et al., 2010]. Telomere length negatively correlates with age whereas the expression of p16, [Song et al., 2010; Takubo et al., 2000]. p16 represents a cell cycle inhibitor that is up-regulated in senescent cells [Alcorta et al., 1996; Stein et al., 1999]. Functional studies on senescent fibroblasts have shown that p16 appears to be upregulated in a p53 and telomere independent manner [Herbig et al., 2004]. Transgenic induction of a telomerase gene in normal human cells extends their lifespan [Bodnar et al., 1998]. Cawthon et al. [Cawthon et al., 2003] showed that individuals with shorter telomeres had significantly poor survival due to higher mortality rate caused by heart and infectious diseases. Progressive shortening of telomeres leads to senescence, apoptotic cell death, or oncogenic transformation of somatic cells in various tissues [Gilley et al., 2005; von Zglinicki et al., 2002]. Telomere length, which can be affected by various lifestyle factors, may determine overall health, lifespan, and the rate at which an individual is aging [Babizhayev et al., 2010].

3.2 Accelerated telomere shortening may increase the pace of aging

As a normal cellular process, telomere length decreases with age [Brouilette et al., 2003; Valdes et al., 2005;]. Telomere length in humans seems to decrease at a rate of 24.8–27.7 base pairs per year [Brouilette et al., 2003; Valdes et al., 2005]. Telomere length is affected by a combination of factors including donor age [Frenck et al., 1998], genetic background, epigenetic make-up, environment [Benetti et al., 2007; Celli et al., 2005; Munoz et al., 2005; Steinert et al., 2004], social and economic status [Adams et al., 2007; Cherkas et al., 2008], exercise [Cherkas et al., 2008], body weight [Nordfjall et al., 2008; Valdes et al., 2005], and smoking [Nawrot et al., 2004; Valdes et al., 2005]. Gender does not seem to have any significant effect on the rate of telomere loss [Brouilette et al., 2003]. When telomere length reaches below a critical limit, the cells undergo senescence and/or apoptosis [Gong et al., 1999; Stiewe et al., 2001]. Certain lifestyle factors such as smoking, obesity, lack of exercise, and consumption of unhealthy diet can increase the pace of telomere shortening, leading to illness and/or premature death.

Accelerated telomere shortening is associated with early onset of many age-associated health problems, including coronary heart disease [Brouilette et al., 2007; Fitzpatrick et al., 2007; Zee et al., 2009], heart failure [Van der Harst et al., 2007], diabetes [Sampson et al., 2006], increased cancer risk [McGrath et al., 2007; Wu et al., 2003], and osteoporosis [Valdes et al., 2007]. The individuals whose leukocyte telomeres are shorter than the corresponding average telomere length have three-fold higher risk to develop myocardial infarction [Brouilette et al., 2003]. Evaluation of telomere length in elders shows that the individuals with shorter telomeres have a much higher rate of mortality than those with longer telomeres [Cawthon et al., 2003]. Excessive or accelerated telomere shortening can affect health and lifespan at multiple levels. Shorter telomeres can also induce genomic instability [Chin et al., 1999; De Lange et al., 2005] by mediating chromosome end-to-end fusions and may contribute to telomere stabilization and development of cancer [Chin et al., 1999; Meeker et al., 2006]. Several studies indicate that shorter telomeres are a risk factor for cancer. Individuals with shorter telomeres seem to have a greater risk for development of lung, bladder, renal cell, gastrointestinal, and head and neck cancers [McGrath et al., 2007; Wu et al., 2003]. Certain individuals may also be born with shorter telomeres or may have genetic disorder leading to shorter telomeres. Such individuals are at a greater risk to develop premature coronary heart disease [Brouilette et al., 2003; Brouilette et al., 2007] and premature aging. Deficiency of telomerase RNA gene in a genetic disorder dyskeratosis congenita leads to shorter telomeres and is associated with premature graying, predisposition to cancer, vulnerability to infections, progressive bone marrow failure, and premature death in adults [Vulliamy et al., 2001].

4. Impact of smoking and obesity on telomeres and aging

Smoking and obesity seem to have adverse effect on telomeres and aging.

4.1 Smoking may accelerate telomere shortening and process of aging

Excessive telomere shortening can also lead to genomic instability [De Lange, 2005; Chin et al., 1999] and tumorigenesis [Chin et al., 1999; Meeker, 2006]. Consistently, the telomeres in most cancer cells are shorter relative to normal cells. Smoking is associated with accelerated telomere shortening [Song et al., 2010]. The dosage of cigarette smoking is shown to negatively correlate with telomere length [Song et al., 2010]. A dose dependent increase in telomere shortening has been observed in blood cells of tobacco smokers [Morla et al., 2006; Valdes et al., 2007]. A study conducted in white blood cells of women indicates that telomeric DNA is lost at an average rate of '25.7–27.7 base pairs' per year and with daily smoking of each pack of cigarettes, an additional '5 base pairs' is lost [Valdes et al., 2005]. Therefore, the telomere attrition caused by smoking one pack of cigarettes a day for a period of 40 years is equivalent to 7.4 years of life [Valdes et al., 2005]. Babizhayev et al. [Babizhayev et al., 2010] have proposed that telomere length can serve as a biomarker for evaluation of the oxidative damage caused by smoking and may also predict the rate at which an individual is aging. The authors also propose that oxidative damage leading to telomere shortening can be prevented by antioxidant therapy [Babizhayev et al., 2010]. In summary, the smoking increases oxidative stress, accelerates telomere shortening, and may increase the pace of aging process.

4.2 Obesity is associated with excessive telomere shortening

Obesity is also associated with increased oxidative stress and DNA damage. Furukawa et al. [Furukawa et al., 2004] showed that the waist circumference and BMI significantly correlate with the elevated plasma and urinary levels of reactive oxygen species. Song et al. [Song et al., 2010] have shown that BMI strongly correlates with biomarkers of DNA damage, independent of age. The obesity related increased oxidative stress is probably due to a deregulated production of adipocytokines. Obese KKAy mice display higher plasma levels of reactive oxygen species and lipid peroxidation, relative to control C57BL/6 mice [Furukawa et al., 2004]. The elevated levels of reactive oxygen species in obese mice were detected in white adipose tissue but not in other tissues, indicating that the oxidative stress detected in plasma could be attributed to oxidizing agents produced in the fat tissue. Moreover, the transcript levels and activities of antioxidant enzymes including catalase and dismutase were significantly lower in white adipose tissue of obese relative to control mice. The authors propose that a lack of antioxidant defense and elevated NADPH oxidase pathway in accrued fat probably led to increased oxidative stress in obese animals. Telomeres are not merely 'cell-division counters'. A proportion of the oxidative damage inflicted upon telomeres remains unrepaired and determines the amount of shortening in the next round of replication. This proportion is related to the total amount of damage in the bulk of the genome. Although most of that damage has been repaired, it is the residual, unrepaired fraction that determines the probability to mutation. Thus, telomere shortening counts not only cell divisions but also the cumulative probability of mutations occurring, and short telomeres trigger senescence in response to oxidative stress and mutational probability [von Zglinicki et al., 2002.].Oxidative stress can induce DNA damage and may therefore accelerate telomere shortening. Telomeres in obese women have been shown to be significantly shorter than those in lean women of the same age group [Valdes et al., 2005]. The excessive loss of telomeres in obese individuals was calculated to be equivalent to 8.8 years of life, an effect which seems to be worse than smoking. Together these data indicate that obesity has a negative impact on telomeres and may unnecessarily expedite the process of aging.

5. Impact of environment, nature of work, and stress on telomeres and aging

Environment, nature of profession, and stress can also affect the rate of telomere shortening and health.

5.1 Exposure to harmful agents and nature of profession may affect telomere shortening

Hoxha et al. [Hoxha et al., 2009] evaluated telomere length in the leukocytes derived from office workers and traffic police officers exposed to traffic pollution. Exposure to pollution was indicated by the levels of toluene and benzene. The investigators found that telomere length in traffic police officers was shorter than that in office workers within each age group,. Similarly the lymphocytes of coke-oven workers, exposed to polycyclic aromatic hydrocarbons, had significantly shorter telomeres and increased evidence of DNA damage and genetic instability, relative to control subjects [Pavanello et al., 2010]. Reduction in telomere length in these workers, although did not correlate with age and markers of DNA damage, significantly correlated with the number of years the workers were exposed to harmful agents. Telomere attrition has been associated with increased cancer risk [Wu et al., 2003; McGrath et al., 2007] and coke-oven workers are at a greater risk to develop lung cancer [Pavanello et al., 2010.]. Telomere attrition in lymphocytes is also associated with aging [Frenck et al., 1998]. Consistently, the reduced telomere length in the lymphocytes of coke oven workers was also associated with hypomethylation of p53 promoter [Pavanello et al, 2010], which may induce the expression of p53 [Esteller et al., 2006], leading to inhibition of growth or induction of apoptosis [Chin et al., 1999]. Thus the exposure to genotoxic agents, which may induce damage to DNA in general or more extensively at telomeres, can increase cancer risk and pace of aging.

Stress increases the pace of telomere shortening and aging [Epel et al., 2004]. The stress is associated with release of glucocorticoid hormones by the adrenal gland. These hormones have been shown to reduce the levels of antioxidant proteins [Patel et al., 2002] and may therefore cause increased oxidative damage to DNA [Irie et al., 2003] and accelerate telomere shortening [Von Zglinicki et al., 2002]. Consistently, women, exposed to stress in their daily life had evidence of increased oxidative pressure, reduced telomerase activity, and shorter telomeres in peripheral blood mononuclear cells than women in the control group [Epel et al., 2004]. Importantly, the difference in telomere length in these two groups of women was equivalent to 10 years of life, indicating that the women under stress were at a risk for early onset of age related health problems. Eventually, stress would adversely affect health and longevity.

6. Impact of diet, dietary restriction, and exercise on telomeres and aging

What we eat and how much we eat can significantly affect our telomeres, health, and longevity.

6.1 Dietary biomarkers and nutritional intake

Unhealthy lifestyles such as smoking [Babizhayev et al., 2010; McGrath et al., 2007; Mirabello et al., 2009; Morla et al., 2006; Nawrot et al., 2010; Valdes et al., 2005], consumption of processed meat products [Nettleton et al., 2008], and high body mass index [Al-Attas et al., 2010; Nordfjall et al., 2008; Lee et al., 2011; O'Callaghan et al., 2009; Zee et al., 2010] have been reported to correlate with the length of the shorter telomeres. Several studies have reported the association between diet and telomere length and human telomerase activity (Gunduz et al., 2005; Avci et al., 2007, 2011; Sahin et al., 2010; Cogulu et al., 2009). Higher plasma vitamin D was associated with increased telomere length in women [Richards et al., 2007]. Another study reported elevated plasma homocysteine is associated with decreased telomere length [Richards et al., 2008], while higher folate was associated with longer telomeres [Paul et al., 2009]. Farzaneh-Far et al. found that in a cohort of patients with coronary artery disease, there was an inverse relationship between baseline levels of marine omega-3 fatty acids and the rate of telomere shortening over the next five years, regardless of other factors [Farzaneh-Far et al., 2010.]. The Sister Study examined the intake of multivitamins [Xu et al., 2009] participants aged 35-74 years and found that multivitamin use is associated with longer telomere length. Specifically, higher intake of vitamins C and E from food associated with long telomere length, even after adjustment for multivitamin use. It should be noted that these studies are observations and most of those studies were biased to the retrospective analysis. In addition, people who take supplements are more likely to lead a healthy lifestyle that includes exercise and a healthy diet. Therefore, the effects of individual nutrients marker of telomere length has to be assessed in this context. There is a need for both intervention studies and for a more systematic analysis of macro-and micronutrients in relation to cell aging. [Paul et al., 2011].

6.2 Impact of fiber, fat, and protein on telomeres

Cassidy et al. [Cassidy et al., 2010] studied the association of leukocyte telomere length with various lifestyle factors in a relatively large group of women. Telomere length positively correlated with dietary intake of fiber and negatively associated with waist circumference and dietary intake of polyunsaturated fatty acids, especially linoleic acid. Reduction in protein intake also seems to increase longevity. Reduction in the protein content of food by 40%, led to a 15% increase in the lifespan of rats. The rats subjected to a protein-restricted diet early in life displayed a long-term suppression of appetite, reduced growth rate, and increased lifespan [Jennings et al., 1999; Jennings et al., 2000], and the increased lifespan in such animals was associated with significantly longer telomeres in kidney [Jennings et al., 1999]. Consistently, the highest life expectancy of Japanese is associated with low protein and high-carbohydrate intake in diet [Matsuzaki et al., 1992].

6.3 Dietary intake of antioxidants reduces the rate of telomere shortening

A study by Farzaneh-Far et al. [Farzaneh-Far et al., 2010] indicates that a diet containing antioxidant omega-3 fatty acids is associated with reduced rate of telomere shortening, whereas a lack of these antioxidants correlates with increased rate of telomere attrition in study participants. The authors followed omega-3 fatty acid levels in blood and telomere length in these individuals over a period of 5 years and found a direct correlation, indicating that antioxidants reduce the rate of telomere shortening. Similarly, the women who consumed a diet lacking antioxidants had shorter telomeres and a moderate risk for development of breast cancer, whereas the consumption of a diet rich in antioxidants such as vitamin E, vitamin C, and betacarotene was associated with longer telomeres and lower risk of breast cancer [Gammon et al., 2009]. Antioxidants can potentially protect telomeric DNA from oxidative damage.

6.4 Dietary restriction reduces the pace of aging

Dietary restriction or eating less has an extremely positive impact on health and longevity. Reducing food intake in animals leads to reduced growth rate [Jennings et al., 1999; Jennings et al., 2000], reduced oxidative burden and reduced damage to DNA [Jennings et al., 2000], and therefore keeps the animals in a biologically younger state and can increase their lifespan by up to 66% [Jennings et al., 2000]. It has been shown that dietary restriction in rodents delays the onset of age-associated diseases and increases the lifespan. Rats subjected to a protein-restricted diet early in life displayed a long-term suppression of appetite, reduced growth rate, and increased lifespan [Jennings et al., 1999; Jennings et al., 2000]. The increased lifespan in such animals was associated with significantly longer telomeres in kidney [Jennings et al., 1999]. Because oxidative stress can substantially accelerate telomere shortening, the reduction in oxidative stress by dietary restriction is expected to preserve telomeres and other cellular components.

7. Exercise may preserve telomeres and reduce the pace of aging

Song et al. [Song et al., 2010] have demonstrated that duration of exercise inversely correlates with biomarkers for damage to DNA and telomeres and with p16 expression, a biomarker for aging human cell. Exercise can reduce harmful fat and help mobilize waste products for faster elimination, leading to reduced oxidative stress and preservation of DNA and telomeres. Werner et al. [Werner et al., 2009] showed that exercise was associated with elevated telomerase activity and suppression of several apoptosis proteins, including p53 and p16, in mice. Consistently, in humans the leukocytes derived from athletes had elevated telomerase activity and reduced telomere shortening than non-athletes [Werner et al., 2009]. Exercise seems to be associated with reduced oxidative stress and elevated expression of telomere stabilizing proteins and may therefore reduce the pace of aging and age-associated diseases.

8. Perceived stress and adverse life events

Severe or chronic psychological stress is known to accelerate biological aging, as defined in broad sense, although the mechanisms by which this occurs have been elusive. A 2004 study by Epel et al. first reported a novel correlation between short telomere length, low telomerase activity and perceived chronic psychological stress in mothers, some who had a healthy child and some who were caregivers of chronically sick children [Epel et al., 2004]. Those who scored high on a 10-item questionnaire assessing their perceived stress level in the past month had shorter telomere length and lower basal telomerase activity in their peripheral blood mononuclear cells (PBMCs). Although the finding was based on cross-sectional analysis, and therefore was not able to establish a cause-effect relationship, the authors found that years of caregiving were inversely related to telomere length, suggesting that the cumulative burden of psychological stress in caregiving may have caused the shorter telomeres observed. This finding was replicated in a different group of caregivers, spouses of Alzheimer's patients [Damjanovic et al., 2007]. In this study, caregivers had significantly shorter telomere lengths in PBMCs as well as in T lymphocytes and monocytes. Caregiving is a prototypical example of chronic life stress, since it is typically full time, demanding, and continues for years. There are many other indices of chronic life stress, and here studies including low socio-economic status (SES), exposure to intimate partner violence, and childhood trauma had been reviewed. Several studies have examined the relationship between adverse socio-economic status and telomere length, but the results so far have been mixed. In one study, 1552 female twins aged 18–75 were compared for their leukocyte telomere length, and it was significantly shorter in lower SES groups. The mean difference in terminal restriction fragment length (TRFL) between non-manual (high SES) and manual SES (low SES) groups was 127 base pairs (bp) (approximating 3–5 years of accelerated shortening), after adjusting for body mass index, smoking and exercise [Cherkas et al., 2006]. A recent study of the Whitehall cohorts found a positive correlation between telomere length and educational attainment, but not current socioeconomic status [Steptoe et al., 2011]. However, Adams et al. [Adams et al, 2007] investigated the association between telomere length and life-course socio-economic status at age 50 in 318 participants in the Newcastle Thousand Families study and did not see correlations between telomere length and multiple measures of socio-economic position. Two other studies - 1542 men in the West of Scotland Coronary Prevention Study and 624 individuals in the National Long Term Care Survey (NTLCS) - also failed to detect a correlation between telomere length and socio-economic status [Batty et al., 2009; Risques et al., 2010]. Moreover, a survey of 958 men and 978 women aged 65 years and over living in Hong Kong showed that - in men only - after adjustment for age and other confounding factors, a higher ranking in community standing was associated with shorter telomere length [Woo et al., 2009], which is the opposite direction of the findings reported by Cherkas et al. and Steptoe et al. Several distinct differences exist between these different reports. First, a larger sample size of 1552 twins in the Twins UK study was studied compared to the 318 participants in Newcastle study and 624 participants National Long Term Care Survey. Given that the Twins UK study found a relative small difference of 127 bp between the low and high SES with a marginal statistical significance of $p < 0.047$, it is probable that Newcastle study and National Long Term Care Survey did not have enough statistical power to capture the small effect even if such a difference existed. The age, sex and racial compositions of each cohort may also play an important role as these factors are all known to be associated with telomere length [Aviv et al., 2002; Aviv et al., 2005; Hunt et al., 2008]. Finally, different socio-economic status markers were used to assess socio-economic status and this may determine whether an association can be found. Exposure to severe psychological trauma, early or late in life, may have lasting effects on hematopoietic stem cell integrity and thus on circulating leukocyte telomere length. Women who had previously experienced inter-partner violence (at least one year before the PBMCs were collected for telomere length measurements) had significantly shorter mean telomere length compared to controls. Length of time in the abusive relationship and having children were associated with telomere shortness after controlling for age and body mass index, suggesting that the stress caused by inter-partner violence and raising children in the abusive relationship causes accelerated telomere shortening [Humphreys et al., 2011]. Several studies show associations between childhood trauma and telomere length. Tyrka and colleagues [Tyrka et al., 2010] evaluated the effects of childhood adversity in a community-based sample of 31 men and women with and without a history of childhood mal-treatment, and with no current depression. Participants reporting a history of maltreatment (mostly neglect rather than abuse) had significantly shorter telomeres than those who did not report such maltreatment independent of the effects of age, gender, smoking, body mass index (BMI), or other demographic factors known to be associated with shortened telomeres. Likewise, Kananen and colleagues [Kananen et al., 2010] also reported that childhood adversity was associated with telomere shortening in adults in the Health 2000 Survey in Finland. Kiecolt-Glaser et al. reported that in 132 healthy older adults including 58 dementia family caregivers and 74 noncaregivers, the presence of multiple childhood adverse events was related to shorter telomeres after controlling for age, caregiving status, gender, body mass index, exercise, and sleep [Kiecolt-Glaser et al., 2011]. In a recent study of young to middle-aged adults with post-traumatic stress (PTSD), those with PTSD had shorter leukocyte telomere length LTL. Early exposure to adverse events may have accounted for the difference in LTL between those with PTSD and controls; all those exposed to multiple events and types of trauma in childhood were in the PTSD group and had shorter LTL than those without such exposure [O'Donovan et al., 2011]. The findings between short telomeres and childhood adverse event were replicated in a large study of ethnically homogenous population of 4441 women of the UK EPIC-Norfolk study [Surtees et al., 2011]. However, one study reported a null finding between physical and/or sexual abuse in childhood and telomere length [Glass et al., 2010]. Here, like the findings for socio-economic status, the specific measurement tool used for assessing childhood trauma may be an important determinant of whether an association with telomere shortness is found. Those reported an association used a broad range of measurements including physical, sexual, emotional abuse, physical and emotional neglect [Kiecolt-Glaser et al., 2011; O'Donovan et al.,2011; Tyrka et al., 2010]. Kananen et al. used a series of 11 questions about the subject's childhood social environment, which has an even broader scope that includes the financial situation of the family, physical and mental health of parents as well as the child, and the conflicts within the family and in school. It should be noted that the most significant childhood adversity in the Kananen et al. study was the person's own chronic or serious illness during childhood. Therefore, it is possible that physiological, rather than psychological adverse events in childhood are associated with shorter telomere length.

8.1 Stress and stress-related psychiatric conditions

PTSD are closely linked and related to, exposure to chronic or severe psychological stress [Wolkowitz et al., 2008]. Several reports have found shorter telomere length in patients with affective disorders, including depression and bipolar depression with and without anxiety [Hartmann et al., 2010; Lung et al., 2007; Simon et al., 2006]. In a small study, Wolkowitz et al. found only slightly shorter telomeres in subjects with major clinical depression compared to controls [Wolkowitz et al., 2011]. There was a significant inverse correlation between telomere length and the total cumulative lifetime period of depression. These results suggest that telomere shortening may develop with longer exposures to depression. Interestingly, depression subjects in Simon et al. studies had an average of 31.8 ± 11.2 years of history, while patients in Wolkowitz study had a shorter mean disease (13.0 ± 11.2 years). It is possible that the lack of correlation between depression and short telomere lengths in Wolkowitz study was due to the short disease duration in some subjects. It is also likely that early trauma and later in life PTSD and MDD may interact to contribute to faster aging of cells.

9. Telomere length and temperament

Damjanovic et al., when examining LTL in older caregivers, found that simply being a caregiver was related to shorter LTL and our recent study on dementia caregivers replicates this finding (O'Donovan et al., under review). However, many studies of stress exposure show individual differences, such as the experience of stress, or personality, those are linked to stress-related physiology. For example, Epel et al.'s 2004 study first demonstrated that level of perceived stress, as opposed to the inherently stressful caregiving situation itself, was correlated with shorter telomere length, suggesting that individual differences in stress vulnerability may be an underlying reason for the differences in telomere length between high and low stress groups. The older age of dementia caregivers may also contribute to vulnerability to stress-induced aging. O'Donovan et al. investigated whether dispositional characteristics are correlated with telomere length and found that pessimism negatively associated with telomere length, regardless of nursing status [O'Donovan et al., 2009]. The personality characteristics assessed in these studies - the experience of stress and pessimism - are relatively stable personality traits and thus may be operating over much of an individual's life, suggesting that they may have cumulative effects on cell aging, as reflected in telomere maintenance, during the relatively long periods.

10. Possible mechanisms mediating relationships between life style factors and telomere length

What potential mechanisms and pathways mediate the relationship between life style factors and telomere length? Research has focused on several interrelated biochemical pathways: stress hormones, inflammation and oxidative stress. Treatment of stimulated T-cells with the stress hormone cortisol in vitro causes decreases in cell proliferation, decreased telomerase activity and lower hTERT mRNA levels after cell activation [Choi et al., 2008]. In vivo, elevated levels of epinephrine, norepinephrine and cortisol were found to be associated with short telomere length in PBMCs [Epel et al., 2006; Parks et al., 2009]. Chronic stress and depression have also been linked to high levels of 8-hydroxy-deoxyguanosine (8-OHdG) and decreases in anti-oxidant enzymes [Forlenza et al., 2006; Irie et al., 2002; Irie et al., 2003; Liu et al., 1999; Tsuboi et al., 2004]. Oxidative stress preferentially damages telomeric versus other genomic DNA regions [Zglinicki et al., 2002] and inhibits telomerase activity in vitro in various cell types [Haendeler et al., 2003; Haendeler et al., 2004]. Micronutrients like vitamin C, E, folate acid and marine omega- 3 fatty acids are associated with anti-oxidative function [Jolly et al., 2001; Romieu et al., 2008], and thereby may be associated with long telomeres due to their anti-oxidative property. Stressed individuals have high levels of proinflammatory cytokines including IL-6 and TNF- alpha [Graham et al., 2006; Kiecolt-Glaser et al., 2003; Kiecolt-Glaser et al., 2005]. IL-6 has been shown to stimulate telomerase activity in cultured cells whereas TNF- alpha negatively regulates telomerase activity [Liu et al., 2010]. The concerted effects of these various biochemical mediators on telomerase may contribute to the observed associations between lifestyle factors and telomere length.

11. Is telomerase activation a compensatory mechanism induced by telomere shortness?

The Epel et al. 2004 study showed that low basal telomerase activity in unstimulated PBMCs is associated with worse stress in women without frank disease. This correlation was confirmed in a more recent study with women caregivers of dementia patients by the same author [Epel et al., 2010] as well as in other studies that showed increases in telomerase activity over a 3 month period were associated with improved health profiles [Ornish et al., 2008; Jacobs et al., 2011]. However, other studies have found the opposite relationship. In a different and older group of caregivers, who were primary caregivers for Alzheimers' patients, unstimulated telomerase activity in PBMC and T cells was higher in caregivers than in controls [Damjanovic et al., 2007]. Telomerase activity was higher in depressed individuals compared to the controls and was directly correlated with depression and stress ratings across both groups of subjects [Wolkowitz et al., 2011]. It was proposed that the elevated PBMC telomerase activity was an unsuccessful attempt of cells to compensate the excessive loss of telomeres in caregivers [Damjanovic et al., 2007]. This appears to support the notion that elevated telomerase activity is reactive to short telomere length. In vitro studies showed that telomerase preferentially add telomeric sequences to short telomeres [Teixeira et al., 2004; Chang et al., 2007; Britt-Compton et al., 2009]. Whether this also happens in vivo remains to be found. Telomerase activity in PBMCs is dynamic in response to acute psychological stress. When a group of post-menopausal women were exposed to a brief laboratory psychological stressor [Kirschbaum et al., 1993], telomerase activity was found to increase within one hour after the acute stressor and this increase was associated with greater cortisol increases in response to the stressor [Epel et al., 2010]. At the organism level, tight regulation of telomerase activity is essential for health as haploinsufficiency of telomerase activity due to genetic mutations is the cause of several human diseases, summarized as the syndromes of telomere shortening reviewed by [Armanios et al., 2009]. However, this does not rule out the possibility of temporal dynamic changes of telomerase activity in response to various stimuli.

12. Future directions

While cross-sectional studies are abundant, there have been very few longitudinal studies of telomere length [Aviv et al., 2009; Ehrlenbach et al., 2009; Epel et al., 2009; Nordfjall et al., 2009; Svenson et al., 2009; Farzaneh-Far et al., 2010]. One consistent finding from the published longitudinal data is that the rate of telomere length change over time is inversely related to the baseline telomere length [Aviv et al., 2009; Svenson et al., 2009; Farzaneh-Far et al., 2010]. The mechanisms that regulate this phenomenon are of great interest. The available studies have shown that telomere length trajectory over time predicts health outcome. For example, in the McArthur aging study, elderly men who showed telomere shortening over a 2.5 year period had a 3-fold higher chance of death from cardiovascular disease in the subsequent 9 years compared with those in the same cohort whose telomere length was maintained or lengthened [Epel et al., 2009]. More studies are clearly needed to establish cause-effect relationships between lifestyle factors, white blood telomere length and health outcomes. A large remaining puzzle in human populations is the relationship of telomerase activity (measured in blood lymphocytes) to life style factors and disease risks and states. As described above, results have been indicative of a complex relationship. Whether the heightened levels of telomerase reflect the cells' unsuccessful attempt to compensate for shorter telomere length, as was first suggested by Damjanovic et al. [Damjanovic et al., 2007], remains to be seen. Many of the studies of telomerase activity in white blood cells have involved a variety of study subject populations, with different disease and other characteristics, making comparisons between these studies difficult. It is known that the rate of telomere length change over time is inversely proportional to the baseline telomere length [Aviv et al., 2009; Svenson et al., 2009; Farzaneh-Far et al., 2010] although whether the rate of change of length is associated with telomerase activity has not been investigated in the population at large. It is also possible that elevated telomerase activity is a response to the proinflammatory cytokine environment associated with immunosenescence [Akiyama et al., 2002; Parish et al., 2009]. Whether epigenetic changes that result from changes in the cellular environments establish more long-lasting changes in telomerase and telomere length regulation is a question open for investigation. How much do lifestyle factors contribute to telomere length differences? Telomere length is determined by the collective effects of genetic, environmental, life experience and lifestyle factors. Several papers have estimated that genetics contribute to 30–80% of the variabilities in telomere length between individuals [Slagboom et al., 1994; Vasa-Nicotera et al., 2005; Andrew et al., 2006], leaving 20–70% of the variability unaccounted for, which presumably comes from external factors including environmental and lifestyle factors. Among these factors, interactions – with additive, synergistic or opposing effects on telomere maintenance – are likely to occur. Lifestyle and environmental factors are potentially modifiable elements in this equation. However, as discussed earlier, stress vulnerability and perception may be shaped by early life experience, such as childhood trauma, and may also partly be genetically predetermined, as in the case of personality traits. Lifestyle changes that have an impact on telomere length are likely to contribute to lower disease incidences and risks and healthy life. Indeed, in at least one elderly study cohort, long telomeres have been associated with years of healthy life [Njajou et al., 2009]. In summary, accelerated cell aging, at least as indexed by short leukocyte telomere length, is emerging as a strong determinant of early onset of diseases of aging. The converging picture from correlational studies of humans shows that cell aging is also intricately related to early life experience, and daily behavior. These studies provide compelling reasons to conduct intervention studies, to examine how much we can capitalize on these malleable relationships to reduce early illness and extend years of healthy living.

As a result, a strong argument can be made to strengthen healthcare on a number of fronts that involve improvements in preventative care and diagnosis, appropriate lifestyle modifications, and the initiation of new investigative platforms to understand the complexities of specific disorders as well as foster new avenues that can promote growth and maturation, mitigate aging-related disorders, and extend longevity.

13. References

A. Aviv, Shay, et al. (2005). The longevity gender gap: are telomeres the explanation? *Sci. Aging Knowl. Environ.* (23) (2005) pe16.

A. Aviv, W. Chen, et al. (2009). Leukocyte telomere dynamics: longitudinal findings among young adults in the Bogalusa Heart Study. *Am. J. Epidemiol.* 169 (3) 323–329.

A. Aviv. (2002). Telomeres, sex, reactive oxygen species, and human cardiovascular aging. *J. Mol. Med.* 80 (11) 689–695.

A. O'Donovan, E. Epel, et al. (2011). Childhood Trauma Associated with Short Leukocyte. Telomere Length in *Posttraumatic Stress Disorder, Biol. Psychiatry.*

A. O'Donovan, J. Lin, et al. (2009). Pessimism correlates with leukocyte telomere shortness and elevated interleukin-6 in post-menopausal women. *Brain Behav.Immun.* 23 (4) 446–449.

A. Steptoe, M. Hamer, et al. (2011). Educational attainment but not measures of current socioeconomic circumstances are associated with leukocyte telomere length in healthy older men and women. *Brain Behav. Immun.*

A.K Damjanovic, Y. Yang, et al. (2007). Accelerated telomere erosion is associated with a declining immune function of caregivers of Alzheimer's disease patients. *J. Immunol.* 179 (6) 4249–4254.

A.M. Valdes, T. Andrew, et al. (2005). Obesity, cigarette smoking, and telomere length in women, *Lancet* 366 (9486) 662–664.

A.R Tyrka, L.H. Price, et al. (2010). Childhood maltreatment and telomere shortening: preliminary support for an effect of early stress on cellular aging. *Biol. Psychiatry* 67 (6) 531–534.

Akiyama M, Hideshima T, Shammas MA, et al. (2003). Molecular sequelae of oligonucleotide N30-P50 phosphoramidate targeting telomerase RNA in human multiple myeloma cells. *Cancer Research*; 63:6187–6194.

Alcorta DA, Xiong Y, Phelps D, Hannon G, Beach D, Barrett JC. (1996). Involvement of the cyclin-dependent kinase inhibitor p16 (INK4a) in replicative senescence of normal human fibroblasts. *Proc Natl Acad Sci U S A. 93*:13742–13747.

Avci CB, Sahin F, Gunduz C, Selvi N, Aydin HH, Oktem G, Topcuoglu N, Saydam G. (2007). Protein phosphatase 2A (PP2A) has a potential role in CAPE-induced apoptosis of CCRF-CEM cells via effecting human telomerase reverse transcriptase activity. *Hematology*. 12(6):519-25.

Avci CB, Yilmaz S, Dogan ZO, Saydam G, Dodurga Y, EH Atakan, Kartal M, Sahin F, Baran Y, Gunduz C. (2011). Quercetin-induced apoptosis involves increased hTERT enzyme activity of leukemic cells. *Hematology*. Sep;16(5):303-7

B. Britt-Compton, R. Capper, et al. (2009). Short telomeres are preferentially elongated by telomerase in human cells. *FEBS Lett.* 583 (18) 3076–3080.

Benetti R, Garcia-Cao M, Blasco MA. (2007). Telomere length regulates the epigenetic status of mammalian telomeres and subtelomeres. *Nat Gene.* 39:243–250.

Bodnar AG, Ouellette M, Frolkis M, et al. (1998). Extension of life-span by introduction of telomerase into normal human cells. *Science.* 279:349–352.

Brouilette S, Singh RK, Thompson JR, et al. (2003). White cell telomere length and risk of prematüre myocardial infarction. *Arterioscler Thromb Vasc Biol;* 23:842–846.

Brouilette SW, Moore JS, McMahon AD, et al. (2007). Telomere length, risk of coronary heart disease, and statin treatment in the West of Scotland Primary Prevention Study: a nested case-control study. *Lancet.* 369:107–114.

C. Kirschbaum, K.M. Pirke, et al. (1993). The 'Trier Social Stress Test' – a tool for investigating psychobiological stress responses in a laboratory setting. *Neuropsychobiology* 28 (1–2) 76–81.

C.A Jolly, A. Muthukumar, et al. (2001). Life span is prolonged in food-restricted autoimmune-prone (NZB×NZW) F(1) mice fed a diet enriched with (n-3) fatty acids. *J. Nutr.* 131 (10) 2753–2760.

C.G. Parks, D.B. Miller, et al. (2009). Telomere length, current perceived stress, and urinary stress hormones in women, *Cancer Epidemiol. Biomarkers Prev.* 18 (2) 551–560.

Cassidy A, De Vivo I, Liu Y, et al. (2010). Associations between diet, lifestyle factors, and telomere length in women. *Am J Clin Nut.* 91:1273–1280.

Cawthon RM, Smith KR, O'Brien E, et al. (2003). Association between telomere length in blood and mortality in people aged 60 years or older. *Lancet*; 361:393–395.

Celli GB, de Lange T. (2005). DNA processing is not required for ATM mediated telomere damage response after TRF2 deletion. *Nat Cell Biol*; 7:712– 718.

Cherkas LF, Hunkin JL, Kato BS, et al. (2008). The association between physical activity in leisure time and leukocyte telomere length. *Arch Intern Med*; 168:154–158.

Chin L, Artandi SE, Shen Q, et al. (1999). p53 deficiency rescues the adverse effects of telomere loss and cooperates with telomere dysfunction to accelerate carcinogenesis. *Cell*; 97:527–538.

Cogulu O, Biray C, Gunduz C, Karaca E, Aksoylar S, Sorkun K, Salih B, Ozkinay F. (2009). Effects of Manisa propolis on telomerase activity in leukemia cells obtained from the bone marrow of leukemia patients. *Int J Food Sci Nutr.* Nov:60(7):601-5.

de Lange T, Shiue L, Myers RM, et al. (1990). Structure and variability of human chromosome ends. *Mol Cell Biol.* 10:518-527.

De Lange T. Telomere-related genome instability in cancer. (2005). *Cold Spring Harb Symp Quant Biol*; 70:197–204.

Dunham MA, Neumann AA, Fasching CL, Reddel RR. (2000). Telomere maintenance by recombination in human cells. *Nat Genet*; 26:447–450.

E.S Epel, J. Lin, et al. (2010). Dynamics of telomerase activity in response to acute psychological stress, *Brain Behav. Immun.* 24 (4) 531–539.

E.S Epel, S.S. Merkin, et al. (2009). The rate of leukocyte telomere shortening predicts mortality from cardiovascular disease in elderly men, *Aging* 1 (1) 81–88.

E.S. Epel, E.H. Blackburn, et al. (2004). Accelerated telomere shortening in response to life stress. *Proc. Natl. Acad. Sci. U.S.A.* 101 (49) 17312–17315.

E.S. Epel, J. Lin, et al. (2006). Cell aging in relation to stress arousal and cardiovascular disease risk factors, *Psychoneuroendocrinology* 31 (3) 277–287.

Epel ES, Blackburn EH, Lin J, et al. (2004). Accelerated telomere shortening in response to life stress. *Proc Natl Acad Sci U S A*; 101:17312–17315.

Esteller M. (2006). Epigenetics provides a new generation of oncogenes and tumoursuppressor genes. *Br J Cancer*; 94:179–183.

F.W. Lung, N.C. Chen, et al. (2007). Genetic pathway of major depressive disorder in shortening telomeric length, *Psychiatr. Genet.* 17 (3) 195–199.

Farzaneh-Far R, Lin J, Epel ES, et al. (2010). Association with marine omega-2-fatty acid levels with telomeric aging in patients with coronary heart disease. *AMA*; 303:250–257.

Fitzpatrick AL, Kronmal RA, Gardner JP, et al. (2007). Leukocyte telomere length and cardiovascular disease in the cardiovascular health study. *Am J Epidemiol;* 165:14–21.

Frenck RW Jr, Blackburn EH, Shannon KM. (1998). The rate of telomere sequence loss in human leukocytes varies with age. *Proc Natl Acad Sci U S A;* 95:5607–5610.

Furukawa S, Fujita T, Shimabukuro M, et al. (2004). Increased oxidative stress in obesity and its impact on metabolic syndrome. *J Clin Invest;* 114:1752- 1761.

G.D Batty, Y. Wang, et al. (2009). Socioeconomic status and telomere length: the West of Scotland Coronary Prevention Study. *J. Epidemiol. Community Health* 63 (10) 839-841.

Gammon SJ, Terry MB, Wang Q, et al. (2009). Telomere length, oxidative damage, and antioxidant breast cancer risk. *Int J Cancer;* 124:1637–1643.

Gilley D, Tanaka H, Herbert BS. (2005). Telomere dysfunction in aging and cancer. *Int J Biochem Cell Biol.* 37:1000–1013.

Gong JG, Costanzo A, Yang HQ, et al. (1999). The tyrosine kinase c-Abl regulates p73 in apoptotic response to cisplatin-induced DNA damage. *Nature;* 399:806–809.

Griffith JD, Comeau L, Rosenfield S, et al. (1999). Mammalian telomeres end in a large duplex loop. *Cell;* 97:503–514.

Gunduz C, Biray C, Kosova B, Yilmaz B, Eroglu Z, Sahin F, Omay SB, Cogulu O. (2005). Evaluation of Manisa propolis effect on leukemia cell line by telomerase activity. *Leuk Res.;* 29: 1343-6.

H. Tsuboi, K. Shimoi, et al. (2004). Depressive symptoms are independently correlated with lipid peroxidation in a female population: comparison with vitamins and carotenoids, *J. Psychosom. Res.* 56 (1) 53–58.

Harley CB, Futcher AB, Greider CW. (1990). Telomeres shorten during ageing of human fibroblasts. *Nature.* 345:458-460.

Herbig U, Jobling WA, Chen BP, Chen DJ, Sedivy JM. (2004). Telomere shortening triggers senescence of human cells through a pathway involving ATM, p53, and p21(CIP1), but not p16(INK4a). *Mol Cell.* 14:501–513.

Hoxha M, Dioni L, Bonzini M, et al. (2009). Association between leukocyte telomere shortening and exposure to traffic pollution: a cross-sectional study on traffic officers and indoor office workers. *Environ Health;* 8:41.

I. Romieu, R. Garcia-Esteban, et al. (2008). The effect of supplementation with omega-3 polyunsaturated fatty acids on markers of oxidative stress in elderly exposed to PM(2.5), *Environ. Health Perspect.* 116 (9) 1237–1242.

Irie M, Asami S, Ikeda M, Kasai H. (2003). Depressive state relates to female oxidative DNA damage via neutrophil activation. *Biochem Biophys Res Commun;* 311:1014–1018.

J. Choi, S.R. Fauce, et al. (2008). Reduced telomerase activity in human T lymphocytes exposed to cortisol, *Brain Behav. Immun.* 22 (4) 600–605.

J. Haendeler, J. Hoffmann, et al. (2003). Hydrogen peroxide triggers nuclear export of telomerase reverse transcriptase via Src kinase family-dependent phosphorylation of tyrosine 707, *Mol. Cell. Biol.* 23 (13) 4598–4610.

J. Haendeler, J. Hoffmann, et al. (2004). Antioxidants inhibit nuclear export of telomerase reverse transcriptase and delay replicative senescence of endothelial cells, *Circ. Res.* 94 (6) 768–775.

J. Humphreys, E.S. Epel, et al. (2011). Telomere shortening in formerly abused and never abused women, *Biol. Res. Nurs.*

J. Liu, A. Mori et al. (1999). Stress, aging, and brain oxidative damage, *Neurochem. Res.* 24(11) 1479–1497.

J. Woo, E.W. Suen, et al. (2009). Older men with higher self-rated socioeconomic status have shorter telomeres, Age *Ageing* 38 (5) 553–558.

J.A. Nettleton, L.M. Steffen, et al. (2008). Associations between microalbuminuria and animal foods, plant foods, and dietary patterns in the Multiethnic Study of Atherosclerosis, *Am. J. Clin. Nutr.* 87 (6) 1825–1836.

J.B Richards, A.M. Valdes, et al. (2007). Higher serum vitamin D concentrations are associated with longer leukocyte telomere length in women, *Am. J. Clin. Nutr.* 86 (5) 1420–1425.

J.B. Richards, A.M. Valdes, et al. (2008). Homocysteine levels and leukocyte telomere length, *Atherosclerosis* 200 (2) 271–277.

J.E Graham, L.M. Christian, et al. (2006). Stress, age, and immune function: toward a lifespan approach, *J. Behav. Med.* 29 (4) 389–400.

J.K Kiecolt-Glaser, J.P. Gouin, et al. (2011). Childhood adversity heightens the impact of later-life caregiving stress on telomere length and inflammation, *Psychosom. Med.* 73 (1) 16–22.

J.K Kiecolt-Glaser, K.J. Preacher, et al. (2003). Chronic stress and age-related increases in the proinflammatory cytokine IL-6, *Proc. Natl. Acad. Sci. U.S.A.* 100 (15) 9090–9095.

J.K. Kiecolt-Glaser, T.J. Loving, et al. (2005). Hostile marital interactions, proinflammatory cytokine production, and wound healing, *Arch. Gen. Psychiatry* 62 (12) 1377–1384.

J.P Liu, S.M. Chen, et al. (2010). Regulation of telomerase activity by apparently opposing elements, *Ageing Res. Rev.* 9 (3) 245–256.

Jennings BJ, Ozanne SE, Dorling MW, Hales CN. (1999). Early growth determines longevity in male rats and may be related to telomere shortening in the kidney. *FEBS Lett*; 448:4–8.

Jennings BJ, Ozanne SE, Hales CN. (2000). Nutrition, oxidative damage, telomere shortening, and cellular senescence: individual or connected agents of aging? *Mol Genet Metab*; 71:32–42.

Jiang H, Schiffer E, Song Z, et al. (2008). Proteins induced by telomere dysfunction and DNA damage represent biomarkers of human aging and disease. *Proc Natl Acad Sci U S A*; 105:11299 11304.

K. Nordfjall, M. Eliasson, et al. (2008). Increased abdominal obesity, adverse psychosocial factors and shorter telomere length in subjects reporting early ageing; the MONICA Northern Sweden Study, *Scand. J. Public Health* 36 (7) 744–752.

K. Nordfjall, M. Eliasson, et al. (2008). Telomere length is associated with obesity parameters but with a gender difference, *Obesity* 16 (12) 2682–2689.

K. Nordfjall, U. Svenson, et al. (2009). The individual blood cell telomere attrition rate is telomere length dependent, *PLoS Genet.* 5 (2)

Kim, N. W., Piatyszek, M. A., Prowse, K. R., Harley, C. B., West, M. D., Ho, P. L., Coviello, G. M., Wright, W. E., Weinrich, S. L. and Shay, J.W. (1994). *Specific association of human telomerase activity with immortal cells and cancer. Science* 266, 2011-2015.

L. Kananen, I. Surakka, et al. (2010). Childhood adversities are associated with shorter telomere length at adult age both in individuals with an anxiety disorder and controls, *PLoS One* 5 (5)

L. Mirabello, W.Y. Huang, et al. (2009). The association between leukocyte telomere length and cigarette smoking, dietary and physical variables, and risk of prostate cancer, *Aging Cell* 8 (4) 405–413.

L. Paul, M. Cattaneo, et al. (2009). Telomere length in peripheral blood mononuclear cells is associated with folate status in men, *J. Nutr.* 139 (7) 1273–1278.

L. Paul. (2011). Diet, nutrition and telomere length, *J. Nutr. Biochem.*

L.F. Cherkas, A. Aviv, et al. (2006). The effects of social status on biological aging as measured by white-blood-cell telomere length, *Aging Cell* 5 (5) 361–365.

M. Akiyama, T. Hideshima, et al. (2002). Cytokines modulate telomerase activity in a human multiple myeloma cell line, *Cancer Res.* 62 (13) 3876–3882.

M. Armanios. (2009). Syndromes of telomere shortening, *Annu. Rev. Genomics Hum. Genet.* 10 45–61.

M. Chang, M. Arneric, et al. (2007). Telomerase repeat addition processivity is increased at critically short telomeres in a Tel1-dependent manner in Saccharomyces cerevisiae, *Genes Dev.* 21 (19) 2485–2494.

M. Irie, S. Asami, et al. (2002). Psychological mediation of a type of oxidative DNA damage, 8-hydroxydeoxyguanosine, in peripheral blood leukocytes of nonsmoking and non-drinking workers, *Psychother. Psychosom.* 71 (2) 90–96.

M. Irie, S. Asami, et al. (2003). Depressive state relates to female oxidative DNA damage via neutrophil activation, *Biochem. Biophys. Res. Commun.* 311 (4) 1014–1018.

M. Lee, H. Martin, et al. (2011). Inverse association between adiposity and telomere length: The fels longitudinal study, *Am. J. Hum. Biol.* 23 (1) 100–106.

M. McGrath, J.Y. Wong, et al. (2007). Telomere length, cigarette smoking, and bladder cancer risk in men and women, *Cancer Epidemiol. Biomarkers Prev.* 16 (4) 815–819.

M. Morla, X. Busquets, et al. (2006). Telomere shortening in smokers with and without COPD, *Eur. Respir. J.* 27 (3) 525–528.

M. Vasa-Nicotera, S. Brouilette, et al. (2005). Mapping of a major locus that determines telomere length in humans, *Am. J. Hum. Genet.* 76 (1) 147–151.

M.A. Babizhayev, Y.E. Yegorov. (2010). Smoking and health: association between telomere length and factors impacting on human disease, quality of life and lifespan in a large population-based cohort under the effect of smoking duration, *Fundam. Clin. Pharmacol.*

M.J Forlenza, G.E. Miller. (2006). Increased serum levels of 8-hydroxy-2′-deoxyguanosine in clinical depression, *Psychosom. Med.* 68 (1) 1–7.

M.T Teixeira, M. Arneric, et al. (2004) Telomere length homeostasis is achieved via a switch between telomerase-extendible and nonextendible states, *Cell* 117 (3) 323–335.

Matsuzaki T. Longevity, diet, and nutrition in Japan.(1992). *Epidemiological studies. Nutr Rev 50*:355–359

McGrath M, Wong JY, Michaud D, et al. (2007). Telomere length, cigarette smoking, and bladder cancer risk in men and women. *Cancer Epidemiol Biomarkers Prev*; 16:815–819.

Meeker AK. (2006). Telomeres and telomerase in prostatic intraepithelial neoplasia and prostate cancer biology. *Urol Oncol*; 24:122–130.

Morla ´ M, Busquets X, Pons J, et al. (2006). Telomere shortening in smokers with and without COPD, *Eur Respir J* 27:525–528.

Munoz P, Blanco R, Flores JM, Blasco MA. (2005). XPF nuclease-dependent telomere loss and increased DNA damage in mice overexpressing TRF2 result in premature aging and cancer. *Nat Genet*; 37:1063–1071.

N. Hartmann, M. Boehner, et al. (2010). Telomere length of patients with major depression is shortened but independent from therapy and severity of the disease, *Depress. Anxiety* 27 (12) 1111–1116.

N.J O'Callaghan, P.M. Clifton, et al. (2009). Weight loss in obese men is associated with increased telomere length and decreased abasic sites in rectal mucosa, *Rejuvenation Res.* 12 (3) 169–176.

N.M Simon, J.W. Smoller, et al. (2006). Telomere shortening and mood disorders: preliminary support for a chronic stress model of accelerated aging, *Biol. Psychiatry* 60 (5) 432–435.

Nawrot TS, Staessen JA, Gardner JP, Aviv A. (2004). Telomere length and possible link to X chromosome. *Lancet*; 363:507–510.

Nordfjall K, Eliasson M, Stegmayr B, et al. (2008). Telomere length is associated with obesity parameters but with a gender difference. *Obesity*; 16:2682–2689.

O.M Wolkowitz, E.S. Epel, et al. (2008). When blue turns to grey: do stress and depression accelerate cell aging? *World J. Biol. Psychiatry* 9 (1) 2–5.

O.M Wolkowitz, S.H. Mellon, et al. (2011). Resting leukocyte telomerase activity is elevated in major depression and predicts treatment response, *Mol. Psychiatry*

O.M. Wolkowitz, S.H. Mellon, et al. (2011). Leukocyte telomere length in majör depression: correlations with chronicity, inflammation and oxidative stress–preliminary findings, *PLoS ONE* 6 (3)

O.S. Al-Attas, N.M. Al-Daghri, et al. (2010). Adiposity and insulin resistance correlate with telomere length in middle-aged Arabs: the influence of circulating adiponectin, *Eur. J. Endocrinol.* 163 (4) 601–607.

O.T Njajou, W.C. Hsueh, et al. (2009). Association between telomere length, specific causes of death, and years of healthy life in health, aging, and body composition, a population-based cohort study, *J. Gerontol. A. Biol. Sci. Med. Sci.* 64 (8) 860–864.

P.E. Slagboom, S. Droog, et al. (1994). Genetic determination of telomere size in humans: a twin study of three age groups, *Am. J. Hum. Genet.* 55 (5) 876–882.

P.G. Surtees, N.W. Wainwright, et al. (2011). Life Stress, Emotional Health, and Mean Telomere Length in the European Prospective Investigation into Cancer (EPIC)-Norfolk Population Study, *J. Gerontol. A. Biol. Sci. Med. Sci.*. D. Glass, L. Parts, et al. (2010). No correlation between childhood maltreatment and telomere length, *Biol. Psychiatry* 68 (6) e23–e24, e21-22; author reply

Patel R, McIntosh L, McLaughlin J, et al. (2002). Disruptive effects of glucocorticoids on glutathione peroxidase biochemistry in hippocampal cultures. *J Neurochem*; 82:118–125.

Pavanello S, Pesatori AC, Dioni L, et al. (2010). Shorter telomere length in peripheral blood lymphocytes of workers exposed to polycyclic aromatic hydrocarbons. *Carcinogenesis;* 31:216–221.

Q. Xu, C.G. Parks, et al. (2009). Multivitamin use and telomere length in women, *Am. J. Clin. Nutr.* 89 (6) 1857–1865.

R. Farzaneh-Far, J. Lin, et al. (2010). Telomere length trajectory and its determinants in persons with coronary artery disease: longitudinal findings from the heart and soul study, *PLoS One* 5 (1) e8612.

R.A. Risques, K.G. Arbeev, et al. (2010). Leukocyte telomere length is associated with disability in older U.S. Population, *J. Am. Geriatr. Soc.* 58 (7) 1289–1298.

R.Y. Zee, A.J. Castonguay, et al. (2010). Mean leukocyte telomere length shortening and type 2 diabetes mellitus: a case-control study, *Transl. Res.* 155 (4) 166–169.

S. Ehrlenbach, P. Willeit, et al. (2009). Influences on the reduction of relative telomere length over 10 years in the population-based Bruneck Study: introduction of a well-controlled high-throughput assay, *Int. J. Epidemiol.* 38 (6) 1725–1734.

S.C. Hunt, W. Chen, et al. (2008). Leukocyte telomeres are longer in african americans than in whites: the national heart, lung, and blood institute family heart studyand the Bogalusa Heart Study, *Aging Cell* 7 (4) 451–458.

S.T Parish, J.E. Wu, et al. (2009). Modulation of T lymphocyte replicative senescence via TNF-{alpha} inhibition: role of caspase-3, *J. Immunol.* 182 (7) 4237–4243.

Sahin F, Avci CB, Gunduz C, Sezgin C, Simsir IY, Saydam G. (2010). Gossypol exert cytotoxic effect on HL-60 leukemic cell line via decreasing activity of protein phosphatase 2A and interacting with human telomerase reverse transcriptase activity. *Hematology.* Jun;15(3):144-50.

Sampson MJ, Winterbone MS, Hughes JC, et al. (2006). Monocyte telomere shortening and oxidative DNA damage in type 2 diabetes. *Diabetes Care;* 29:283–289.

Shammas MA, Shmookler Reis RJ, Koley H, et al. (2009). Dysfunctional homologous recombination mediates genomic instability and progression in myeloma. *Blood;* 113:2290–2297.

Shin JS, Hong A, Solomon MJ, Lee CS. (2006). The role of telomeres and telomerase in the pathology of human cancer and aging. *Pathology;* 38:103–113.

Song Z, von Figura G, Liu Y, et al. (2010). Lifestyle impacts on the aging-associated expression of biomarkers of DNA damage and telomere dysfunction in human blood. *Aging Cell;* 9:607–615.

Starr JM, McGurn B, Harris SE, Whalley LJ, Deary IJ, Shiels PG. (2007). Association between telomere length and heart disease in a narrow age cohort of older people. *Exp Gerontol* 42(6):571-3.

Stein GH, Drullinger LF, Soulard A, Dulić V. (1999). Differential roles for cyclin-dependent kinase inhibitors p21 and p16 in the mechanisms of senescence and differentiation in human fibroblasts. *Mol Cell Biol.* 19:2109–2117.

Steinert S, Shay JW, Wright WE. (2001). Modification of subtelomeric DNA. Mol Cell Biol 2004; 24:4571–4580.

Stiewe T, Putzer BM. p73 in apoptosis. *Apoptosis;* 6:447–452.

T. Andrew, A. Aviv, et al. (2006). Mapping genetic loci that determine leukocyte telomere length in a large sample of unselected female sibling pairs, *Am. J. Hum. Genet.* 78 (3) 480–486.

T. von Zglinicki. (2002). Oxidative stress shortens telomeres, *Trends Biochem. Sci.* 27(7) 339–344.

T.S. Nawrot, J.A. Staessen, et al. (2010). Telomere length and its associations with oxidized-LDL, carotid artery distensibility and smoking, *Front Biosci.* 2 1164–1168.

Takubo K, Nakamura K, Izumiyama N, et al. (2000). Telomere shortening with aging in human liver. *J Gerontol A Biol Sci Med Sci*; 55:B533–B536.

U. Svenson, B. Ljungberg, et al. (2009). Telomere length in peripheral blood predicts survival in clear cell renal cell carcinoma, *Cancer Res.* 69 (7) 2896–2901.

Valdes AM, Andrew T, Gardner JP, et al. (2005). Obesity, cigarette smoking, and telomere length in women. *Lancet*; 366:662–664.

Valdes AM, Richards JB, Gardner JP, et al. (2007). Telomere length in leukocytes correlates with bone mineral density and is shorter in women with osteoporosis. *Osteoporos Int*; 18:1203–1210.

Van der Harst P, van der Steege G, de Boer RA, et al. (2007). Telomere length of circulating leukocytes is decreased in patients with chronic heart failure. *J Am Coll Cardiol*; 49:1459–1464.

Van Steensel B, Smogorzewska A, de Lange T. (1998). TRF2 protects human telomeres from end-to-end fusions. *Cell*; 92:401–413.

Von Zglinicki T. (2002). Oxidative stress shortens telomeres. *Trends Biochem Sci.*; 27:339–344.

Vulliamy T, Marrone A, Goldman F, et al. (2001). The RNA component of telomerase is mutated in autosomal dominant dyskeratosis congenita. *Nature*; 413:432–435.

Werner C, Fu ¨ rster T, Widmann T, et al. (2009). Physical exercise prevents cellular senescence in circulating leukocytes and in the vessel wall. *Circulation* 120:2438–2447.

Wright, W. E., Piatyszek, M. A., Rainey, W. E., Byrd, W. and Shay, J. W. (1996). Telomerase activity in human germline and embryonic tissues and cells. *Dev. Genet.* 18, 173-179.

Wu X, Amos CI, Zhu Y, et al. (2003). Telomere dysfunction: a potential cancer predisposition factor. *J Natl Cancer Inst*; 95:1211–1218.

Zee RY, Michaud SE, Germer S, Ridker PM. (2009). Association of shorter mean telomere length with risk of incident myocardial infarction: a prospective, nested case-control approach. *Clin Chim Acta*; 403:139–141.

8

Telomere as an Important Player in Regulation of Microbial Pathogen Virulence

Bibo Li
Cleveland State University
USA

1. Introduction

Telomeres are nucleoprotein complexes located at the ends of linear chromosomes. In most eukaryotic cells, telomere DNA consists of simple repetitive TG-rich sequences, with the TG-rich strand running 5′ to 3′ towards the chromosome ends. Telomere DNA contains both the duplex region and a 3′ G-rich single-stranded overhang at the very end. In human, mouse, a hypotrichous ciliate, and trypanosomes, the single-stranded telomere G-overhang invades the double-stranded region and forms a T-loop structure (Griffith et al. 1999; Munoz-Jordan et al. 2001; Murti & Prescott 1999; Nikitina & Woodcock 2004), which has been proposed to play an important role in chromosome end protection (de Lange 2002).

A number of proteins have been identified to specifically associate with the telomere DNA, and this telomere complex appears to be largely conserved from protozoa to mammals. The telomere protein complex termed "Shelterin" is well characterized in mammalian cells (Fig. 1) (de Lange 2005). Within the complex, TTAGGG Repeat binding Factor 1 (TRF1) and TRF2 are duplex telomere DNA binding factors (Bilaud et al. 1997; Broccoli et al. 1997; Chong et al. 1995), Protection of Telomeres 1 (POT1) is a single-stranded telomere DNA binding factor (Baumann & Cech 2001), while Repressor Activator Protein 1 (RAP1) (Li et al. 2000), TRF1-Interacting Nuclear factor 2 (TIN2) (Kim et al. 1999), and TPP1 (previously known as POT1-interacting protein PIP1 (Ye et al. 2004), TIN2 interacting protein TINT1 (Houghtaling et al. 2004), or POT1- and TIN2-interacting factor PTOP (Liu et al. 2004)) do not directly contact telomere DNA but tightly associate with TRFs or POT1. Very recently, a trimeric CST complex containing Conserved Telomere maintenance Component 1 (CTC1), STN1, and TEN1 have also been identified in human cells to bind the single-stranded telomere DNA (Miyake et al. 2009; Wan et al. 2009).

In fission yeast *Schizosaccharomyces pombe,* SpTaz1 (a TRF homolog), SpRap1, SpPot1, SpPoz1 (a TIN2 homolog), SpTpz1 (a TPP1 homolog), SpTen1, and SpStn1 have been identified (Fig. 1), and the complex is very similar to that in mammalian cells (Dehe & Cooper 2010). Recent studies in our lab has led to the identification of TRF (Li et al. 2005), RAP1 (Yang et al. 2009), and TIN2 (Jehi S. & Li B., unpublished data) homologues in *Trypanosoma brucei*, a protozoan parasite belongs to the kinetoplastids group (Fig. 1), although no specific single-stranded telomere DNA binding proteins has been identified in this organism. These studies indicated that the TRF-RAP1-TIN2-TPP1-POT1 complex is at least partially conserved from protozoan to mammalian cells. However, the telomere complex in budding yeast

Saccharomyces cerevisiae is much less conserved (Fig. 1). ScRap1, instead of a TRF homolog, binds the duplex telomere DNA (Longtine et al. 1989b), while TIN2, TPP1, and POT1 homologs appear to have been lost, and the ScCdc13/ScTen1/ScStn1 complex binds the single-stranded telomere DNA (Grandin et al. 1997, 2001; Nugent et al. 1996).

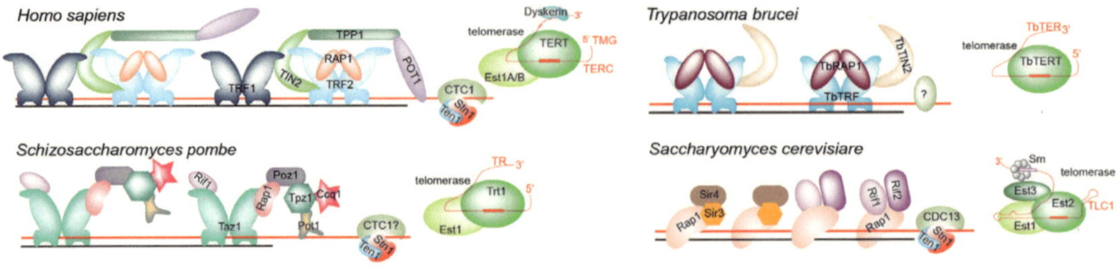

Fig. 1. The telomere complexes in human cells, budding and fission yeasts, and a protozoan parasite, *Trypanosoma brucei*. Proteins specifically associate with the telomeres are shown and marked. The telomerase holoenzyme is also shown. In human cells, TERT and TERC are the protein and the RNA component, respectively. Est1A/B is part of the holoenzyme, while Dyskerin interacts with TERC and plays an important role for TERC maturation. The telomerase (Trt1 and TR) and its associated Est1 has been identified in *S. pombe*. In *S. cerevisiae*, the core telomerase (Est2 and TLC1) is associated with Est1 and Est3, while TLC1 interacts with Sm proteins to maintain its stability.

Telomeres have two essential functions. First, binding of telomere proteins masks the natural chromosome ends so that telomeres are not recognized as DNA double strand breaks (DSB) and are protected from illegitimate DNA degradation, repair, and recombination processes (Stewart et al. 2011). Hence, the telomere structure is essential for genome integrity. Second, conventional DNA polymerases are incapable of fully replicate the ends of linear DNA molecules, and telomeres are expected to shorten progressively after each round of DNA replication (Levy et al. 1992). Fortunately, a specialized reverse transcriptase called telomerase can synthesize *de novo* the telomere G-rich strand DNA according to its internal RNA template and effectively solve this "end replication problem" (Greider & Blackburn 1987; Zvereva et al. 2010). Both chromosome end protection and telomere maintenance are complicated processes and are regulated at multiple levels. For more comprehensive reviews on these topics, please refer to (Cifuentes-Rojas & Shippen 2011; Palm & de Lange 2008; Stewart et al. 2011)

It is worth to point out that recombination mechanisms can be activated to maintain the telomere length when telomerase is absent in many organisms including yeasts and mammals (Bryan et al. 1995; Hande et al. 1999; Lendvay et al. 1996; Lundblad & Szostak 1989; Nabetani & Ishikawa 2011; Niida et al. 2000; Singer & Gottschling 1994). In *S. cerevisiae*, when telomerase is dysfunctional, a *RAD51*-dependent recombination pathway can amplify the subtelomeric Y' element to generate Type I survivors (Le et al. 1999; Teng & Zakian 1999), and a *RAD50*-dependent recombination pathway can amplify the telomere repeats to give rise to Type II survivors (Le et al. 1999; Lundblad & Blackburn 1993; McEachern & Blackburn 1996; Teng & Zakian 1999; Teng et al. 2000). Both pathways depend on *RAD52*, indicating that recommendation events are involved. In ~10% of human tumor cells, telomeres are maintained by a telomerase-independent mechanisms termed ALT (Reddel et al. 1997). In the ALT cells, telomere lengths are typically very heterogeneous, ranging from <3 kb to >50 kb (Bryan et al.

1995, 1997; Grobelny et al. 2000; Murnane et al. 1994; Opitz et al. 2001). Telomere maintenance in ALT cells appears to also involve recombination between different telomeres: when a plasmid tag was targeted into a telomere in a clonal ALT cell, with increasing population doubling, a progressive increase in the number of chromosomes containing the tagged telomeres was observed by FISH analysis (Dunham et al. 2000). Using a Chromosome Oriented-FISH (CO-FISH) analysis (Bailey et al. 2001), a detailed analysis of a number of mortal cell strains, *in vitro* immortalized cell lines, and cancer-derived cell lines showed that postreplicative exchanges involving a telomere and another TTAGGG-repeat tract occurred frequently in ALT cells but only rarely or never in non–ALT cells (Bailey et al. 2004; Londono-Vallejo et al. 2004), further suggesting that telomere recombination is a main pathway for telomere maintenance in ALT cells. In addition, one unusual telomere maintenance has been observed in telomerase negative *Trypanosoma brucei* cells (Dreesen & Cross 2006b). At least for a subset of telomeres that are marked with subtelomeric silent *VSG* expression sites (see below), the telomere can be as short as ~40 bp. Yet, these telomeres can be maintained stably for several tens of population doublings. However, the underlying mechanism is completely unknown.

2. Telomere position effect (TPE)

2.1 The phenomenon of TPE

Telomere position effect or TPE has been observed in a number of organisms, where the telomere structure exerts a variegated repressive effect on the transcription of genes located at subtelomeric regions.

TPE was first observed in *D. melanogaster* as a phenomenon of position effect variegation (PEV), which is a silencing effect on a gene located near a heterochromatic region in general (Gehring et al. 1984; Hazelrigg et al. 1984; Levis et al. 1985). A few years later, TPE was observed in *S. cerevisiae* (Gottschling et al. 1990): When a *URA3* marker together with a short TG_{1-3} telomere seed sequence is inserted to the left arm of chromosome VII at the subtelomeric region, the original VII-L telomere breaks off, and a new telomere forms from the seed ~1.1 kb from the *URA3* transcription starting site. This *URA3* gene can be expressed, allowing cells to grow on uracil lacking medium, but it can also be suppressed, allowing cells to grow on 5-FOA-containing medium (5-FOA will be converted to a toxic compound by the functional *URA3* gene product). Therefore, the silencing effect is variegated and its regulation appears to be epigenetic. Similarly, a subtelomeric *ADE2* marker can be either expressed (colonies are white when growing on low adenine medium) or silenced (colonies are red). In addition, the transcriptional state is quite stable, inheritable for a number of generations, giving rise to yeast colonies with red and white sectors.

A fundamental aspect of TPE is position dependent, which reflects that the silencing machinery works in a *cis*-acting fashion - association of the machinery with the telomere is necessary for an effect on subtelomeric genes. Studies in several organisms revealed a common theme: telomere DNA is the anchor, and one or two telomere binding proteins would recruit the silencing machinery to the telomere to establish TPE.

2.2 TPE in *S. cerevisiae*

Extensive studies in the last couple of decades have led to a fairly good understanding of TPE in *S. cerevisiae*. One of the key players for TPE in *S. cerevisiae* is Rap1 (Kyrion et al. 1993), which binds telomere DNA directly (Giraldo & Rhodes 1994; Konig et al. 1996; Longtine et al. 1989a) and recruits Sir3 and Sir4 silencers to the telomere through its C-terminal RCT domain (Buck & Shore 1995; Chen et al. 2011; Cockell et al. 1995; Feeser & Wolberger 2008; Hecht et al. 1996; Liu & Lustig 1996; Luo et al. 2002; Moretti & Shore 2001; Moretti et al. 1994).

S. cerevisiae Rap1 has a central myb domain that is quite similar to the classical myb DNA binding motif, with the three helices forming a helix-turn-helix structure (Fig. 2) (Konig et al. 1996). In addition, ScRap1 also has a myb-like domain baring an atypical long insertion between its first and second helices (Konig et al. 1996). Nevertheless, the myb and myb-like domains are able to coordinate with each other and enable ScRap1 to bind the duplex telomere DNA directly (Konig et al. 1996). It is interesting to note that human RAP1 appears to contain only one myb domain (Li et al. 2000), whose third helix presents a negatively charged surface (Hanaoka et al. 2001), so it does not interact with telomere DNA directly. Rather, human RAP1 is tethered to the telomeres through its interaction with TRF2, a duplex telomere DNA binding factor. Similarly, *S. pombe* Rap1 seems to rely on SpTaz1, the duplex telomere DNA binding factor in *S. pombe* and a TRF homolog (Cooper et al. 1997; Li et al. 2000), to recruit it to the telomere. In support of this, SpRap1 is rarely found to localized at the telomere in SpTaz1 null cells (Cooper et al. 1997; Kanoh & Ishikawa 2001). However, it is not clear whether residue amount of SpRap1 may still be associated with the telomere independent of SpTaz1. The RAP1 homolog has also been identified in *Trypanosoma brucei*, a protozoan parasite, and it seems to have both the myb and myb-like domains (Yang et al. 2009). Preliminary structural analysis of the myb-like domain suggests that TbRAP1 may have some weak sequence non-specific DNA binding activities (Zhao Y. & Li, B. unpublished data), but more careful analyses are necessary before a clear conclusion can be drawn.

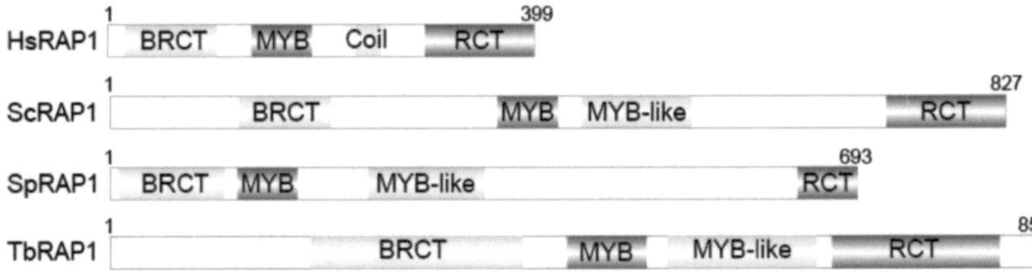

Fig. 2. Domain structure of RAP1 homologs. All RAP1s have a BRCT, a myb, and an RCT domain. In addition, except human RAP1, which has a Coil domain, all other RAP1 homologs have a myb-like domain next to the myb domain.

Other than the myb domain, RAP1 homologs have an N-terminal BRCA1 C Terminus (BRCT) domain at the N-terminal half of the protein (Bork et al. 1997; Callebaut & Mornon 1997; Li et al. 2000; Yang et al. 2009), which is usually found in proteins involved in DNA damage response or cell cycle checkpoint and is often capable of binding proteins with phosphorylated peptide (Bork et al. 1997; Callebaut & Mornon 1997; Glover et al. 2004). However, the function of BRCT domain in RAP1 homologs is still unknown. The very C-terminal region of RAP1 homologs is also conserved and termed RAP1 C-terminus (RCT) domain, which appears to be a protein-interacting domain, too (Li et al. 2000). Human RAP1 has an additional coiled-coil domain next to the myb domain, which may also have a protein-protein interaction function (Li et al. 2000; O'Connor et al. 2004). Therefore, one striking feature of RAP1 is that it has several protein interacting domains, suggesting that this protein has a "recruiter" function that tethers various proteins to telomeres.

In addition to ScRap1, the yKu70/80 dimer is another factor that can recruit silencing factors to the telomere in the budding yeast (Boulton & Jackson 1998; Laroche et al. 1998; Tsukamoto et al. 1997). Ku70/80 is a heterodimer complex that binds DNA ends in a sequence-independent manner (Riha et al. 2006). They were originally identified in mammalian V(D)J recombination process and play an essential function in the classical NHEJ pathway (Critchlow & Jackson 1998; Weaver et al. 1995). The function of Ku homolog at telomeres varies in different organisms, and deletion of yKu leads to multiple defects including heat sensitivity, shortened telomere length, longer telomere G-overhang, abolished TPE, and mislocalization of ScRap1 in nucleus (Boulton & Jackson 1996, 1998; Driller et al. 2000; Smith et al. 2008).

Recruitment of Sir2, Sir3, and Sir4 to telomeres is essential for establishment of the heterochromatic structure at the subtelomeric regions and TPE (Aparicio et al. 1991). Unlike Sir2 and Sir3, Sir4 remains telomere-bound when other Sir proteins are absent (Bourns et al. 1998; Luo et al. 2002), and Sir2/4 binds to chromatin independently of deacetylation at H4K16 and loss of Sir3 interaction in an *in vitro* analysis (Johnson et al. 2009), suggesting that Sir4 is the first one to be recruited to the telomere to initiate the silencing. Either ScRap1 or yKu can recruit Sir4 to the telomere, and ScRap1 can also recruit Sir3 (Luo et al. 2002; Martin et al. 1999; Moretti & Shore 2001; Moretti et al. 1994; Tsukamoto et al. 1997). Together, Sir3 and Sir4 can recruit Sir2 (Bourns et al. 1998; Buchberger et al. 2008; Martino et al. 2009; Moazed et al. 1997; Strahl-Bolsinger et al. 1997), which is an NAD^+-dependent histone deacetylase (Landry et al. 2000; Smith et al. 2000; Tanny et al. 1999). Sir2 activity and the interaction between Sir3/4 and histone tails are necessary for propagating of the heterochromatic structure from telomere to chromosome internal regions (Hoppe et al. 2002).

Sir2 can remove the acetyl group from histone H3 at K9 and K14 residues and from histone H4K16 (Imai et al. 2000). Particularly, unacetylated H4K16 can be recognized by Sir3 (Hecht et al. 1995). Binding of Sir3 on H4K16 will block Dot1 (Altaf et al. 2007), which specifically methylates histone H3K79 (Feng et al. 2002; Lacoste et al. 2002; Ng et al. 2002; van Leeuwen et al. 2002). As an antagonizing effect, methylation of H3K79 by Dot1 will prevent Sir3 from binding the nucleosome (Ng et al. 2002). Similarly, Set1 and Set2 methylates H3 on K4 and K36 residues, respectively (Krogan et al. 2002; Nagy et al. 2002; Roguev et al. 2001; Strahl et al. 2002), and methylated histone H3 prevents Sir4 from binding the nucleosome (Tompa & Madhani 2007; Venkatasubrahmanyam et al. 2007). Therefore, binding of Sir3 and Sir4 recruits Sir2, which deacetylates neighboring histone tails and allows subsequent binding of Sir3 and Sir4 to neighboring nucleosome. Repetitive Sir3 and Sir4 binding and Sir2 action effectively propagate the heterochromatin structure (Rusche et al. 2002). Finally, Sir2 activity can be counteracted by Sas2-dependent acetylation of H4K16 (Ehrenhofer-Murray et al. 1997; Kimura et al. 2002; Reifsnyder et al. 1996; Suka et al. 2002). In fact, a gradient of acetylated H4K16 has been observed where internal chromosomal regions are hyperacetylated while telomeric regions are hypoacetylated, which also corresponds to an inverse gradient of Sir3 binding to chromatin (Kimura et al. 2002).

TPE in *S. cerevisiae* appears to depend on the length of the telomere tract: the longer the telomere, the stronger the silencing effect (Eugster et al. 2006; Kyrion et al. 1993; Renauld et al. 1993). Presumably, longer telomeres are bound by more ScRap1 proteins, which in turn recruit more Sir proteins to the telomere and lead to stronger silencing.

In *S. cerevisiae,* TPE levels at different telomeres vary dramatically, particularly at native telomeres (Loney et al. 2009; Pryde & Louis 1999). This is largely because different telomeres have different composition of subtelomeric elements (Zakian & Blanton 1988). *S. cerevisiae* has two subtelomeric elements, X (contains a core X element) and Y′ (Fig. 3) (Louis 1995; Zakian & Blanton 1988). The X element is present at all yeast telomeres, and core X has an ARS consensus sequence (ACS) that is bound by the ORC complex (which is the DNA replication origin recognition complex) and an ABF1 binding site (Diffley & Stillman 1989; Foss et al. 1993; Marahrens & Stillman 1992; Micklem et al. 1993; Rao et al. 1994; Wyrick et al. 2001). The core X element can reinforce silencing when located near a master silencer such as the telomere, but itself does not convey any silencing effect (Lieb et al. 2001). Therefore, core X is considered as a protosilencer (Boscheron et al. 1996; Lebrun et al. 2001). The X-ACS (ORC binding site) and the ABF1 binding sites of the core X both contribute to silencing at XI-L telomere (Diffley & Stillman 1989; Wyrick et al. 1999). In addition, Sir1, which is not required for TPE at the truncated telomeres (Aparicio et al. 1991), participates in silencing at XI-L telomere (Fourel et al. 1999; Pryde & Louis 1999), presumably by interaction with ORC (Triolo & Sternglanz 1996). The Y′ element is not ubiquitous at all yeast telomere. Only 50–70% of telomeres are marked with 1–4 copies of subtelomeric Y′ elements, which always reside between the X element and the telomere (Chan & Tye 1983a, b; Zakian & Blanton 1988) (Fig. 3). Y′ has two open reading frames (ORF), an ARS, and a SubTelomeric Antisilencing Region (STAR) element adjacent the telomere repeats. Within the X and Y′ elements, there is a small domain of repression centering on the X-ACS, but limited repression is observed through out the Y′ (Pryde & Louis 1999). Therefore, TPE at X-only telomeres is usually stronger.

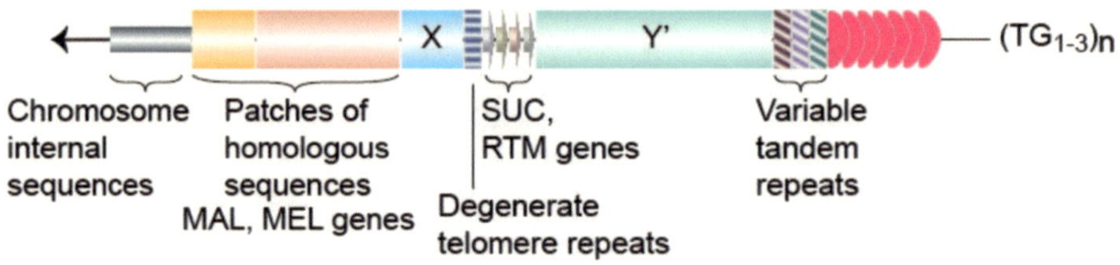

Fig. 3. The subtelomere elements in *S. cerevisiae*. The telomere-proximal region of *S. cerevisiae* subtelomere contains a ubiquitous Core X element and 0-4 copies of Y′ elements. Degenerated telomere repeats and *SUC/RTM* gene families separates the X and Y′ elements, while variable tandem repeats separate the Y′ and the telomere TG_{1-3} repeats. The telomere-distal part of yeast subtelomere consist of *MAL* and *MEL* gene families as large patches of homologous sequences.

At truncated telomeres with targeted reporter genes, TPE levels decrease exponentially with increased distance to the telomere, and the silencing effect spreads inward continuously (Gottschling et al. 1990; Renauld et al. 1993). This is not always true at the native telomeres. Regions closer to telomeres may not be affected by TPE because of the STAR boundaries, while regions more distal to telomeres may resume TPE because of nearby protosilencers such as the core X (Pryde & Louis 1999). Therefore, TPE may not spread continuously along a native telomere.

In *S. cerevisiae,* telomeres are clustered into several foci and are mainly located at the periphery of the nucleus (Gotta et al. 1996). Esc1 is a protein that localizes at the nuclear periphery and plays an important role in the association of telomeres with nuclear envelope (Taddei & Gasser 2004). First, Esc1 interacts with the PAD4-domain of Sir4. Second, Esc1 can also interact with yKu in the S phase, which contributes to the periphery localization of telomeres independently (Taddei & Gasser 2004). Although nuclear periphery localization is not strictly required for TPE (Gartenberg et al. 2004), artificial tethering a reporter gene flanked by silencers to nuclear periphery facilitates the silencing (Andrulis et al. 1998). It is therefore hypothesized that the telomere-clustering site might be a subnuclear compartment that is concentrated with silencing factors such as Sir proteins.

2.3 TPE in *S. pombe*

Silencing has been observed at pericentromeric loci, mating type loci, and telomeres/subtelomeres in *S. pombe* (Grewal & Jia 2007). These loci all have the same signature heterochromatic structure - methylated H3K9 that is bound by Swi6 (HP1 homolog) (Ekwall et al. 1995; Nakayama et al. 2001). Methylation of H3K9 by Clr4 and subsequent Swi6 binding at pericentric and mating type loci are mediated by RNAi-RITS complex (Cam et al. 2005; Hall et al. 2002; Noma et al. 2004; Petrie et al. 2005; Sadaie et al. 2004; Volpe et al. 2002). For a comprehensive review about the RNAi-mediated gene silencing in *S. pombe,* please refer to (Creamer & Partridge 2011). TPE in *S. pombe* is mediated through at least two independent pathways: an SpTaz1-dependent and an RNAi RITS-dependent pathway (Kanoh et al. 2005; Park et al. 2002; Sugioka-Sugiyama & Sugiyama 2011). The SpTaz1-dependent pathway relies on the telomere repeat DNA. SpTaz1, SpRap1, SpPoz1, SpTpz1, SpCcq1, and SpPot1 interact one with another and form the core telomere protein complex at the *S. pombe* telomere (Dehe & Cooper 2010). SpCcq1 also interacts with SHREC, which promotes the Clr4-dependent methylation of H4K9 (Sugiyama et al. 2007). As a separate mechanism, a cenH-like sequence is found at the subtelomeric regions of *S. pombe* telomeres, which is used by RNAi-RITS pathway for establishment of Swi6 heterochromatin (Kanoh et al. 2005). Therefore, TPE depends on not only the telomere sequence but also subtelomeric elements in *S. pombe.*

2.4 TPE in *D. melanogaster*

D. melanogaster is the first organism in which TPE was observed (Gehring et al. 1984; Hazelrigg et al. 1984; Levis et al. 1985), and its telomere consists of reverse transposon elements instead of the simple repetitive TG-rich sequences (Pardue & DeBaryshe 2008), which is very different from most other eukaryotes (see Chapter 5). At the very end of the reverse transposon arrays (including *HeT-A*, *TART*, and *TAHRE*, or the HTT array (Abad et al. 2004; Biessmann et al. 1992; Levis et al. 1993)) lies the cap, which is bound by sequence-nonspecific proteins such as HP1 and HOAP to protect the very end of the chromosome independent of HTT array (Cenci et al. 2003; Fanti et al. 1998). At regions immediately internal to the HTT array lie the telomere-associated sequences (TAS), which contain several kilobases of complex satellite repetitive DNA sequences (Karpen & Spradling 1992; Walter et al. 1995).

Not only is *D. melanogaster* telomere sequence unusual, but also has TPE in *D. melanogaster* some unique features. First, TAS, rather than HTT array, is the telomere silencer (Biessmann et al. 2005). Reporter genes targeted inside TAS or in HTT close to TAS are repressed, while those targeted inside HTT array but more than 5 kb away from TAS are not (Boivin et al. 2003). This may be partly because the transposon elements contain transcribed ORFs (Biessmann et al. 1994). Second, although usually both methylated H3K9 and methylated H3K27 are markers for inactive chromatin, methylated H3K9 is found at HTT but not at TAS while methylated H3K27 is absent from HTT but present at TAS and the cap (Andreyeva et al. 2005). E(Z) is a histone methyltransferase that modifies H3K27, and it is also found to be enriched at TAS. However, although HP1 usually binds methylated H3K9, it does not associate with the HTT array (Frydrychova et al. 2008). Furthermore, silencing level depends on TAS array length and orientation (Mason et al. 2003), but the spreading of silencing varies among different telomeres, possibly because of different HTT and TAS composition at various telomeres (Cryderman et al. 1999; Wallrath & Elgin 1995).

2.5 TPE in mammalian cells

TPE has been observed in human and mouse cells (Baur et al. 2001; Koering et al. 2002; Pedram et al. 2006). By transfecting a linear plasmid carrying a selective marker and a luciferase gene adjacent to a 1.6 kb telomere repeat seed into the telomerase positive Hela cells, a new telomere was formed next to the markers, and the luciferase gene was expressed at a level on average ten-fold lower than when it is at non-telomeric sites. Human TPE is similar to that in yeast – it is variegated and spreads from the telomere inwardly. The silencing strength is also dependent on the length of the telomere, although there is no simple correlation between telomere length and TPE level in both human and yeast (Baur et al. 2001; Koering et al. 2002). TPE in human cells appears to be mediated by the heterochromatic chromatin structure, as treatment with Trichostatin A, an inhibitor of class I and II histone deacetylases, led to decreased TPE. Normally, all three HP1 paralogs associate with telomeres (Koering et al. 2002). However, after Trichostatin A treatment, both histone H3 methylation and the amount of telomere-associated HP1 decrease (Koering et al. 2002). Human subtelomeric elements are much more complicated than that in yeast (Fig. 4). Although some studies suggested that certain subtelomeric elements are important for telomeric silencing, no consistent observations have been made.

3. Telomere and subtelomere recombination

As mentioned above, telomere recombination can serve as an important means for telomere maintenance when telomerase is absent in yeast and mammalian cells (McEachern & Haber 2006; Nabetani & Ishikawa 2011). in addition, telomere recombination can participate in telomere length regulation in telomerease positive cells, too. In *S. cerevisiae*, abnormally long telomeres are observed to shorten in an apparently single-step process called telomere rapid deletion (TRD) (Li & Lustig 1996). TRD depends on *RAD52*, indicating that DNA recombination is involved. Further analysis showed that it is an intrachromatid telomere recombination event and depends on telomere clustering. However, telomere recombination appears to be a low frequent event in wild-type cells. As discussed above, in mammalian cells, sister telomere exchanges and extrachromosomal telomere circles resulted from introchromatid telomere recombination are rarely observed in non-ALT cells (Londono-Vallejo et al. 2004), which is presumably because telomere recombination events are normally inhibited by telomere specific proteins: Both the N-terminus deletion mutant of

TRF2 and depletion of RAP1 led to an elevated telomere sister chromatid exchanges when analyzed by CO-FISH, and the N-terminus deletion mutation of TRF2 also led to an increased extrachromosomal telomere circles presumably as a result of elevated intrachromatid telomere recombination (Martinez et al. 2010; Sfeir et al. 2010; Wang et al. 2004).

Subtelomeric repeats are the sequences located next to telomeres. They are defined as patchworks of blocks that are duplicated near the ends of multiple chromosomes and are highly dynamic with very heterogeneous sequences, sizes, and copy numbers (Mefford & Trask 2002). However, similar organization of subtelomere elements have been observed in organisms that are distantly related such as *Homo sapiens, S. cerevisiae,* and *Plasmodium falciparum.*

Although a detailed sequence database is still lacking for human subtelomere elements on all chromosome ends, recent studies have revealed a common structure (Fig. 4): a proximal and a distal subtelomeric domain is separated by a stretch of degenerate TTAGGG repeats (Mefford & Trask 2002). The telomere-proximal (closer to telomere) domain usually contains short repetitive sequences that can be found at many chromosome ends, while the telomere-distal (more chromosome internal) domain usually consist of longer blocks of homologous sequences that are only found at a few chromosome ends (Brown et al. 1990; Cross et al. 1990; de Lange et al. 1990; Ijdo et al. 1992; Wilkie et al. 1991). In addition, genes belonging to the olfactory receptor family have been found in subtelomeric region (Trask et al. 1998). Olfactory receptor is a membrane-spanning receptor in the sensory neuroepithelium of the nose that bind volatile odorants. Upon binding the ligand, the receptor initiates a signaling cascade that results in transmission of an electrical signal to the brain (DeMaria & Ngai 2010). In any olfactory receptor cell, only one type of olfactory receptor is expressed (Serizawa et al. 2004; Shykind 2005), which is not unlike the monoallelic expression of surface antigen genes in several microbial pathogens (see below).

The subtelomeres of *S. cerevisiae* also consist of two domains that are separated by the Core X element (Fig. 3) and often a stretch of degenerate telomere repeats (Louis 1995). The Core X element is present at all telomeres with a 57–92% of sequence identity across different chromosomes (Louis & Haber 1991; Louis et al. 1994). The telomere-proximal domain consist of 0–4 repeats of Y′ elements, which are highly conserved (98-99% sequence identity) across all chromosomes (Louis & Haber 1992). The telomere-distal domain contains sequence blocks that are only homologous to a few subtelomeres and includes gene families that function in the use of different carbon sources such as MAL (α-glucosidase/maltose permease) and MEL (α-glactosidase) (Carlson & Botstein 1983; Carlson et al. 1985; Charron & Michels 1988; Charron et al. 1989; Louis & Haber 1992; Naumov et al. 1992; Ness & Aigle 1995; Turakainen et al. 1993; Viswanathan et al. 1994).

In *Plasmodium falciparum* that causes malaria in humans, subtelomeres are also arranged into two major domains (Fig. 5A) (Scherf et al. 2001): The telomere-proximal domain consists of six Telomere-Associated Repetitive Elements (TAREs), which are variable tandem repeats (De Bruin et al. 1994; Figueiredo et al. 2002; Pizzi & Frontali 2001), and a couple of these elements are transcribed as long non-coding RNA (Broadbent et al. 2011). The telomere-distal domain consists of a number of gene families including *rif* and *var* genes that encode virulence factors expressed at the surface of the infected host cells and involved in antigenic variation (see below) (Cheng et al. 1998; Rubio et al. 1996).

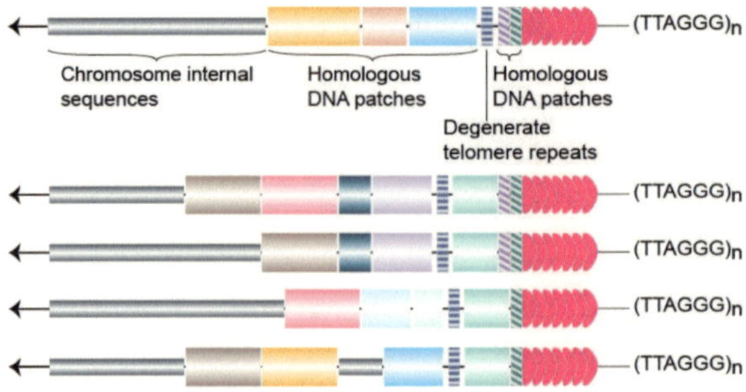

Fig. 4. The organization of subtelomere elements on human chromosomes. The telomere-proximal region usually consists of short patches of homologous DNA sequences that are common at multiple chromosome ends. The telomere-distal region, on the other hand, consists of longer patches of homologous DNA sequences, and degenerated telomere repeats separate the distal and proximal regions.

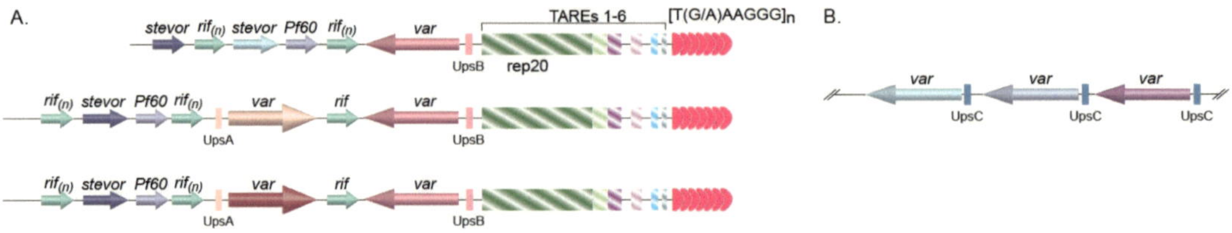

Fig. 5. (A) The organization of subtelomere elements in *P. falciparum*. Immediately internal to the telomere tract are six Telomere-Associated Repeat Elements (TAREs 1-6), with the largest one, *rep20*, located furthest away from the telomere repeats. One or two *var* genes are usually found immediately upstream of *rep20*, followed by the *rifin*, *stevor*, and *Pf60* gene families. Depending on the upstream flanking sequences, three classes of *var* genes have been identified. The ones with associated UpsB and UpsA are located at subtelomeric regions and transcribed in opposite directions as drawn, while the ones with associated UpsC are located as gene arrays in chromosome-internal loci (B).

Subtelomere sequences from many organisms appear to have been duplicated and dispersed among many chromosome ends. It has been hypothesized that translocation recombination events may lead to swapping of chromosome ends, gene conversion events may lead to replacement of all or part of a subtelomeric region by another, and transposition-like events may lead to duplications (Mefford & Trask 2002). In addition, many of these events appear to occur recently because subtelomeric content of a given chromosome varies markedly among individuals. In human cells, FISH analysis revealed high degree of recent genomic rearrangement in human subtelomeres, and sequencing analysis showed that for the two homologous alleles of 16p, sequence identity decreases from 99.8% at unique chromosomal sequence region to 93% at subtelomeric region (Linardopoulou et al. 2005). These studies suggested a two-step event contributed to subtelomere organization: initial interchromosomal translocation events predominantly mediated by NHEJ created new blocks of homologous sequences, and subsequent mutations or homology-directed sequence transfers further enhance sequence variations and spread the subtelomeric elements to other chromosomes (Linardopoulou et al. 2005). The human subtelomere regions therefore exchange sequences at a remarkably high rate and represent recombination hot spots. In *S. cerevisiae*, although subtelomeres are poor substrates for meiotic recombination because chiasmata formed near the ends of chromosomes are much less efficient at promoting homologous chromosome segregation (Su et al. 2000), a high level of nucleotide divergence among *Saccharomyces* yeasts has been observed at the subtelomeres (Teytelman et al. 2008). In *S. pombe*, mutations disrupting heterochromatin led to elevated subtelomeric duplication and rearrangements that are *RAD50*-dependent, indicating that subtelomeres are susceptible to high rate of homologous recombination but the heterochromatic telomere structure can help suppress these events (Bisht et al. 2008).

The subtelomere elements do not seem to have any essential functions (Corcoran et al. 1988; Murray & Szostak 1983; Pologe & Ravetch 1988; Thompson et al. 1997), but they can be useful in more than one way. Recombination at subtelomere regions can contribute to telomere maintenance (McEachern & Haber 2006; Nabetani & Ishikawa 2011). As described above, in telomerase negative *S. cerevisiae* cells, Type I survivors amplify subtelomeric elements using a *RAD51*-dependent mechanism (Le et al. 1999; Teng & Zakian 1999). In addition, subtelomeric DNA recombination appears to be a major factor for genome plasticity, which may help to diversify the sequences of subtelomeric genes (Corcoran et al. 1988; De Bruin et al. 1994; Louis 1995; Pologe & Ravetch 1988; Trask et al. 1998). Particularly for several microbial pathogens, subtelomere recombination appears to play important roles in antigenic variations (see below).

4. Telomere functions in regulation of microbial pathogen virulence

4.1 Antigenic variation and phenotypic switch in microbial pathogens

Living organisms, either unicellular or multicellular, have evolved sophisticated ways to adjust to their living environment for a better survival. Many microbial pathogens that infect mammals have adopted antigenic variation to avoid eradication by the host immune system so that they can maintain persistent infections and enhance the chances of being transmitted to new hosts (Deitsch et al. 2009).

Antigenic variation is the phenomenon that a pathogen changes its surface antigen presented to the host immune system regularly and much more frequently than spontaneous gene mutation. The term of antigenic variation usually encompasses both phase variation (the expression of an individual antigen switches between "on" or "off" states) and true antigenic variation (the expression of a certain antigen switches among different forms). In the latter case, the antigen is usually expressed in a mutually exclusive manner - a single gene from a multi-copy gene family is expressed at any time. In addition, many microbial pathogens can go through phenotypic switching in response to environmental conditions - change of gene expression patterns that leads to a change in organismal phenotypes, which, in turn, can also contribute to the virulence of the pathogen. For example, expression of a different type of certain surface molecule may enhance or weaken adhesion of the pathogen to the host and therefore affect the virulence of the pathogen. In general, both antigenic variation and phenotypic switching can occur through two general types of mechanisms: genetic and epigenetic (Deitsch et al. 2009). A genetic event involves changes in DNA sequences of an antigen encoding gene or its regulatory elements so that either its expression level or its gene product is changed. An epigenetic event only affects a gene expression level but does not change its DNA sequences. However, recent studies suggest that epigenetic changes such as chromatin remodeling may also influence genetic events such as DNA recombination (Benetti et al. 2007; Bisht et al. 2008).

Antigenic variation occurs widely among various microbial pathogens including virus, bacteria, fungi, and parasites (Deitsch et al. 2009). Common mechanisms of antigenic variation have been evolved in different pathogens, including bacteria, fungi, and parasites, possibly due to similar selection pressure exerted from the mammalian immune responses. However, in this chapter, we will focus on those mechanisms that are influenced by the telomere structure.

4.2 TPE participates in the regulation of *EPA* expression in *C. glabrata*

Candida glabrata is part of the normal human mucosal flora and usually commensal. It is a prevalent yeast pathogen, ranking only second to *Candida albicans*, and like *C. albicans*, it can cause opportunistic mucosal and bloodstream infections in immunocompromised individuals. During infection, binding of the pathogen to host cells, host cell proteins, or microbial competitors would help to reduce the chance of clearance by the host. Therefore, the adherence of *C. glabrata* to host cells has been proposed to play an important role in its virulence (Kaur et al. 2005).

When cultured human epithelial cells are used, 95% of *in vitro C. glabrata* adherence depends on an adhesin molecule encoded by the *EPA1* gene (Kapteyn et al. 1999), which binds the host N-acetyl lactosamine-containing glycoconjugates (Castano et al. 2005). The *EPA1* gene belongs to the *EPA* gene family. So far, a total of 23 putative *EPA* genes and pseudogenes have been identified in *C. glabrata* strain BG2 based on their sequence similarity (Kaur et al. 2005). Seven *EPA* genes encode full-length GPI-anchored proteins, among which Epa1 is a lectin (Cormack et al. 1999), Epa6 and Epa7 are confirmed to be adhesins (Castano et al. 2005), while Epa2 and Epa3 are predicted to be cell wall proteins (De Las Penas et al. 2003). All seven *EPA* genes located at subtelomeric regions (Fig. 6) (Castano et al. 2005; De Las Penas et al. 2003; Iraqui et al. 2005). *EPA1*, *EPA2* and *EPA3* are at the same subtelomere, and *EPA1* is the furthest from the telomere (De Las Penas et al. 2003). *EPA4* and *EPA5* are located on a different subtelomere as near-perfect inverted repeats (De Las Penas et al. 2003). *EPA6* and *EPA7* are located on yet two other subelomeres, both are only ~2.5 kb from the telomere tracts (Castano et al. 2005).

Normally, only *EPA1* gene is active, while *EPA2–7* genes are silenced by TPE (Castano et al. 2005; De Las Penas et al. 2003). Like *S. cerevisiae*, TPE in *C. glabrata* dependents on telomere DNA binding factor Rap1. Deletion of the C-terminal 28 amino acids of Rap1 led to derepression of *EPA4–7* and in another case, also *EPA2* and *EPA3* (De Las Penas et al. 2003). This *rap1* allele is equivalent to *rap1-21* mutant allele in *S. cerevisiae* (Liu & Lustig 1996), which causes similar loss of TPE phenotype. Silencing of subtelomeric *EPA* genes also depends on Sir proteins (Castano et al. 2005; De Las Penas et al. 2003). Deletion of *SIR3* led to hyper expression of *EPA1* and derepression of *EPA2–7*, although the derepression of *EPA2* and *EPA3* is very mild, and derepression of *EPA4/5* is also not as strong as that of *EPA6* and *EPA7*. Deletion of *SIR4* also led to derepression of *EPA6*. In addition, deletion of *RIF1* led to elongated telomeres and dererepssion of *EPA4–7*, but not *EPA2* or *EPA3* (Castano et al. 2005). The different derepression of different *EPA* genes indicated that TPE at different telomeres varies, which is the same as in *S. cerevisiae* at native telomeres. In the case of deletion of *SIR3* or *RIF1*, expression of *EPA6* and *EPA7* appears to be the reason or at least one of the reasons for hyper-adherent phenotype, demonstrating that TPE can be directly involved in regulation of pathogen virulence (Castano et al. 2005). Interestingly, Epa6 expression is associated with the ability of *C. glabrata* cells to form biofilm on plastic surface (Iraqui et al. 2005). Biofilm formed by microbial pathogens can increase infection probability and is of great clinical importance because microorganisms adopting this life form is more tolerant or resistant to host defense machinery and anti-microbial agents than free cells.

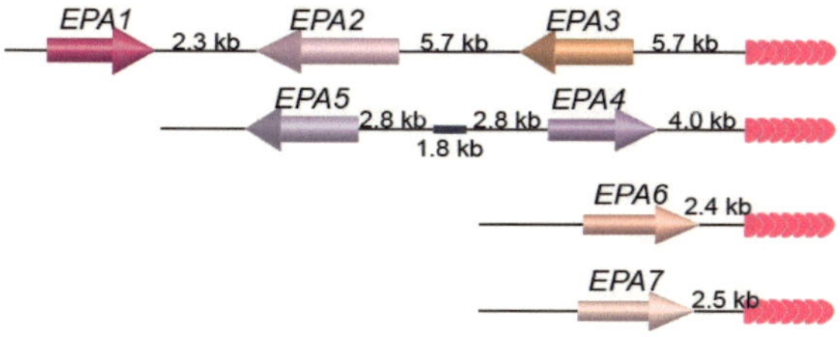

Fig. 6. *EPA1–7* are located at subtelomeric loci in *C. glabrata*. The positions of seven *EPA* genes at their respective chromosome end loci are shown. *EPA1* is furthest away from the telomere and is the only one that is expressed normally, while *EPA 2–7* are usually silenced by TPE.

This TPE regulated adhesin gene expression is well exploited by *C. glabrata* to sense a particular host environment. *C. glabrata* is an nicotinic acid (NA or vitamin niacin) auxotroph, as it lost all the *BNA* genes involved in the NA synthesis except *BNA5* (Domergue et al. 2005). When growing in urine, where NA is limited, the activity of Sir2, an NAD^+-dependent histone deacetylase, decreases correspondingly since NA is the precursor of NAD^+. As a consequence, TPE level decreases and *EPA1, 6,* and *7* genes are highly expressed (Domergue et al. 2005). This effect can be reverted by adding NA or a related compound nicotinamide (NAM). Most importantly, when using an established murine model of urinary track infection, transurethrally inoculated *C. glabrata* has an elevated colonization frequency in bladder and kidney, which is dependent on *EPA1, 6* and *7* gene expression, and mice fed with high-NA diet are no longer susceptible for high rate of colonization of *C. glabrata* (Domergue et al. 2005). Therefore, in *C. glabrata*, TPE plays an important role in regulation of expression of virulence genes.

A similar regulatory role of TPE has also been observed in *S. cerevisiae*, which is not a human pathogen. In *S. cerevisiae*, 5 flocculin genes of the *FLO* family encode cell-wall glycoproteins that regulate cell-cell and cell-surface adhesion, which are important for cell flocculation (Reynolds & Fink 2001; Van Mulders et al. 2009). In this family, *FLO11* is located at a non-telomeric locus and is usually expressed, while *FLO1, 5, 9,* and *10* are at subtelomeric regions (10–40 kb from the telomere repeats) and are normally silenced (Halme et al. 2004). Silencing of *FLO10* requires Sir3 and yKu, suggesting that *FLO* gene silencing and TPE share some common mechanisms. However, silencing of *FLO10* does not require Sir2 and is promoter dependent, indicating that this silencing is not identical to TPE.

4.3 Sir2-mediated TPE plays an essential role in manoallelic expression of *var* genes in *P. falciparum*

Plasmodium falciparum is a protozoan parasite in the Apicomplexa phylum that causes the most severe form of malaria, which is a debilitating and sometimes fatal disease mostly found in tropical and subtropical regions of the world and is most common in Africa. After *P. falciparum* cells being injected into a mammalian host by a female Anopheline mosquito, the sporozoites first invade hepatocytes. At this liver stage, parasites undergo asexual multiplication and differentiate into merozoites, which eventually burst from the hepatocyte and invade erythrocytes (red blood cells). While inside the erythrocytes, individual merozoite enlarges and differentiates into mononucleated ring trophozoites. The trophozoite's nucleus then divides asexually to produce a schizont with several nuclei. Subsequently, schizont divides and produces more mononucleated merozoites. When the erythrocyte erupts eventually, more merozoites and toxins are released to the host bloodstream. The released merozoites will infect more erythrocytes, and the synchronous rupture of the infected erythrocytes is the reason for the periodical fever and chills, typical symptoms of malaria. Some merozoites differentiate into sexual gametocytes inside the erythrocytes. These can be taken up by another mosquito and sexual reproduction is completed inside the insect intestine wall, after which, sporozoites are formed and migrated to the salivary gland of the mosquito, ready to infect next mammalian host when the mosquito takes another blood meal.

One major reason why it is very difficult to eliminate *Plasmodium* parasites once an infection is established is that *P. falciparum* undergoes antigenic variation at the erythrocyte stage (Dzikowski & Deitsch 2009). Merozoites produce *P. falciparum* erythrocyte membrane protein 1 (PfEMP1), which is encoded by *var* genes and is transported to the infected erythrocyte membrane (Baruch et al. 1995; Smith et al. 1995; Su et al. 1995). Expression of PfEMP1 on the infected cell surface allows the infected erythrocyte to adhere to the endothelium of the post-capillary venules and avoid circulation through the spleen, where the infected cells will be destroyed (Baruch 1999). Therefore, expression of PfEMP1 on host cell surface is critical for prolonged parasite infection. However, PfEMP1 is also susceptible to host antibody recognition and subsequent immune attack. As an important pathogenesis mechanism, *P. falciparum* regularly switches the expressed PfEMP1, therefore effectively evading the host immune attack (Roberts et al. 1992). Other proteins encoded by *rif* and *stevor* genes appear to be also important for *P. falciparum* virulence (Kaviratne et al. 2002; Khattab & Meri 2011; Kyes et al. 1999), but *var* gene switching is by far the best understood.

There are ~60 *var* genes in the *P. falciparum* genome (Gardner et al. 2002). However, only one *var* gene is expressed at any moment (Roberts et al. 1992). Based on its upstream regulatory elements, *var* genes can be classified into three groups (Fig. 5) (Kraemer & Smith 2003; Lavstsen et al. 2003). Those with UpsA and transcribed towards the telomere and those with UpsB and transcribed away from the telomere are located at subtelomeric loci (Fig. 5A), while the ones with UpsC are located at chromosome internal loci (Fig. 5B) (Gardner et al. 2002; Kraemer & Smith 2003; Lavstsen et al. 2003; Voss et al. 2000). Monoallelic expression of *var* gene is regulated at the DNA level, affected by epigenetic factors such as the chromatin structure, and depends on its subnuclear localization (Dzikowski & Deitsch 2009). Telomeres appear to be important in the latter two mechanisms.

All *var* genes contain a larger exon 1, an intron of ~800 bp, a smaller exon 2, and two promoters (Calderwood et al. 2003; Su et al. 1995). The promoter located upstream of exon 1 drives the expression of the *var* gene, which is subject to mutually exclusive expression regulation and hence only one is active at any time, while the promoter located within the intron appears to be active in most if not all *var* genes (Epp et al. 2009). Studies have shown that proper silencing of the *var* gene relies on the intron promoter activity, the pairing of the upstream and intron promoters, and passing through at least one cell cycle (Calderwood et al. 2003; Deitsch et al. 2001; Dzikowski et al. 2007; Frank et al. 2006). The detailed mechanism underlying the regulatory role of the intron promoter is still unknown. However, it has been proposed that the sterile transcripts resulted from the intron promoter may contribute to *var* gene silencing in a similar way as how non-coding RNA is involved in chromatin-mediated silencing and the inactivation of genes (Ralph & Scherf 2005).

Other studies have shown that epigenetic factors also contribute to *var* gene expression regulation. For example, acetylated histone H3 and methylated H3K27 are found at active *var* gene promoters, while tri-methylation of H3K9 is found at silent *var* gene promoters (Chookajorn et al. 2007; Duraisingh et al. 2005; Freitas-Junior et al. 2005; Lopez-Rubio et al. 2007). Particularly relevant to this chapter, TPE has been shown to play an important role in *var* gene expression regulation (Duraisingh et al. 2005; Freitas-Junior et al. 2005; Tonkin et al. 2009). TPE was first observed in *P. falciparum* by targeting a reporter gene to the rep20 repeats located at the subtelomeric regions (Fig. 5A) (Duraisingh et al. 2005). Rep20 is the most telomere-distal TARE and is usually adjacent to the subtelomeric *var* gene promoter. TPE in *P. falciparum* is similar to that in *S. cerevisiae* in that it depends on Sir2 (Duraisingh et al. 2005; Freitas-Junior et al. 2005; Tonkin et al. 2009). However, PfSir2 is both a histone deacetylase and an ADP-ribosyltransferase (Chakrabarty et al. 2008; Merrick & Duraisingh 2007), and the Sir2-dependent TPE spreads much further away along the chromosome in *P. falciparum* (~55 kb) than in *S. cerevisiae* (~3 kb). PfSir2 is localized at the telomeres, and histones H4 acetylation is absent from the telomeres (Freitas-Junior et al. 2005). By examining subnuclear localization of a number of genetic markers along chromosome 2 in FISH, it is also inferred that chromatin structure is more condensed for telomere-proximal regions than telomere-distal ones (Freitas-Junior et al. 2005). The direct evidence of involving TPE in *var* gene regulation came from the observation that deletion of PfSir2 led to a significant increase in transcription of a subset of *var* genes, particularly the *var* genes with UpsA and at the subtelomere regions (Duraisingh et al. 2005).

Telomeres appear to be involved in another layer of *var* gene expression regulation - specific subnuclear localization (Dzikowski & Deitsch 2009). Several studies showed that silent *var* genes and active *var* genes are located in different compartments of the nucleus (Ralph et al. 2005). Specifically for *var2csa* located at a subtelomeric locus, when it is silent, it is predominantly colocalized with telomere clusters (84%) at the nuclear periphery. However, when *var2csa* is active, it moves to a different nuclear periphery location away from the telomere clusters (Mok et al. 2008; Salanti et al. 2003). It is therefore hypothesized that telomeres are generally clustered in a heterochromatic region of the nuclear periphery where silent *var* genes are also located. Upon activation, *var* genes will leave the heterochromatic region and move to a euchromatic region in the nuclear periphery, allowing transcription to occur (Ralph et al. 2005). However, contrary observations were made for episomal located *var* genes, which tend to co-localize with the telomere cluster when activated (Voss et al. 2006). In addition, chromosome internally located *var* genes appear to co-localize with the telomere clusters independently of their transcriptional status (Voss et al. 2006). Nevertheless, it is clear that active *var* gene is relocated to a specialized peri-nuclear compartment for its proper transcription. In addition, *var* genes located at subtelomeres or chromosome internal loci appear to be differently regulated regarding their subnuclear localization. Apparently, in addition to telomeres, other genome environment factors are involved in *var* gene expression regulation.

4.4 RAP1-mediated silencing is essential for monoallelic expression of *VSG* in *T. brucei*

The kinetoplastids are a group of flagellated protozoa. Three members of kinetoplastids are of great clinical importance because they cause human diseases: *Trypanosoma brucei* causes human African trypanosomiasis or sleeping sickness, *Trypanosoma cruzi* causes South America trypanosomiasis or Chagas Disease, and several *Leishmania* species cause leishmaniasis. Of these three trypanosomatids (the kinetoplastid organisms that only have a single flagellum), only *T. brucei* undergoes antigenic variation, which is an important mechanism of its pathogenesis and one of its most interesting physiological aspects (Barry & McCulloch 2001).

Trypanosoma brucei is transmitted between its mammalian hosts by its insect vector, tsetse (*Glossina* spp.). *T. brucei* has several different life forms through its life cycle (Matthews 2005). While inside the mid-gut of a tsetse fly, *T. brucei* cells are in the procyclic form (PF), which is a non-virulent proliferative stage. After *T. brucei* cells migrate into the salivary gland of the tsetse fly, they differentiate into the metacyclic form. At this stage, *T. brucei* cells stop proliferating and acquire virulence. When a tsetse fly takes a blood meal, *T. brucei* cells can be injected into a mammalian host. *T. brucei* cells stay in the bloodstream or extracellular spaces in its mammalian host, and they quickly differentiate into bloodstream form (BF). The slender bloodstream form is proliferative, while the stumpy bloodstream form is quiescent, non-proliferative. When a tsetse fly takes a blood meal from the infected mammalian host, stumpy bloodstream form *T. brucei* cells can quickly differentiate into the procyclic form, ending the life cycle. Throughout its life cycle, *T. brucei* cells are covered with surface glycoproteins. At the PF stage, several Procyclic Acidic Repetitive Proteins (PARPs, or procyclins) are expressed at its surface, while the metacyclic form and bloodstream form cells express variant surface glycoproteins (VSGs) as their surface glycoprotein (Mehlert et al. 1998).

Because *T. brucei* cells stay in extracellular spaces in its mammalian host, they are exposed to the host's immune system and are not only vulnerable to the innate immune response (inflammations, complements, etc.) but also constantly threatened by the adaptive immune responses (antibody, killer T cells, etc.). However, *T. brucei* has evolved a sophisticated antigenic variation mechanism and regularly switches its surface VSG coat, thus effectively evading the host's immune attack (Barry & McCulloch 2001).

Antigenic variation in *T. brucei* has two essential aspects: switch to express a different *VSG* gene (*VSG* switching) and monoallelic expression of *VSG*. Although there are ~1,500 *VSG* genes and pseudogenes in the *T. brucei* genome (Berriman et al. 2005), only one type of VSG is expressed at any time. After a new *VSG* gene is turned on, it is essential to turn off the previously active *VSG* so that the old surface antigen is no longer presented to the host immune system. In addition, expressing only one *VSG* gene at a time would allow the *VSG* gene pool to be used for a maximum period of time, enabling a persistent infection. Therefore, both *VSG* switching and monoallelic expression of *VSG* are critical for antigenic variation and have been the focus of intensive research for several decades.

T. brucei has many unusual intriguing physiological aspects. In addition to the fact that it undergoes antigenic variation (Barry & McCulloch 2001), most of *T. brucei* genes are arranged in polycistronic transcription units (Johnson et al. 1987; Mottram et al. 1989), and

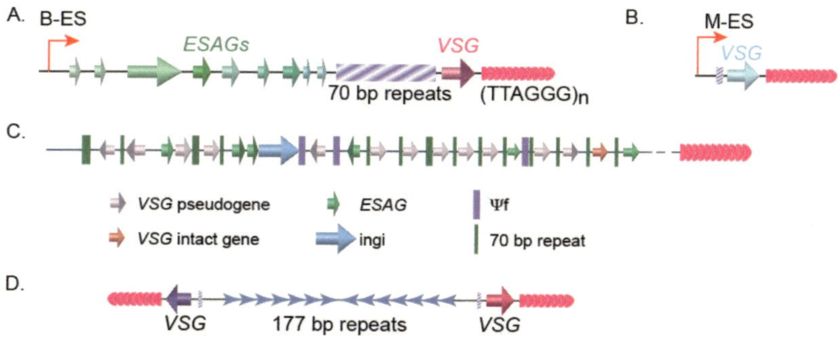

Fig. 7. Distribution of *VSG* genes in *T. brucei* genome. (A) In a bloodstream form *VSG* expression site (B-ES), the *VSG* gene is the last one in the large polycistronic transcription unit and is located within 2 kb from the telomere repeats. A stretch of 70 bp repeats with various length is located upstream of the *VSG* gene followed by a number of ES associated genes (*ESAGs*). (B) The metacyclic *VSG* expression site (M-ES) is a monocyctronic transcription unit also located at subtelomeric region. (C) Most *VSG* genes (and some *ESAG* genes) are found in gene arrays located at subtelomeric regions on megabase chromosomes. Short stretches of 70 bp repeats are found upstream of each gene. (D) On minichromosomes, single *VSG* genes and upstream 70 bp repeats are also found at subtelomeric regions.

the large polycistronic transcripts are trans-spliced so that each mature RNA molecule has a common 5′ end spliced leader element (Liang et al. 2003). In BF *T. brucei* cells, *VSGs* are expressed exclusively from bloodstream form *VSG* expression sites (B-ESs), which are RNA polymerase I (RNAP I)-transcribed, polycistronic transcription units located at subtelomere loci (Fig. 7A) (de Lange & Borst 1982; Gunzl et al. 2003). B-ESs usually consists of a number of *Expression Sites-Associated Genes* (*ESAGs*) upstream of the *VSG* gene, which is the last in the unit and usually within 1.5 kb from the telomere repeats, while the promoter is often 40–60 kb upstream of the *VSG* (Hertz-Fowler et al. 2008). In contrast, at the metacyclic stage, *VSGs* are expressed from metacyclic *VSG* expression sites (M-ESs), which are monocistronic transcription units located at the subtelomeric regions (Fig. 7B), with the promoter located only ~ 5 kb from the telomere (Cornelissen et al. 1985; Lenardo et al. 1984). Although the M-ESs have much simpler organizations than the B-ESs, much less is understood about metacyclic than bloodstream *VSG* expression regulation. *T. brucei* has multiple B-ESs (e.g. Lister 427 has 15 different B-ESs), usually carrying different *VSGs*, but all B-ESs have very similar genomic organization with ~90% sequence identity (Hertz-Fowler et al. 2008). Earlier studies focused on B-ES promoters also showed that they are almost always identical (Pham et al. 1996; Zomerdijk et al. 1990, 1991). Therefore, how *T. brucei* manages to fully express only one B-ES and *VSG* had been a great puzzle for more than a couple of decades.

A number of studies in the last decade have shown that *VSG* expression is regulated at multiple levels. First, transcription elongation from B-ES promoter appears to be regulated. Silent B-ES promoters are actually mildly active (Vanhamme et al. 2000). Transcription is initiated from these "silent" promoters, but transcription elongation is quickly attenuated after a few kilobases, effectively stopping transcription long before the *VSG* genes. Second, chromatin structure is very different from the active to silent B-ESs. The active B-ES has very few nucleosomes while silent ESs are packed with nucleosomes (Figueiredo & Cross 2010; Stanne & Rudenko 2010). A number of studies also showed that chromatin remodeling plays an important role, particularly in regulating the B-ES promoter activity: Depletion of a Swi/Snf homolog, TbISWI, led to an elevated transcription from the silent ES promoters, although *VSG* expression is not affected (Hughes et al. 2007; Stanne et al. 2011); Deletion of the histone H3K79 methyltransferase TbDot1b led to a 10-fold increase in transcription throughout the silent ESs (Janzen et al. 2006); Of the three *T. brucei* histone deacetylase homologs, DAC3 is required for B-ES promoter silencing at both BF and PF stages, and DAC1 antagonizes basal telomeric silencing in BF cells without affecting B-ES transcription (Wang et al. 2010); And depletion of TbSpt16, a subunit of the FACT chromatin remodeling complex, also led to an ~20-fold increase in silent B-ES promoter transcription in both BF and PF cells (Denninger et al. 2010). Third, ever since the discovery that *VSGs* are exclusively expressed from subtelomeric regions (de Lange & Borst 1982), it has been proposed that telomeres may play an important role in *VSG* expression regulation (Dreesen et al. 2007). This hypothesis was supported by the fact that *T. brucei* also has TPE (Glover & Horn 2006; Horn & Cross 1997). When a *neo* reporter gene driven by a B-ES promoter or an rDNA promoter (both are transcribed by RNAP I) is inserted into a silent B-ES, repression of the *neo* gene is observed to be stronger at loci immediately upstream or downstream the *VSG* gene than at loci 7 or 16 kb upstream of the telomere repeats (Horn & Cross 1997). In a later study, the *neo* reporter gene with an rDNA promoter was integrated to a telomere not marked with any B-ES. Again, higher *neo* expression is detected at a locus 5 kb upstream of the telomere than at a locus only 2 kb from the telomere in both BF and PF cells, further confirming that TPE exist in *T. brucei* regulation (Glover & Horn 2006). Interestingly, when the same reporter cassette is inserted in a silent B-ES at the same distance from the telomere as in a non-ES telomere, stronger silencing effect is detected in the silent B-ES, suggesting that in addition to TPE, other factors are involved in B-ES expression regulation (Glover & Horn 2006).

Although the earlier studies provided promising evidence for TPE, direct evidence linking TPE and *VSG* silencing was lacking for a long time. In addition, although the *T. brucei* Sir2 homolog plays an essential role in TPE at reporter marked telomeres without native B-ESs, its deletion does not affect *VSG* silencing at all (Alsford et al. 2007). Furthermore, Glover et al. was able to target an I-Sce I digestion site together with a *neo* reporter gene downstream of the *VSG* gene and immediately upstream of the telomere in a telomerase null background. Induction of ectopic I-Sce I expression led to immediate cleavage and loss of the marked telomere. Within 9 hours, degradation of the reporter gene and the subtelomeric *VSG* gene was also observed. Although a mild derepression of the reporter gene was observed shortly before it was degraded, the *VSG* gene was not derepressed at all (Glover et al. 2007). These observations raised a great deal of doubts whether telomeres are indeed necessary for proper *VSG* silencing.

It was difficult to exam the roles of the telomere in antigenic variation directly without identifying any telomere specific proteins. Earlier attempts to identify telomere DNA binding factors in *T. brucei* using biochemical approaches led to the identification of a couple of telomere DNA binding activities without identification of the responsible proteins (Eid & Sollner-Webb 1995, 1997).

Approximately nine years ago, the nearly completed *T. brucei* genome database allowed us to use an *in silico* approach to identify potential telomere protein homologs in *T. brucei* (Li et al. 2005). Because *T. brucei* telomere DNA consists of the same TTAGGG repeats as vertebrates, it was reasoned that the duplex telomere binding protein in *T. brucei* is likely to have a conserved functional domain for recognizing the double-stranded TTAGGG repeats as mammalian TRF homologs. Indeed, a *T. brucei* TRF homolog with a C-terminal conserved myb domain was identified in the genome database and was subsequently proved to bind the duplex TTAGGG repeats directly both *in vitro* and *in vivo*.

Although the initial study found that depletion of TbTRF does not affect *VSG* expression, a yeast 2-hybrid screen using TbTRF as bait led to the identification of *T. brucei* RAP1 homolog (Yang et al. 2009). Subsequent co-IP, immunofluorescence (IF), and Chromatin IP (ChIP) analyses further confirmed that TbRAP1 is an integral component of the *T. brucei* telomere complex. Extensive studies on *S. cerevisiae* Rap1 showed that it has a major function in establishment and maintenance of TPE (Kyrion et al. 1993; Liu et al. 1994). To determine whether TbRAP1 has a conserved function in TPE, we depleted TbRAP1 in BF cells using an RNAi approach (Shi et al. 2000), as TbRAP1 is essential for cell viability. As soon as the protein level of TbRAP1 started to decrease, a derepression of silent B-ES-linked *VSGs* can be detected (Yang et al. 2009). Using quantitative RT-PCR analysis, it was shown that all B-ES-linked silent *VSGs* had an elevated expression level upon depletion of TbRAP1, although the level of derepression varies among different *VSGs*, ranging from 8–56 fold. This is similar to situations in *S. cerevisiae*, where different levels of TPE are observed at different native telomeres (Pryde & Louis 1999). Subsequently, it was confirmed by IF that multiple VSGs are expressed simultaneously in individual cells on cell surface (Yang et al. 2009). In addition, such *VSG* derepression effect is TbRAP1-specific, as depletion of TbTRF did not affect *VSG* silencing at all. Most importantly, the TbRAP1-mediated silencing is position dependent. First, only subtelomeric B-ES-linked *VSGs* were affected. Genes located in chromosome internal regions including RNAP I transcribed rDNA and RNAP II transcribed telomerase protein gene, a ribosomal protein gene, and a glycolytic protein gene were not affected. Second, along a same B-ES, the telomere-adjacent *VSG* gene is almost always derepressed at a higher level than a *VSG* pseudogene located 7–20 kb away from the telomere. The silencing effect spreads 40–60 kb away from the telomere and can cause derepression of a reporter gene targeted immediately downstream of the B-ES promoter. It is therefore convinced that the TbRAP1-mediated silencing originates from the telomere, demonstrating for the first time that the telomere structure indeed plays an essential role in *VSG* expression regulation.

Recent work from our lab has led to further understanding of the underlying mechanisms of TbRAP1-mediated *VSG* silencing. First, silencing appears to depend on the association of TbRAP1 with the local chromatin, as more TbRAP1 proteins seem to associate with silent B-ESs than the active B-ES in the same BF cells when analyzed by ChIP (Unnati P. & Li B., unpublished data). This is consistent with the observation that proximity to telomeres leads to stronger TbRAP1-mediated silencing, as TbRAP1 is an intrinsic part of the telomere complex. Second, depletion of TbRAP1 resulted in more loosely packed chromatin structure at the silent B-ESs in PF cells: using a FAIRE (Formaldehyde-Assisted Isolation of Regulatory Elements) approach, more silent B-ES-linked *VSG* DNA can be extracted after depletion of TbRAP1 than in wild-type cells, indicating fewer nucleosomes are packed in the chromatin after B-ESs are derepressed. Although the details of histone modifications at the silent or derepressed B-ESs are unknown, this finding suggests that the TbRAP1-mediated *VSG* silencing is similar to ScRap1-mediated TPE in yeast, both involves establishment of heterochromatin structure at the telomere vicinity.

Therefore, studies on the functions of *T. brucei* telomere proteins have finally proved the hypothesis and clearly shown that the telomere structure is important for subtelomeric *VSG* silencing. However, the involvement of telomere in *VSG* expression regulation does not necessarily exclude other mechanisms mentioned above. In fact, TbRAP1-mediated silencing appears to block the elongation of the basal level transcription from the silent B-ES promoters, because in TbRAP1 deficient cells, derepressed *VSGs* are expressed at a level that is still ~100 fold lower than when the same *VSG* is in a fully active B-ES (Yang et al. 2009). Therefore, the observed quick attenuation of transcription elongation along silent B-ESs may well be the combined effect of a basal level transcription initiated from silent B-ES promoters and a TbRAP1-mediated TPE. The fact that derepressed *VSGs* are not expressed at its fullest potential also suggests that B-ES promoters are regulated by additional factors other than TPE. This is consistent with the observations that a number of chromatin remodeling factors are involved in B-ES promoter regulation as mentioned above.

Recent studies have made great contributions to our understanding of how *VSG* expression is silenced. However, how is allelic-exclusive expression of *VSG* achieved is not fully understood. It has been proposed that sufficient amount of RNAP I machinery, which is responsible for high level *VSG* transcription, may be accessible for only one B-ES, which would effectively ensure its monoallelic expression (Horn & McCulloch 2010). In an IF analysis, Navarro and Gull found that in BF *T. brucei* cells, RNAP I forms a small nuclear focus in addition to the large focus inside the nucleolus, where it transcribes rRNA. By labeling nascent RNA with Br-UTP, they confirmed that the extranucleolar RNAP I was transcriptionally active. Furthermore, by tagging the active B-ES with an array of Lac operator sequences and expressing an ectopic GFP-Lac I fusion protein, they were able to visualize that the active B-ES but not the silent ones is co-localized with RNAP I in this extranucleolar body termed ES body (ESB), which only exists in BF but not PF cells (Navarro & Gull 2001). It is therefore hypothesized that ESB, enriched with RNAP I, can only accommodate one B-ES, which would effectively limit the number of active B-ES to one. In support of this view, when two different B-ESs were tagged with selective markers immediately downstream of their respective promoters and forced to be active simultaneously, the two B-ESs appear to switch back and force rapidly and locate next to each other in the nucleus, presumably competing for available RNAP I at ESB (Chaves et al. 1999).

4.5 Telomere proteins influence *VSG* switching frequency in *T. brucei*

As mentioned above, antigenic variation in *T. brucei* has two major aspects: monoallelic *VSG* expression and *VSG* switching. We have discussed about monoallelic *VSG* expression regulation above. Here we will review mechanisms involved in *VSG* switching and its regulation.

VSG switching can occur through several different pathways (Fig. 8) (Barry & McCulloch 2001). In the so-called *in situ* switch, a silent B-ES promoter is turned fully active while the originally active B-ES promoter is turned off. This type of switch does not involve any DNA rearrangements, only B-ES promoter activities change. There are 15 B-ESs carrying distinctive *VSGs* in the *T. brucei* Lister 427 cells, providing a small number of possible *in situ* switch opportunities (Hertz-Fowler et al. 2008). However, *in situ VSG* switching is usually a rare event, and *VSG* switching involving DNA recombination events are much more prevalent (Robinson et al. 1999). *T. brucei* has more than 1,500 *VSG* genes and pseudogenes in its genome (Fig. 7), providing a large gene pool for the homologous recombination-mediated *VSG* switching (Berriman et al. 2005).

There are 11 pairs of megabase chromosomes (0.9–5.7 Mb), several intermediate chromosomes (300–900 kb), and ~100 copies of minichromosomes (50–100 kb) in *T. brucei* genome (Alsford et al. 2001; Berriman et al. 2005; Melville et al. 2000). The majority of *VSG* genes are found in long tandem arrays of repeated genes at subtelomeric locations on megabase chromosomes (Fig. 7C). Approximately 200 copies of *VSG* genes are found immediately upstream of telomeres of the minichromosomes, which carry besides the *VSG* genes, only repetitive sequences, including 177 bp repeats in the chromosome internal region and telomere repeats at the chromosome ends (Fig. 7D) (Alsford et al. 2001). The rest of *VSGs* are found in *VSG* expression sites. In addition to the 15–20 copies of B-ESs located at megabase and intermediate chromosomes that express *VSG* at the bloodstream form stage (Fig. 7A), there are several hundred copies of metacyclic *VSG* ESs (M-ESs), and 1–2% of which are expressed at the metacyclic stage (Fig. 7B) (Graham et al. 1998; Turner et al. 1988). Similar to B-ESs, M-ESs are located at subtelomeric regions of megabase chromosomes. However, unlike B-ESs, M-ESs are monocistronic transcription units, and their individual promoter is only ~5 kb upstream of the telomere repeats (Pedram & Donelson 1999). The *VSG* genes found in subtelomeric gene arrays and at minichromsome subtelomeres are often referred to as basic *VSG* copies because these loci are transcriptional silent. However, these basic *VSG* genes can be copied into the active B-ES via DNA recombination (Fig. 8).

In gene conversion events, a silent *VSG* is copied into the active B-ES while the originally active *VSG* is lost. In this event, the donor can be any functional *VSG* gene in the genome. There is almost always a stretch of 70 bp repeats upstream of a *VSG* gene, in which homologous recombination can initiate as DNA double strand breaks (Boothroyd et al. 2009). In rare occasions, several *VSG* donors have been identified in a single *VSG* switching event, where each donor contributes only a fragment of the gene, generating a new mosaic *VSG* gene product (Marcello & Barry 2007). Such mechanism has been proposed to be useful in late stage of persistent infection. More often, a silent B-ES is used as a donor possibly because long stretch of 70 bp repeats (2 to >14 kb) and telomere repeats (3 to 20 kb) are found to flank the *VSG* gene in any B-ES, and efficient homologous recombination can initiate from these sites. In fact, all B-ESs have very similar genome organization and are ~90% identical in sequences, so gene conversion event can initiate at places upstream of 70 bp repeats and often a whole silent B-ES can be copied to replace the active B-ES (Hertz-Fowler et al. 2008; Pays et al. 1983b). Therefore, the terms of *VSG* gene conversion and ES gene conversion are used to differentiate different types of gene conversion events (Kim & Cross 2010). In addition to gene conversion, reciprocal crossover event can occur in a *VSG* switching (Rudenko et al. 1996). In this case, the crossover usually occurs at the 70 bp repeats, and the silent and active *VSGs* (often together with their respective downstream telomeres) simply trade places without deletion of large fragments of genetic information. It is worth to note that in a crossover switching, the originally silent *VSG* often comes from a silent B-ES, but it can also be from a minichromosome subtelomere.

It has been shown that some key players in the homologous DNA recombination pathway including TbRAD51 and TbBRCA2 are important for *VSG* switching in *T. brucei* (McCulloch & Barry 1999). In homologous recombination, searching for DNA sequence homology and

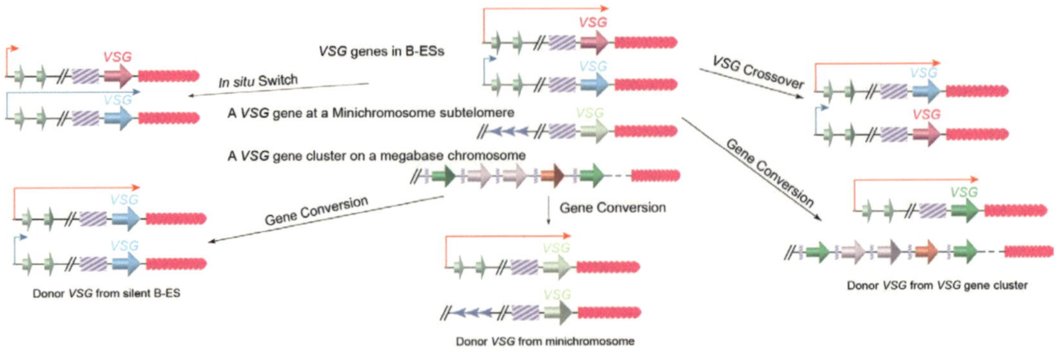

Fig. 8. *VSG* switching can occur through *in situ* switch, gene conversion, or crossover. Top Middle, before switching, an active B-ES (with a longer red arrows extended from its promoter), a silent B-ES (with a shorter blue arrow extended from its promoter), a *VSG* gene at a minichromosome subtelomere, and an array of *VSG* genes and pseudogenes on a megabase chromosome are shown. *In situ* switch (top left) results from turning on (longer blue arrow) of the silent B-ES and turning off (shorter red arrow) of the active B-ES simultaneously without any DNA rearrangements. In gene conversion, a silent *VSG* gene is duplicated into the active B-ES, and the originally active *VSG* gene is lost. The *VSG* donor can come from a silent B-ES (bottom-left), a minichromosome subtelomere (bottom-middle), or a *VSG* gene array (bottom-right). In *VSG* cross-over (top-right), the active *VSG* and a silent *VSG* (most often from a silent B-ES) exchange their loci reciprocally, resulting in a new *VSG* gene in the active B-ES without losing any genetic information. The cross-over site is often found within the 70 bp repeats upstream of the *VSG* genes, although it can locate more upstream because all B-ES have high sequence homology.

subsequent strand-invasion is a key step. In eukaryotes, the RecA homolog RAD51 is the key player in this step (Holthausen et al. 2010). RAD51 polymerizes around ssDNA to assemble a nucleoprotein helical filament (Holloman 2011). With the help of ATP, RAD51 extends the DNA structure and carries out the strand exchange process. After ATP is hydrolyzed, the extended state is relieved and the filament is disassembled. Factors contributing to filament assembly and disassembly thus provide a means for regulating homologous recombination. When ssDNA is coated with RPA (a single strand-specific DNA binding protein), it will not be accessible by RAD51 without the help of a mediator, such as BRCA2 (Holloman 2011). In *T. brucei*, six RAD51 related proteins have been identified: RAD51, DMC1, RAD51-3, RAD51-4, RAD51-5, and Rad51-6 (Proudfoot & McCulloch 2005). Among these, deletion of TbRAD51 and TbRAD51-3 led to a decrease in *VSG* switching rate while deletion of TbRAD51-5 did not have any effect (Proudfoot & McCulloch 2005). In addition, deletion of TbBRCA2 also led to a similar decreased *VSG* switching rate (Hartley & McCulloch 2008).

Homologous recombination is important for the repair of ssDNA gaps, double-strand breaks, and stalled replication forks that arise during DNA synthesis. However, aberrant and inappropriate mitotic homologous recombination, such as high frequency of sister chromatid exchanges, posts a threat to genome stability. The RecQ helicase BLM (or Sgs1 in yeast) forms a complex with type 1A topoisomerase TOPO III (or Top3 in yeast) and an OB fold containing RMI1 (Mankouri & Hickson 2007). This so-called RTR complex has been shown to suppress aberrant and inappropriate homologous recombination. It has been shown recently that in *T. brucei*, the homologues of TOPO3 and RMI1 also form a complex (Kim & Cross 2011). In addition, both TbTOPO3α and TbRMI1 are involved in regulation of *VSG* switching (Kim & Cross 2010, 2011). Deletion of TbTOPO3α or TbRMI1 led to 10–40 or ~4 fold of increase, respectively, in *VSG* switching frequency. Particularly, the *VSG* gene conversion frequency was increased more than 10 fold in either TbTOPO3α null or TbRMI1 null cells. These observations suggest that the TbTOPO3α and TbRMI1 complex is important to suppress aberrant homologous recombination to maintain integrity of the active *VSG* B-ES.

Apparently, homologous recombination is a major pathway for *VSG* switching. In fact, it has been shown that gene conversion is the preferred mechanism for *VSG* switching (Robinson et al. 1999). However, exactly how *VSG* switching is regulated is less clear. Several recent studies now indicate that the telomere structure can also influence *VSG* switching greatly.

It has been shown that the active *VSG*-marked telomere is less stable than the silent telomeres (Bernards et al. 1983; Horn & Cross 1997; Myler et al. 1988; Pays et al. 1983a; van der Ploeg et al. 1984). Rapidly shortened active telomere arises frequently, which is quite similar to the TRD observed in yeast cells carrying abnormally long telomeres (Li & Lustig 1996). Presumably the active transcription of the telomere is a major cause for the brittle telomere (Rudenko & Van der Ploeg 1989). With the presence of telomerase, shortened telomeres are elongated quickly (Horn et al. 2000). With frequent truncation and elongation, telomere length at the active chromosome end is often much more heterogeneous than those at silent telomeres (Bernards et al. 1983). However, in the absence of telomerase, the truncated active telomere remains short, allowing the isolation of clones baring extremely short active telomere in a relatively short culturing period (Dreesen & Cross 2006a). Interestingly, when such telomerase negative clones were obtained that carry extremely short active telomere, these clones tend to switch to express a new *VSG* (Dreesen & Cross 2006a). This observation led to the hypothesis that shorter telomeres may cause higher *VSG* switching rate (Dreesen et al. 2007). It is speculated that all active telomeres are prone to large telomere fragment deletions due to its active transcription state, but shorter telomeres is more likely to have a deletion landed in the subtelomeric region and to cause damage in the active *VSG* gene, which will force the parasite to go through *VSG* switching. Introducing a break at the I-SCE I site targeted immediately upstream of the active *VSG* gene led to a 250-fold increase in *VSG* switching frequency, confirming part of this theory that damage to the active *VSG* gene will force the parasite to switch (Boothroyd et al. 2009). In consistent with this observation, deplete the active *VSG* using the RNAi approach also led to elevated *VSG* switching rate (Aitcheson et al. 2005).

Whether telomere length plays a direct role in *VSG* switching is harder to confirm. In consistence with the hypothesis, several *T. brucei* strains with only limited propagation in a laboratory (usually called pleomorphic strains) have much higher *VSG* switching rate (10^{-4} to 10^{-2} per population doubling) and relatively shorter telomeres (3–12 kb long, with an average of 8–10 kb) (Dreesen & Cross 2008). In contrast, the 427 Lister strain has been extensively propagated in the laboratory, has a *VSG* switch rate of 10^{-6} per generation, and has telomeres ranging 3–20 kb with an average of 15 kb (Munoz-Jordan & Cross 2001). More direct evidence supporting this theory came from a recent study using newly developed MACS-based *VSG* switching analysis: in 427 Lister strain, in telomerase null cells that most telomeres are very short (less than 2 kb), the *VSG* switching frequency was increased ~10 fold compared to wild-type cells carrying long telomeres, confirming that the telomere length does influence *VSG* switching (Cross GAM & Papavasiliou FN, personal communications). However, telomere length is probably only one of many reasons for the high *VSG* switching rate in the pleomorphic strains: The telomerase null 427 strain has extremely short telomeres (as short as ~40 bp), but the *VSG* switching rate is only 10 fold elevated; The telomeres in the pleomorphic strains are only a little shorter than those in the 427 strain (8–10 kb vs 15 kb on average), but the *VSG* switching rate is 100–10,000 fold higher in pleomorphic cells than in the 427 strain.

In addition to telomere length, our recent studies indicated that telomere-specific proteins play important roles in antigenic variation. Using a double-marked cell line established by Kim and Cross (Kim & Cross 2010), we were able to estimate *VSG* switching rate and examine switching pathways in *T. brucei* cells depleted of individual telomere proteins. In this switching reporter cell line, a blasticidin-resistance gene (*BSD*) had been inserted at the promoter driving the *VSG2* B-ES and a puromycin-resistance gene fused to the *Herpes simplex* virus thymidine kinase (*PUR-TK*) downstream of the 70-bp repeats in the same B-ES (Fig. 9). *VSG* switchers are expected to lose the *PUR-TK* marker or repress *PUR-TK* expression, making cells resistant to ganciclovir (GCV). After *VSG* switching, the mechanism of switching can also be determined by examination of various markers. *In-situ* switching occurs by inactivating the active B-ES and activating one of silent B-ESs. Therefore, *in-situ* switchers will preserve *BSD* and *VSG2* genes but repress their expression. ES gene conversion occurs through recombination near the B-ES promoter, which allows duplication and translocation of an entire silent B-ES to the *VSG2* subtelomere. These switchers will lose *BSD* and *VSG2* genes. Recombination near *VSGs* can result in either duplicative gene conversion of a new *VSG* to the *VSG2* B-ES (*VSG* gene conversion) or in *VSG* crossover switching. In both cases, the *BSD* gene will be at the active promoter, but these two recombinants can be distinguished by *VSG2* absence (*VSG* gene conversion) or presence (crossover).

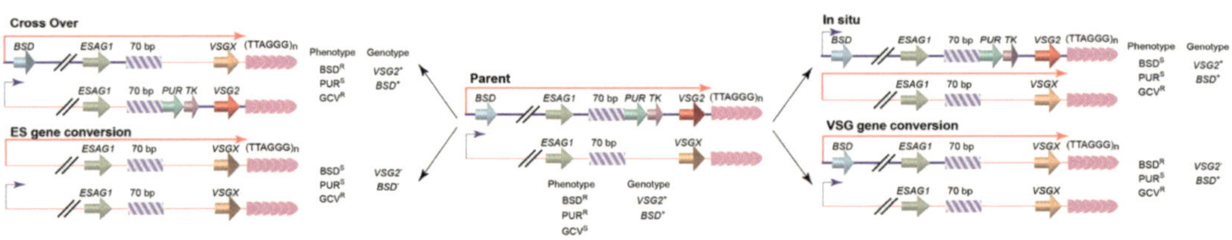

Fig. 9. Strategy for analyzing *VSG* switching in a double-marked *T. brucei* cell line. The parent cell line is shown in the center. Several different switching events are shown on either side.

In *T. brucei*, TbTRF is the duplex telomere DNA binding factor (Li et al. 2005), and it associates with TbTIN2. TbTIN2 was also observed to be localized at telomeres by IF and ChIP analyses, and TbTIN2 interacts with TbTRF *in vivo* in co-IP experiments, indicating that TbTIN2 is an intrinsic component of the *T. brucei* telomere complex (Jehi S. & Li B. unpublished data). Using the above described *VSG* switching assay, we observed that a transient depletion of TbTIN2 led to an ~3.8 fold increase in *VSG* switching frequency. In addition, 93% of all switching events are ES gene conversion in TbTIN2 deficient cells compared to 80% of the switchers were resulted from ES gene conversion in wild-type cells. Because TbTIN2 is essential for cell viability, it is only transiently depleted in the experiment so that switchers can be recovered. Therefore, the phenotype in true TbTIN2 null cells is expected to be more severe. TbTRF appears to have a similar influence on *VSG* switching (Benmerzouga I. & Li B., unpublished data). We have established viable cell lines that express a single TbTRF allele with a point mutation in its DNA binding myb domain. *In vitro* Isothermal Titration Calorimetry (ITC) analysis and *in vivo* ChIP analysis both confirmed that the mutant TbTRF has a severely reduced telomere DNA binding activity (Zhao Y., Benmerzouga I. & Li B., unpublished data). *VSG* switching frequency is ~3 fold higher in the TbTRF mutant than in wild-type cells. In the TbTRF mutant, 41% of the switchers were *VSG* gene conversion events compared to only 8% in wild-type cells. Depletion of another telomere protein, TbRAP1, also led to >7 fold of increase in *VSG* switching frequency, and 65% of all switchers resulted from *VSG* gene conversions, but only 30% of switchers resulted from ES gene conversion (Nanavaty V. & Li B., unpublished data). Depleting of TbRAP1 also led to derepression of subtelomeric *VSGs* (Yang et al. 2009), which is not observed in TbTRF or TbTIN2 deficient cells. Therefore, TbRAP1 appears to regulate *VSG* expression and *VSG* switching differently from TbTRF and TbTIN2.

These preliminary data indicate that the telomere structure is not only important for proper *VSG* silencing but also plays an important role in regulating *VSG* switching rate. It is possible that disruption of the heterochromatic telomere structure, especially in the case of depletion of TbRAP1, elevated subtelomeric homologous recombination and led to higher *VSG* switching rate, similar to what was observed in *S. pombe* (Bisht et al. 2008).

4.6 Does telomere affect switching of subtelomere-located surface antigen in *P. carinii* and *B. burgdorferi*?

Pneumocystis carinii is a fungus that solely dwells in the lung tissue of mammals. Normally, *P. carinii* infection does not cause any symptom, but in immunocompromised individuals it can cause pneumonia. The complete life cycle of *P. carinii* is still not very well defined, mainly because of the lack of a continuous cultivation system. However, it is obvious that *P. carinii* can survive in the lower respiratory tract where strong and effective defense systems normally work to eliminate invaders, and the reason for persistent and effective *P. carinii* infection is that it undergoes antigenic variation at a high frequency (Cushion & Stringer 2010).

The major surface glycoprotein (MSG) is one of the major surface molecules of *P. carinii* that is involved in antigenic variation (Stringer 2005). MSG is encoded by the *MSG* gene family. So far 73 *MSG* genes have been identified, all are located at the subtelomeric loci (Fig. 10) (Keely & Stringer 2009). There are 17 chromosomes in *P. carinii* (Hong et al. 1990), indicating that on average at least 2 *MSG* genes are at each telomere, which is often the case in cloned terminal fragments from various chromosomes (Keely et al. 2005; Wada & Nakamura 1996). Similar to the situation in *T. brucei*, only one *MSG* gene is transcribed at any time. Transcribed *MSG* messengers always contained an upstream conserved sequence (UCS) (Edman et al. 1996; Sunkin & Stringer 1997; Wada & Nakamura 1996; Wada et al. 1995), which has only one copy in the *P. carinii* genome (Edman et al. 1996; Wada et al. 1995), suggesting that *MSG* is transcribed from a specific expression site marked with the unique UCS element. In addition, translation initiation codon on an *MSG* mRNA is located in the sequence transcribed from the UCS (Edman et al. 1996; Wada et al. 1995). Therefore, transcribing MSG from UCS-containing expression site is essential for proper MSG translation. Furthermore, the UCS encoded peptide contains a signal sequence that targets the pre-MSG protein into the endoplasmic reticulum, where it can be cleaved and glycosylated, then deposited on the cell surface (Sunkin et al. 1998). Hence the UCS peptide is also essential for MSG function, although it is not present on MSG found on the cell surface because it is likely removed in the endoplasmic reticulum.

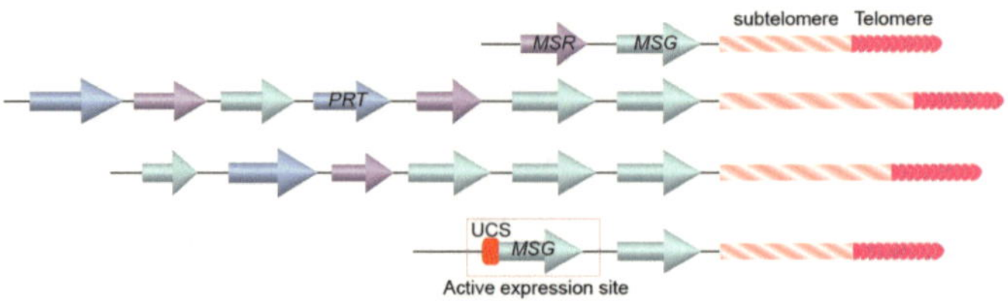

Fig. 10. Gene arrays at the ends of three *Pneumocystis carinii* chromosomes. *MSG* genes (cyan colored arrows) are located closest to the telomere and subtelomeric repetitive sequences. A single copy UCS is found in the active *MSG* expression site immediately upstream of the *MSG* gene.

If *P. carinii* contains only one UCS-containing *MSG* expression site, how does it achieve antigenic variation? Computational analysis of *MSG* gene sequences suggested that these genes commonly undergo recombination (Keely & Stringer 2009; Keely et al. 2005; Wada & Nakamura 1996), which is not unlike the *VSG* switching in *T. brucei*. Similar to *VSG*, *MSG* is also the last transcribed gene on the chromosome (Keely et al. 2005; Wada & Nakamura 1996). The proximity of *MSG* genes to telomeres suggests that the *MSG* switching events might also be regulated by the telomere structure, although this has not be investigated at all.

In a different microbial pathogen *Borrelia burgdorferi*, the spirochete that causes the Lyme disease, the gene encoding variant surface antigen is found at a subtelomere region on a linear plasmid (Zhang et al. 1997). *B. burgdorferi* also undergoes antigenic variation, and the liproprotein VlsE is the variant surface protein (Norris 2006; Schwan et al. 1991; Steere et al. 2004; Zhang & Norris 1998a; Zhang et al. 1997). VlsE is encoded by the *vls* gene family located on the linear plasmid lp28-1 (Fig. 11). Immediately next to the telomere is the active *vlsE* expression site. More upstream is the silent *vls* gene cluster (Zhang et al. 1997). Bacteria lost the lp28-1 exhibit an intermediate infectivity phenotype where it is hard to establish a persistent infection in the mouse model (Bankhead & Chaconas 2007). Deletion of *vlsE* and silent *vls* cassettes also led to reduced persistent infection, indicating that antigenic variation through *vls* switching is an important virulence mechanism in *B. burgdorferi* (Bankhead & Chaconas 2007; Labandeira-Rey & Skare 2001; Purser & Norris 2000; Zhang et al. 1997). The *vlsE* and the silent *vls* genes are highly homologous at the sequence level, and most of the sequence differences within the cassette regions are concentrated in six variable regions, VR1–VR6 (Zhang & Norris 1998b). Segmental gene conversion between the silent cassettes and the *vlsE* cassette region occurs as early as 4 days after infection in mice, and appears to continue throughout the course of infection (Zhang & Norris 1998a). Because these recombination events appear to involve random segments of any silent cassette and occur continuously during infection, an almost unlimited number of *VlsE* amino acid sequence permutations are theoretically possible (Zhang & Norris 1998b). Apparently, *vls* switching is not so unlike the *VSG* switching in *T. brucei* or *MSG* switching in *P. carinii*. However, nothing is known about the telomere structure at the ends of lp28 or any protein(s) associated with it. Therefore, it is unclear whether the nearby telomere structure might exhibit any influence to *vls* switching.

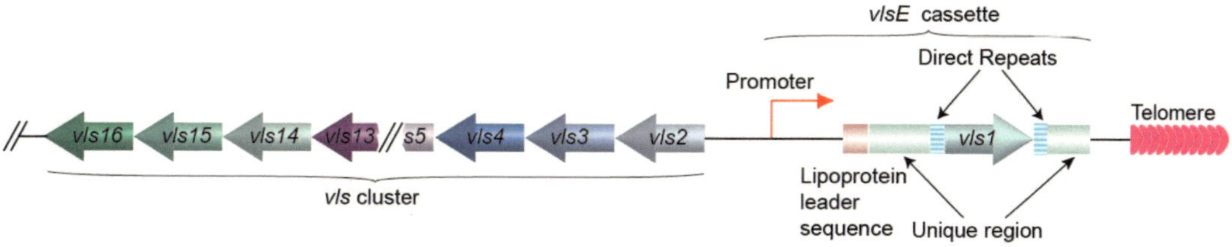

Fig. 11. The organization of *vlsE* and the array of silent *vls* genes on lp28 linear plasmid of *B. burgdorferi*. The *vls1* gene (moss colored arrow) is expressed from the *vlsE* expression site next to the telomere (pink arrows). The direct repeats (barred boxes) and the unique regions (green boxes) flanking the *vls1* gene and the lipoprotein leader sequence (rouge box) upstream of *vls1* are marked. The silent array includes *vls 2–16* genes (various colored arrows) going to the opposite direction from *vls1* are located at the internal region of the linear plasmid.

5. Conclusions

In many organisms, telomere forms a specialized heterochromatic structure that can influence the expression of genes located nearby. It appears that a number of microbial pathogens have conveniently taken advantage of this telomere position effect to regulate expression of surface antigen-encoding gene families at subtelomeric regions. Further studies of the telomere structure and telomere specific proteins in these microbial pathogens should provide more insight about the allelic exclusion expression of surface antigen genes. Similarly, the subtelomeric region in many eukaryotic cells appear to be a recombination hot spot, which has been proposed to contribute to gene diversity. This could be one of the reasons why many gene families encoding virulence factors are located at subtelomeric loci. One cannot help to speculate that the intrinsic plastic nature of the subtelomeres might facilitate antigenic variation. On the other hand, unchecked homologous recombination could cause hazardous genome instability, and the telomere structure with telomere-specific proteins appears to suppress subtelomeric recombination to maintain a relatively stable genome organization.

6. References

Abad, J. P.; De Pablos, B.; Osoegawa, K.; De Jong, P. J.; Martin-Gallardo, A. et al. 2004. TAHRE, a novel telomeric retrotransposon from Drosophila melanogaster, reveals the origin of Drosophila telomeres. *Mol Biol Evol* 21: 1620-1624.

Aitcheson, N.; Talbot, S.; Shapiro, J.; Hughes, K.; Adkin, C. et al. 2005. VSG switching in Trypanosoma brucei: antigenic variation analysed using RNAi in the absence of immune selection. *Mol Microbiol* 57: 1608-1622.

Alsford, S.; Kawahara, T.; Isamah, C. & Horn, D. 2007. A sirtuin in the African trypanosome is involved in both DNA repair and telomeric gene silencing but is not required for antigenic variation. *Mol Microbiol* 63: 724-736.

Alsford, S.; Wickstead, B.; Ersfeld, K. & Gull, K. 2001. Diversity and dynamics of the minichromosomal karyotype in *Trypanosoma brucei*. *Mol. Biochem. Parasitol.* 113: 79-88.

Altaf, M.; Utley, R. T.; Lacoste, N.; Tan, S.; Briggs, S. D. et al. 2007. Interplay of chromatin modifiers on a short basic patch of histone H4 tail defines the boundary of telomeric heterochromatin. *Mol Cell* 28: 1002-1014.

Andreyeva, E. N.; Belyaeva, E. S.; Semeshin, V. F.; Pokholkova, G. V. & Zhimulev, I. F. 2005. Three distinct chromatin domains in telomere ends of polytene chromosomes in Drosophila melanogaster Tel mutants. *J Cell Sci* 118: 5465-5477.

Andrulis, E. D.; Neiman, A. M.; Zappulla, D. C. & Sternglanz, R. 1998. Perinuclear localization of chromatin facilitates transcriptional silencing. *Nature* 394: 592-595.

Aparicio, O. M.; Billington, B. L. & Gottschling, D. E. 1991. Modifiers of position effect are shared between telomeric and silent mating-type loci in S. cerevisiae. *Cell* 66: 1279-1287.

Bailey, S. M.; Cornforth, M. N.; Kurimasa, A.; Chen, D. J. & Goodwin, E. H. 2001. Strand-specific Postreplicative Processing of Mammalian Telomeres. *Science* 2462-2465.

Bailey, S. M.; Brenneman, M. A. & Goodwin, E. H. 2004. Frequent recombination in telomeric DNA may extend the proliferative life of telomerase-negative cells. *Nucleic Acids Res* 32: 3743-3751.

Bankhead, T. & Chaconas, G. 2007. The role of VlsE antigenic variation in the Lyme disease spirochete: persistence through a mechanism that differs from other pathogens. *Mol Microbiol* 65: 1547-1558.

Barry, J. D. & McCulloch, R. 2001. Antigenic variation in trypanosomes: enhanced phenotypic variation in a eukaryotic parasite. *Adv Parasitol* 49: 1-70.

Baruch, D. I.; Pasloske, B. L.; Singh, H. B.; Bi, X.; Ma, X. C. et al. 1995. Cloning the P. falciparum gene encoding PfEMP1, a malarial variant antigen and adherence receptor on the surface of parasitized human erythrocytes. *Cell* 82: 77-87.

Baruch, D. I. 1999. Adhesive receptors on malaria-parasitized red cells. *Baillieres Best Pract Res Clin Haematol* 12: 747-761.

Baumann, P. & Cech, T. R. 2001. Pot1, the putative telomere end-binding protein in fission yeast and humans. *Science* 292: 1171-1175.

Baur, J. A.; Zou, Y.; Shay, J. W. & Wright, W. E. 2001. Telomere position effect in human cells. *Science* 292: 2075-2077.

Benetti, R.; Gonzalo, S.; Jaco, I.; Schotta, G.; Klatt, P. et al. 2007. Suv4-20h deficiency results in telomere elongation and derepression of telomere recombination. *J Cell Biol* 178: 925-936.

Bernards, A.; Michels, P. A. M.; Lincke, C. R. & Borst, P. 1983. Growth of chromosome ends in multiplying trypanosomes. *Nature* 303: 592-597.

Berriman, M.; Ghedin, E.; Hertz-Fowler, C.; Blandin, G.; Renauld, H. et al. 2005. The genome of the African trypanosome *Trypanosoma brucei*. *Science* 309: 416-422.

Biessmann, H.; Valgeirsdottir, K.; Lofsky, A.; Chin, C.; Ginther, B. et al. 1992. HeT-A, a transposable element specifically involved in "healing" broken chromosome ends in Drosophila melanogaster. *Mol Cell Biol* 12: 3910-3918.

Biessmann, H.; Kasravi, B.; Bui, T.; Fujiwara, G.; Champion, L. E. et al. 1994. Comparison of two active HeT-A retroposons of Drosophila melanogaster. *Chromosoma* 103: 90-98.

Biessmann, H.; Prasad, S.; Semeshin, V. F.; Andreyeva, E. N.; Nguyen, Q. et al. 2005. Two distinct domains in Drosophila melanogaster telomeres. *Genetics* 171: 1767-1777.

Bilaud, T.; Brun, C.; Ancelin, K.; Koering, C. E.; Laroche, T. et al. 1997. Telomeric localization of TRF2, a novel human telobox protein. *Nat. Genet.* 17: 236-239.

Bisht, K. K.; Arora, S.; Ahmed, S. & Singh, J. 2008. Role of heterochromatin in suppressing subtelomeric recombination in fission yeast. *Yeast* 25: 537-548.

Boivin, A.; Gally, C.; Netter, S.; Anxolabehere, D. & Ronsseray, S. 2003. Telomeric associated sequences of Drosophila recruit polycomb-group proteins in vivo and can induce pairing-sensitive repression. *Genetics* 164: 195-208.

Boothroyd, C. E.; Dreesen, O.; Leonova, T.; Ly, K. I.; Figueiredo, L. M. et al. 2009. A yeast-endonuclease-generated DNA break induces antigenic switching in *Trypanosoma brucei*. *Nature* 459: 278-281.

Bork, P.; Hofmann, K.; Bucher, P.; Neuwald, A. F.; Altschul, S. F. et al. 1997. A superfamily of conserved domains in DNA damage-responsive cell cycle checkpoint proteins. *FASEB J.* 11: 68-76.

Boscheron, C.; Maillet, L.; Marcand, S.; Tsai-Pflugfelder, M.; Gasser, S. M. et al. 1996. Cooperation at a distance between silencers and proto-silencers at the yeast HML locus. *EMBO J* 15: 2184-2195.

Boulton, S. J. & Jackson, S. P. 1998. Components of the Ku-dependent non-homologous end-joining pathway are involved in telomeric length maintenance and telomeric silencing. *EMBO J.* 17: 1819-1828.

———. 1996. Identification of a *Saccharomyces cerevisiae* Ku80 homologue: roles in DNA double strand break rejoining and in telomeric maintenance. *Nucleic Acids Res* 24: 4639-4648.

Bourns, B. D.; Alexander, M. K.; Smith, A. M. & Zakian, V. A. 1998. Sir proteins, Rif proteins, and Cdc13p bind *Saccharomyces telomeres* in vivo. *Mol Cell Biol* 18: 5600-5608.

Broadbent, K. M.; Park, D.; Wolf, A. R.; Van Tyne, D.; Sims, J. S. et al. 2011. A global transcriptional analysis of Plasmodium falciparum malaria reveals a novel family of telomere-associated lncRNAs. *Genome Biol* 12: R56.

Broccoli, D.; Smogorzewska, A.; Chong, L. & de Lange, T. 1997. Human telomeres contain two distinct Myb-related proteins, TRF1 and TRF2. *Nat. Genet.* 17: 231-235.

Brown, W. R.; MacKinnon, P. J.; Villasante, A.; Spurr, N.; Buckle, V. J. et al. 1990. Structure and polymorphism of human telomere-associated DNA. *Cell* 63: 119-132.

Bryan, T. M.; Englezou, A.; Gupta, J.; Bacchetti, S. & Reddel, R. R. 1995. Telomere elongation in immortal human cells without detectable telomerase activity. *Embo J* 14: 4240-4248.

Bryan, T. M.; Englezou, A.; Dalla-Pozza, L.; Dunham, M. A. & Reddel, R. R. 1997. Evidence for an alternative mechanism for maintaining telomere length in human tumors and tumor-derived cell lines [see comments]. *Nat Med* 3: 1271-1274.

Buchberger, J. R.; Onishi, M.; Li, G.; Seebacher, J.; Rudner, A. D. et al. 2008. Sir3-nucleosome interactions in spreading of silent chromatin in Saccharomyces cerevisiae. *Mol Cell Biol* 28: 6903-6918.

Buck, S. W. & Shore, D. 1995. Action of a RAP1 carboxy-terminal silencing domain reveals an underlying competition between HMR and telomeres in yeast. *Genes Dev* 9: 370-384.

Calderwood, M. S.; Gannoun-Zaki, L.; Wellems, T. E. & Deitsch, K. W. 2003. Plasmodium falciparum var genes are regulated by two regions with separate promoters, one upstream of the coding region and a second within the intron. *J Biol Chem* 278: 34125-34132.

Callebaut, I. & Mornon, J. P. 1997. From BRCA1 to RAP1: a widespread BRCT module closely associated with DNA repair. *FEBS Lett.* 400: 25-30.

Cam, H. P.; Sugiyama, T.; Chen, E. S.; Chen, X.; FitzGerald, P. C. et al. 2005. Comprehensive analysis of heterochromatin- and RNAi-mediated epigenetic control of the fission yeast genome. *Nat Genet* 37: 809-819.

Carlson, M. & Botstein, D. 1983. Organization of the SUC gene family in Saccharomyces. *Mol Cell Biol* 3: 351-359.

Carlson, M.; Celenza, J. L. & Eng, F. J. 1985. Evolution of the dispersed SUC gene family of Saccharomyces by rearrangements of chromosome telomeres. *Mol Cell Biol* 5: 2894-2902.

Castano, I.; Pan, S. J.; Zupancic, M.; Hennequin, C.; Dujon, B. et al. 2005. Telomere length control and transcriptional regulation of subtelomeric adhesins in *Candida glabrata*. *Mol Microbiol* 55: 1246-1258.

Cenci, G.; Siriaco, G.; Raffa, G. D.; Kellum, R. & Gatti, M. 2003. The Drosophila HOAP protein is required for telomere capping. *Nat Cell Biol* 5: 82-84.

Chakrabarty, S. P.; Saikumari, Y. K.; Bopanna, M. P. & Balaram, H. 2008. Biochemical characterization of Plasmodium falciparum Sir2, a NAD+-dependent deacetylase. *Mol Biochem Parasitol* 158: 139-151.

Chan, C. S. M. & Tye, B.-K. 1983a. Organization of DNA sequences and replication origins at yeast telomeres. *Cell* 33: 563-573.

Chan, C. S. M. & Tye, B.-K. 1983b. A family of Saccharomyces cerevisiae repetitive autonomously replicating sequences that have very similar genomic environments. *JMB* 168: 505-524.

Charron, M. J. & Michels, C. A. 1988. The naturally occurring alleles of MAL1 in Saccharomyces species evolved by various mutagenic processes including chromosomal rearrangement. *Genetics* 120: 83-93.

Charron, M. J.; Read, E.; Haut, S. R. & Michels, C. A. 1989. Molecular evolution of the telomere-associated MAL loci of Saccharomyces. *Genetics* 122: 307-316.

Chaves, I.; Rudenko, G.; Dirks-Mulder, A.; Cross, M. & Borst, P. 1999. Control of variant surface glycoprotein gene-expression sites in *Trypanosoma brucei*. *EMBO J* 18: 4846-4855.

Chen, Y.; Rai, R.; Zhou, Z. R.; Kanoh, J.; Ribeyre, C. et al. 2011. A conserved motif within RAP1 has diversified roles in telomere protection and regulation in different organisms. *Nat Struct Mol Biol*

Cheng, Q.; Cloonan, N.; Fischer, K.; Thompson, J.; Waine, G. et al. 1998. stevor and rif are Plasmodium falciparum multicopy gene families which potentially encode variant antigens. *Mol Biochem Parasitol* 97: 161-176.

Chong, L.; van Steensel, B.; Broccoli, D.; Erdjument-Bromage, H.; Hanish, J. et al. 1995. A human telomeric protein. *Science* 270: 1663-1667.

Chookajorn, T.; Dzikowski, R.; Frank, M.; Li, F.; Jiwani, A. Z. et al. 2007. Epigenetic memory at malaria virulence genes. *Proc Natl Acad Sci U S A* 104: 899-902.

Cifuentes-Rojas, C. & Shippen, D. E. 2011. Telomerase regulation. *Mutat Res*

Cockell, M.; Palladino, F.; Laroche, T.; Kyrion, G.; Liu, C. et al. 1995. The carboxy termini of Sir4 and Rap1 affect Sir3 localization: Evidence for a multicomponent complex required for yeast telomeric silencing. *J Cell Biol* 129: 909-924.

Cooper, J. P.; Nimmo, E. R.; Allshire, R. C. & Cech, T. R. 1997. Regulation of telomere length and function by a Myb-domain protein in fission yeast. *Nature* 385: 744-747.

Corcoran, L. M.; Thompson, J. K.; Walliker, D. & Kemp, D. J. 1988. Homologous recombination within subtelomeric repeat sequences generates chromosome size polymorphisms in P. falciparum. *Cell* 53: 807-813.

Cormack, B. P.; Ghori, N. & Falkow, S. 1999. An adhesin of the yeast pathogen Candida glabrata mediating adherence to human epithelial cells. *Science* 285: 578-582.

Cornelissen, A. W.; Bakkeren, G. A.; Barry, J. D.; Michels, P. A. & Borst, P. 1985. Characteristics of trypanosome variant antigen genes active in the tsetse fly. *NAR* 13: 4661-4676.

Creamer, K. M. & Partridge, J. F. 2011. RITS-connecting transcription, RNA interference, and heterochromatin assembly in fission yeast. *Wiley Interdiscip Rev RNA* 2: 632-646.

Critchlow, S. E. & Jackson, S. P. 1998. DNA end-joining: from yeast to man. *TIBS* 23: 394-398.

Cross, S.; Lindsey, J.; Fantes, J.; McKay, S.; McGill, N. et al. 1990. The structure of a subterminal repeated sequence present on many human chromosomes. *Nucleic Acids Res* 18: 6649-6657.

Cryderman, D. E.; Morris, E. J.; Biessmann, H.; Elgin, S. C. & Wallrath, L. L. 1999. Silencing at Drosophila telomeres: nuclear organization and chromatin structure play critical roles. *EMBO J* 18: 3724-3735.

Cushion, M. T. & Stringer, J. R. 2010. Stealth and opportunism: alternative lifestyles of species in the fungal genus Pneumocystis. *Annu Rev Microbiol* 64: 431-452.

De Bruin, D.; Lanzer, M. & Ravetch, J. V. 1994. The polymorphic subtelomeric regions of Plasmodium falciparum chromosomes contain arrays of repetitive sequence elements. *Proc Natl Acad Sci Usa* 91: 619-623.

de Lange, T. & Borst, P. 1982. Genomic environment of the expression-linked extra copies of genes for surface antigens of *Trypanosoma brucei* resembles the end of a chromosome. *Nature* 299: 451-453.

de Lange, T.; Shiue, L.; Myers, R. M.; Cox, D. R.; Naylor, S. L. et al. 1990. Structure and variability of human chromosome ends. *Mol. Cell. Biol.* 10: 518-527.

de Lange, T. 2002. Protection of mammalian telomeres. *Oncogene* 21: 532-540.

———. 2005. Shelterin: the protein complex that shapes and safeguards human telomeres. *Genes Dev* 19: 2100-2110.

De Las Penas, A.; Pan, S. J.; Castano, I.; Alder, J.; Cregg, R. et al. 2003. Virulence-related surface glycoproteins in the yeast pathogen *Candida glabrata* are encoded in subtelomeric clusters and subject to RAP1- and SIR-dependent transcriptional silencing. *Genes Dev* 17: 2245-2258.

Dehe, P. M. & Cooper, J. P. 2010. Fission yeast telomeres forecast the end of the crisis. *FEBS Lett* 584: 3725-3733.

Deitsch, K. W.; Calderwood, M. S. & Wellems, T. E. 2001. Malaria - Cooperative silencing elements in var genes. *Nature* 412: 875-876.

Deitsch, K. W.; Lukehart, S. A. & Stringer, J. R. 2009. Common strategies for antigenic variation by bacterial, fungal and protozoan pathogens. *Nat Rev Microbiol* 7: 493-503.

DeMaria, S. & Ngai, J. 2010. The cell biology of smell. *J Cell Biol* 191: 443-452.

Denninger, V.; Fullbrook, A.; Bessat, M.; Ersfeld, K. & Rudenko, G. 2010. The FACT subunit TbSpt16 is involved in cell cycle specific control of VSG expression sites in *Trypanosoma brucei*. *Mol Microbiol* 78: 459-474.

Diffley, J. F. & Stillman, B. 1989. Similarity between the transcriptional silencer binding proteins ABF1 and RAP1. *Science* 246: 1034-1038.

Domergue, R.; Castano, I.; De Las Penas, A.; Zupancic, M.; Lockatell, V. et al. 2005. Nicotinic acid limitation regulates silencing of Candida adhesins during UTI. *Science* 308: 866-870.

Dreesen, O. & Cross, G. A. 2006a. Consequences of telomere shortening at an active VSG expression site in telomerase-deficient Trypanosoma brucei. *Eukaryot. Cell* 5: 2114-2119.

———. 2006b. Telomerase-independent stabilization of short telomeres in Trypanosoma brucei. *Mol. Cell. Biol.* 26: 4911-4919.

Dreesen, O.; Li, B. & Cross, G. A. M. 2007. Telomere structure and function in trypanosomes: a proposal. *Nat Rev Microbiol* 5: 70-75.

Dreesen, O. & Cross, G. A. M. 2008. Telomere length in *Trypanosoma brucei*. *Exp Parasitol* 118: 103-110.

Driller, L.; Wellinger, R. J.; Larrivee, M.; Kremmer, E.; Jaklin, S. et al. 2000. A short C-terminal domain of Yku70p is essential for telomere maintenance. *J Biol Chem* 275: 24921-24927.

Dunham, M. A.; Neumann, A. A.; Fasching, C. L. & Reddel, R. R. 2000. Telomere maintenance by recombination in human cells. *Nat Genet* 26: 447-450.

Duraisingh, M. T.; Voss, T. S.; Marty, A. J.; Duffy, M. F.; Good, R. T. et al. 2005. Heterochromatin silencing and locus repositioning linked to regulation of virulence genes in *Plasmodium falciparum*. *Cell* 121: 13-24.

Dzikowski, R.; Li, F.; Amulic, B.; Eisberg, A.; Frank, M. et al. 2007. Mechanisms underlying mutually exclusive expression of virulence genes by malaria parasites. *EMBO Rep* 8: 959-965.

Dzikowski, R. & Deitsch, K. W. 2009. Genetics of antigenic variation in Plasmodium falciparum. *Curr Genet* 55: 103-110.

Edman, J. C.; Hatton, T. W.; Nam, M.; Turner, R.; Mei, Q. et al. 1996. A single expression site with a conserved leader sequence regulates variation of expression of the Pneumocystis carinii family of major surface glycoprotein genes. *DNA Cell Biol* 15: 989-999.

Ehrenhofer-Murray, A. E.; Rivier, D. H. & Rine, J. 1997. The role of Sas2, an acetyltransferase homologue of Saccharomyces cerevisiae, in silencing and ORC function. *Genetics* 145: 923-934.

Eid, J. E. & Sollner-Webb, B. 1995. ST-1, a 39-kilodalton protein in Trypanosoma brucei, exhibits a dual affinity for the duplex form of the 29-base-pair subtelomeric repeat and its C-rich strand. *Mol Cell Biol* 15: 389-397.

———. 1997. ST-2, a telomere and subtelomere duplex and G-strand binding protein activity in Trypanosoma brucei. *J Biol Chem* 272: 14927-14936.

Ekwall, K.; Javerzat, J. P.; Lorentz, A.; Schmidt, H.; Cranston, G. et al. 1995. The chromodomain protein Swi6: a key component at fission yeast centromeres. *Science* 269: 1429-1431.

Epp, C.; Li, F.; Howitt, C. A.; Chookajorn, T. & Deitsch, K. W. 2009. Chromatin associated sense and antisense noncoding RNAs are transcribed from the var gene family of virulence genes of the malaria parasite Plasmodium falciparum. *RNA* 15: 116-127.

Eugster, A.; Lanzuolo, C.; Bonneton, M.; Luciano, P.; Pollice, A. et al. 2006. The finger subdomain of yeast telomerase cooperates with Pif1p to limit telomere elongation. *Nat Struct Mol Biol* 13: 734-739.

Fanti, L.; Giovinazzo, G.; Berloco, M. & Pimpinelli, S. 1998. The heterochromatin protein 1 prevents telomere fusions in Drosophila. *Mol Cell* 2: 527-538.

Feeser, E. A. & Wolberger, C. 2008. Structural and functional studies of the Rap1 C-terminus reveal novel separation-of-function mutants. *J Mol Biol* 380: 520-531.

Feng, Q.; Wang, H.; Ng, H. H.; Erdjument-Bromage, H.; Tempst, P. et al. 2002. Methylation of H3-lysine 79 is mediated by a new family of HMTases without a SET domain. *Curr Biol* 12: 1052-1058.

Figueiredo, L. M.; Freitas-Junior, L. H.; Bottius, E.; Olivo-Marin, J. C. & Scherf, A. 2002. A central role for *Plasmodium falciparum* subtelomeric regions in spatial positioning and telomere length regulation. *EMBO Journal* 21: 815-824.

Figueiredo, L. M. & Cross, G. A. M. 2010. Nucleosomes are depleted at the VSG expression site transcribed by RNA polymerase I in African trypanosomes. *Eukaryot Cell* 9: 148-154.

Foss, M.; McNally, F. J.; Laurenson, P. & Rine, J. 1993. Origin recognition complex (ORC) in transcriptional silencing and DNA replication in S. cerevisiae. *Science* 262: 1838-1844.

Fourel, G.; Revardel, E.; Koering, C. E. & Gilson, E. 1999. Cohabitation of insulators and silencing elements in yeast subtelomeric regions. *Embo J* 18: 2522-2537.

Frank, M.; Dzikowski, R.; Costantini, D.; Amulic, B.; Berdougo, E. et al. 2006. Strict pairing of var promoters and introns is required for var gene silencing in the malaria parasite Plasmodium falciparum. *J Biol Chem* 281: 9942-9952.

Freitas-Junior, L. H.; Hernandez-Rivas, R.; Ralph, S. A.; Montiel-Condado, D.; Ruvalcaba-Salazar, O. K. et al. 2005. Telomeric heterochromatin propagation and histone acetylation control mutually exclusive expression of antigenic variation genes in malaria parasites. *Cell* 121: 25-36.

Frydrychova, R. C.; Mason, J. M. & Archer, T. K. 2008. HP1 is distributed within distinct chromatin domains at Drosophila telomeres. *Genetics* 180: 121-131.

Gardner, M. J.; Hall, N.; Fung, E.; White, O.; Berriman, M. et al. 2002. Genome sequence of the human malaria parasite Plasmodium falciparum. *Nature* 419: 498-511.

Gartenberg, M. R.; Neumann, F. R.; Laroche, T.; Blaszczyk, M. & Gasser, S. M. 2004. Sir-mediated repression can occur independently of chromosomal and subnuclear contexts. *Cell* 119: 955-967.

Gehring, W. J.; Klemenz, R.; Weber, U. & Kloter, U. 1984. Functional analysis of the white gene of Drosophila by P-factor-mediated transformation. *EMBO J* 3: 2077-2085.

Giraldo, R. & Rhodes, D. 1994. The yeast telomere-binding protein RAP1 binds to and promotes the formation of DNA quadruplexes in telomeric DNA. *Embo J* 13: 2411-2420.

Glover, J. N.; Williams, R. S. & Lee, M. S. 2004. Interactions between BRCT repeats and phosphoproteins: tangled up in two. *Trends Biochem Sci* 29: 579-585.

Glover, L.; Alsford, S.; Beattie, C. & Horn, D. 2007. Deletion of a trypanosome telomere leads to loss of silencing and progressive loss of terminal DNA in the absence of cell cycle arrest. *Nuc Acids Res* 35: 872-880.

Glover, L. & Horn, D. 2006. Repression of polymerase I-mediated gene expression at *Trypanosoma brucei* telomeres. *EMBO Rep* 7: 93-99.

Gotta, M.; Laroche, T.; Formenton, A.; Maillet, L.; Scherthan, H. et al. 1996. The clustering of telomeres and colocalization with Rap1, Sir3, and Sir4 proteins in wild-type *Saccharomyces cerevisiae. Journal of Cell Biology* 134: 1349-1363.

Gottschling, D. E.; Aparicio, O. M.; Billington, B. L. & Zakian, V. A. 1990. Position effect at *S. cerevisiae* telomeres: reversible repression of pol II transcription. *Cell* 63: 751-762.

Graham, S. V.; Wymer, B. & Barry, J. D. 1998. Activity of a trypanosome metacyclic variant surface glycoprotein gene promoter is dependent upon life cycle stage and chromosomal context. *Molecular & Cellular Biology* 18: 1137-1146.

Grandin, N.; Reed, S. I. & Charbonneau, M. 1997. Stn1, a new *Saccharomyces cerevisiae* protein, is implicated in telomere size regulation in association with cdc13. *Genes & Development* 11: 512-527.

Grandin, N.; Damon, C. & Charbonneau, M. 2001. Ten1 functions in telomere end protection and length regulation in association with Stn1 and Cdc13. *Embo J* 20: 1173-1183.

Greider, C. W. & Blackburn, E. H. 1987. The telomere terminal transferase of Tetrahymena is a ribonucleoprotein enzyme with two kinds of primer specificity. *Cell* 51: 887-898.

Grewal, S. I. & Jia, S. 2007. Heterochromatin revisited. *Nat Rev Genet* 8: 35-46.

Griffith, J. D.; Comeau, L.; Rosenfield, S.; Stansel, R. M.; Bianchi, A. et al. 1999. Mammalian telomeres end in a large duplex loop. *Cell* 97: 503-514.

Grobelny, J. V.; Godwin, A. K. & Broccoli, D. 2000. ALT-associated PML bodies are present in viable cells and are enriched in cells in the G(2)/M phase of the cell cycle. *J Cell Sci* 113 Pt 24: 4577-4585.

Gunzl, A.; Bruderer, T.; Laufer, G.; Schimanski, B.; Tu, L. C. et al. 2003. RNA polymerase I transcribes procyclin genes and variant surface glycoprotein gene expression sites in *Trypanosoma brucei*. *Eukaryot Cell* 2: 542-551.

Hall, I. M.; Shankaranarayana, G. D.; Noma, K.; Ayoub, N.; Cohen, A. et al. 2002. Establishment and maintenance of a heterochromatin domain. *Science* 297: 2232-2237.

Halme, A.; Bumgarner, S.; Styles, C. & Fink, G. R. 2004. Genetic and epigenetic regulation of the FLO gene family generates cell-surface variation in yeast. *Cell* 116: 405-415.

Hanaoka, S.; Nagadoi, A.; Yoshimura, S.; Aimoto, S.; Li, B. et al. 2001. NMR structure of the hRap1 Myb motif reveals a canonical three-helix bundle lacking the positive surface charge typical of Myb DNA-binding domains. *J Mol Biol* 312: 167-175.

Hande, M. P.; Samper, E.; Lansdorp, P. & Blasco, M. A. 1999. Telomere length dynamics and chromosomal instability in cells derived from telomerase null mice. *J Cell Biol* 144: 589-601.

Hartley, C. L. & McCulloch, R. 2008. *Trypanosoma brucei* BRCA2 acts in antigenic variation and has undergone a recent expansion in BRC repeat number that is important during homologous recombination. *Mol Microbiol* 68: 1237-1251.

Hazelrigg, T.; Levis, R. & Rubin, G. M. 1984. Transformation of white locus DNA in drosophila: dosage compensation, zeste interaction, and position effects. *Cell* 36: 469-481.

Hecht, A.; Laroche, T.; Strahl-Bolsinger, S.; Gasser, S. M. & Grunstein, M. 1995. Histone H3 and H4 N-termini interact with SIR3 and SIR4 proteins: A molecular model for the formation of heterochromatin in yeast. *Cell* 80: 583-592.

Hecht, A.; Strahl-Bolsinger, S. & Grunstein, M. 1996. Spreading of transcriptional repressor SIR3 from telomeric heterochromatin. *Nature* 383: 92-96.

Hertz-Fowler, C.; Figueiredo, L. M.; Quail, M. A.; Becker, M.; Jackson, A. et al. 2008. Telomeric expression sites are highly conserved in *Trypanosoma brucei*. *PLoS ONE* 3: e3527.

Holloman, W. K. 2011. Unraveling the mechanism of BRCA2 in homologous recombination. *Nat Struct Mol Biol* 18: 748-754.

Holthausen, J. T.; Wyman, C. & Kanaar, R. 2010. Regulation of DNA strand exchange in homologous recombination. *DNA Repair (Amst)* 9: 1264-1272.

Hong, S. T.; Steele, P. E.; Cushion, M. T.; Walzer, P. D.; Stringer, S. L. et al. 1990. Pneumocystis carinii karyotypes. *J Clin Microbiol* 28: 1785-1795.

Hoppe, G. J.; Tanny, J. C.; Rudner, A. D.; Gerber, S. A.; Danaie, S. et al. 2002. Steps in assembly of silent chromatin in yeast: Sir3-independent binding of a Sir2/Sir4 complex to silencers and role for Sir2-dependent deacetylation. *Mol. Cell. Biol.* 22: 4167-4180.

Horn, D. & McCulloch, R. 2010. Molecular mechanisms underlying the control of antigenic variation in African trypanosomes. *Curr Opin Microbiol* 13: 700-705.

Horn, D. & Cross, G. A. M. 1997. Position-dependent and promoter-specific regulation of gene expression in *Trypanosoma brucei*. *EMBO J* 16: 7422-7431.

———. 1997. Analysis of *Trypanosoma brucei vsg* expression site switching *in vitro*. *Mol. Biochem. Parasitol.* 84: 189-201.

Horn, D.; Spence, C. & Ingram, A. K. 2000. Telomere maintenance and length regulation in *Trypanosoma brucei*. *EMBO J.* 19: 2332-2339.

Houghtaling, B. R.; Cuttonaro, L.; Chang, W. & Smith, S. 2004. A Dynamic Molecular Link between the Telomere Length Regulator TRF1 and the Chromosome End Protector TRF2. *Curr Biol* 14: 1621-1631.

Hughes, K.; Wand, M.; Foulston, L.; Young, R.; Harley, K. et al. 2007. A novel ISWI is involved in *VSG* expression site downregulation in African trypanosomes. *EMBO J* 26: 2400-2410.

Ijdo, J. W.; Lindsay, E. A.; Wells, R. A. & Baldini, A. 1992. Multiple variants in subtelomeric regions of normal karyotypes. *Genomics* 14: 1019-1025.

Imai, S.; Armstrong, C. M.; Kaeberlein, M. & Guarente, L. 2000. Transcriptional silencing and longevity protein Sir2 is an NAD- dependent histone deacetylase. *Nature* 403: 795-800.

Iraqui, I.; Garcia-Sanchez, S.; Aubert, S.; Dromer, F.; Ghigo, J. M. et al. 2005. The Yak1p kinase controls expression of adhesins and biofilm formation in Candida glabrata in a Sir4p-dependent pathway. *Mol Microbiol* 55: 1259-1271.

Janzen, C. J.; Hake, S. B.; Lowell, J. E. & Cross, G. A. 2006. Selective di- or trimethylation of histone H3 lysine 76 by two DOT1 homologs is important for cell cycle regulation in Trypanosoma brucei. *Mol Cell* 23: 497-507.

Johnson, A.; Li, G.; Sikorski, T. W.; Buratowski, S.; Woodcock, C. L. et al. 2009. Reconstitution of heterochromatin-dependent transcriptional gene silencing. *Mol Cell* 35: 769-781.

Johnson, P. J.; Kooter, J. M. & Borst, P. 1987. Inactivation of transcription by UV irradiation of *T. brucei* provides evidence for a multicistronic transcription unit including a VSG gene. *Cell* 51: 273-281.

Kanoh, J.; Sadaie, M.; Urano, T. & Ishikawa, F. 2005. Telomere binding protein Taz1 establishes Swi6 heterochromatin independently of RNAi at telomeres. *Curr Biol* 15: 1808-1819.

Kanoh, J. & Ishikawa, F. 2001. spRap1 and spRif1, recruited to telomeres by Taz1, are essential for telomere function in fission yeast. *Curr Biol* 11: 1624-1630.

Kapteyn, J. C.; Van Den Ende, H. & Klis, F. M. 1999. The contribution of cell wall proteins to the organization of the yeast cell wall. *Biochim Biophys Acta* 1426: 373-383.

Karpen, G. H. & Spradling, A. C. 1992. Analysis of subtelomeric heterochromatin in the Drosophila minichromosome Dp1187 by single P element insertional mutagenesis. *Genetics* 132: 737-753.

Kaur, R.; Domergue, R.; Zupancic, M. L. & Cormack, B. P. 2005. A yeast by any other name: Candida glabrata and its interaction with the host. *Curr Opin Microbiol* 8: 378-384.

Kaviratne, M.; Khan, S. M.; Jarra, W. & Preiser, P. R. 2002. Small variant STEVOR antigen is uniquely located within Maurer's clefts in Plasmodium falciparum-infected red blood cells. *Eukaryot Cell* 1: 926-935.

Keely, S. P.; Renauld, H.; Wakefield, A. E.; Cushion, M. T.; Smulian, A. G. et al. 2005. Gene arrays at Pneumocystis carinii telomeres. *Genetics* 170: 1589-1600.

Keely, S. P. & Stringer, J. R. 2009. Complexity of the MSG gene family of Pneumocystis carinii. *BMC Genomics* 10: 367.

Khattab, A. & Meri, S. 2011. Exposure of the Plasmodium falciparum clonally variant STEVOR proteins on the merozoite surface. *Malar J* 10: 58.

Kim, H. S. & Cross, G. A. M. 2010. TOPO3alpha influences antigenic variation by monitoring expression-site-associated VSG switching in *Trypanosoma brucei*. *PLoS Pathog* 6: e1000992.

Kim, H. S. & Cross, G. A. 2011. Identification of Trypanosoma brucei RMI1/BLAP75 homologue and its roles in antigenic variation. *PLoS One* 6: e25313.

Kim, S. H.; Kaminker, P. & Campisi, J. 1999. TIN2, a new regulator of telomere length in human cells. *Nat Genet* 23: 405-412.

Kimura, A.; Umehara, T. & Horikoshi, M. 2002. Chromosomal gradient of histone acetylation established by Sas2p and Sir2p functions as a shield against gene silencing. *Nat Genet* 32: 370-377.

Koering, C. E.; Pollice, A.; Zibella, M. P.; Bauwens, S.; Puisieux, A. et al. 2002. Human telomeric position effect is determined by chromosomal context and telomeric chromatin integrity. *EMBO Rep* 3: 1055-1061.

Konig, P.; Giraldo, R.; Chapman, L. & Rhodes, D. 1996. The crystal structure of the DNA-binding domain of yeast RAP1 in complex with telomeric DNA. *Cell* 85: 125-136.

Kraemer, S. M. & Smith, J. D. 2003. Evidence for the importance of genetic structuring to the structural and functional specialization of the Plasmodium falciparum var gene family. *Mol Microbiol* 50: 1527-1538.

Krogan, N. J.; Dover, J.; Khorrami, S.; Greenblatt, J. F.; Schneider, J. et al. 2002. COMPASS, a histone H3 (Lysine 4) methyltransferase required for telomeric silencing of gene expression. *J Biol Chem* 277: 10753-10755.

Kyes, S. A.; Rowe, J. A.; Kriek, N. & Newbold, C. I. 1999. Rifins: a second family of clonally variant proteins expressed on the surface of red cells infected with Plasmodium falciparum. *Proc Natl Acad Sci U S A* 96: 9333-9338.

Kyrion, G.; Liu, K.; Liu, C. & Lustig, A. J. 1993. RAP1 and telomere structure regulate telomere position effects in *Saccharomyces cerevisiae*. *Genes Dev* 7: 1146-1159.

Labandeira-Rey, M. & Skare, J. T. 2001. Decreased infectivity in Borrelia burgdorferi strain B31 is associated with loss of linear plasmid 25 or 28-1. *Infect Immun* 69: 446-455.

Lacoste, N.; Utley, R. T.; Hunter, J. M.; Poirier, G. G. & Cote, J. 2002. Disruptor of telomeric silencing-1 is a chromatin-specific histone H3 methyltransferase. *J Biol Chem* 277: 30421-30424.

Landry, J.; Sutton, A.; Tafrov, S. T.; Heller, R. C.; Stebbins, J. et al. 2000. The silencing protein SIR2 and its homologs are NAD-dependent protein deacetylases. *Proceedings of the National Academy of Sciences of the United States of America* 97: 5807-5811.

Laroche, T.; Martin, S. G.; Gotta, M.; Gorham, H. C.; Pryde, F. E. et al. 1998. Mutation of yeast Ku genes disrupts the subnuclear organization of telomeres. *Curr Biol* 8: 653-656.

Lavstsen, T.; Salanti, A.; Jensen, A. T.; Arnot, D. E. & Theander, T. G. 2003. Sub-grouping of Plasmodium falciparum 3D7 var genes based on sequence analysis of coding and non-coding regions. *Malar J* 2: 27.

Le, S.; Moore, J. K.; Haber, J. E. & Greider, C. W. 1999. RAD50 and RAD51 define two pathways that collaborate to maintain telomeres in the absence of telomerase. *Genetics* 152: 143-152.

Lebrun, E.; Revardel, E.; Boscheron, C.; Li, R.; Gilson, E. et al. 2001. Protosilencers in Saccharomyces cerevisiae subtelomeric regions. *Genetics* 158: 167-176.

Lenardo, M. J.; Rice-Ficht, A. C.; Kelly, G.; Esser, K. M. & Donelson, J. E. 1984. Characterization of the genes specifying two metacyclic variable antigen types in Trypanosoma brucei rhodesiense. *PNAS* 81: 6642-6646.

Lendvay, T. S.; Morris, D. K.; Sah, J.; Balasubramanian, B. & Lundblad, V. 1996. Senescence mutants of Saccharomyces cerevisiae with a defect in telomere replication identify three additional EST genes. *Genetics* 144: 1399-1412.

Levis, R.; Hazelrigg, T. & Rubin, G. M. 1985. Effects of genomic position on the expression of transduced copies of the white gene of Drosophila. *Science* 229: 558-561.

Levis, R. W.; Ganesan, R.; Houtchens, K.; Tolar, L. A. & Sheen, F. M. 1993. Transposons in place of telomeric repeats at a Drosophila telomere. *Cell* 75: 1083-1093.

Levy, M. Z.; Allsopp, R. C.; Futcher, A. B.; Greider, C. W. & Harley, C. B. 1992. Telomere end-replication problem and cell aging. *J Mol Biol* 225: 951-960.

Li, B.; Oestreich, S. & de Lange, T. 2000. Identification of human Rap1: implications for telomere evolution. *Cell* 101: 471-483.

Li, B.; Espinal, A. & Cross, G. A. M. 2005. Trypanosome telomeres are protected by a homologue of mammalian TRF2. *Mol Cell Biol* 25: 5011-5021.

Li, B. & Lustig, A. J. 1996. A novel mechanism for telomere size control in *Saccharomyces cerevisiae*. *Genes Dev* 10: 1310-1326.

Liang, X. H.; Haritan, A.; Uliel, S. & Michaeli, S. 2003. trans and cis splicing in trypanosomatids: mechanism, factors, and regulation. *Eukaryot Cell* 2: 830-840.

Lieb, J. D.; Liu, X.; Botstein, D. & Brown, P. O. 2001. Promoter-specific binding of Rap1 revealed by genome-wide maps of protein-DNA association. *Nat Genet* 28: 327-334.

Linardopoulou, E. V.; Williams, E. M.; Fan, Y.; Friedman, C.; Young, J. M. et al. 2005. Human subtelomeres are hot spots of interchromosomal recombination and segmental duplication. *Nature* 437: 94-100.

Liu, C.; Mao, X. & Lustig, A. J. 1994. Mutational analysis defines a C-terminal tail domain of RAP1 essential for telomeric silencing in Saccharomyces cerevisiae. *Genetics* 138: 1025-1040.

Liu, C. & Lustig, A. J. 1996. Genetic analysis of Rap1p/Sir3p interactions in telomeric and HML silencing in *Saccharomyces cerevisiae*. *Genetics* 143: 81-93.

Liu, D.; Safari, A.; O'Connor, M. S.; Chan, D. W.; Laegeler, A. et al. 2004. PTOP interacts with POT1 and regulates its localization to telomeres. *Nat Cell Biol* 6: 673-680.

Londono-Vallejo, J. A.; Der-Sarkissian, H.; Cazes, L.; Bacchetti, S. & Reddel, R. R. 2004. Alternative lengthening of telomeres is characterized by high rates of telomeric exchange. *Cancer Res* 64: 2324-2327.

Loney, E. R.; Inglis, P. W.; Sharp, S.; Pryde, F. E.; Kent, N. A. et al. 2009. Repressive and non-repressive chromatin at native telomeres in Saccharomyces cerevisiae. *Epigenetics Chromatin* 2: 18.

Longtine, M. S.; Wilson, N. M.; Petracek, M. E. & Berman, J. 1989a. A yeast telomere binding activity binds to two related telomere sequence motifs and is indistinguishable from RAP1. *Curr. Genet.* 16: 225-239.

Longtine, M. S.; Wilson, N. M.; Petracek, M. E. & Berman, J. 1989b. A yeast telomere binding activity binds to two related telomere sequence motifs and is indistinguishable from RAP1. *Curr Genet* 16: 225-239.

Lopez-Rubio, J. J.; Gontijo, A. M.; Nunes, M. C.; Issar, N.; Hernandez Rivas, R. et al. 2007. 5' flanking region of var genes nucleate histone modification patterns linked to phenotypic inheritance of virulence traits in malaria parasites. *Mol Microbiol* 66: 1296-1305.

Louis, E. J. & Haber, J. E. 1991. Evolutionarily recent transfer of a group I mitochondrial intron to telomere regions in Saccharomyces cerevisiae. *Curr Genet* 20: 411-415.

———. 1992. The structure and evolution of subtelomeric Y' repeats in Saccharomyces cerevisiae. *Genetics* 131: 559-574.

Louis, E. J.; Naumova, E. S.; Lee, A.; Naumov, G. & Haber, J. E. 1994. The chromosome end in yeast: its mosaic nature and influence on recombinational dynamics. *Genetics* 136: 789-802.

Louis, E. J. 1995. The chromosome ends of Saccharomyces cerevisiae. *Yeast* 11: 1553-1573.

Lundblad, V. & Szostak, J. W. 1989. A mutant with a defect in telomere elongation leads to senescence in yeast. *Cell* 57: 633-643.

Lundblad, V. & Blackburn, E. H. 1993. An alternative pathway for yeast telomere maintenance rescues est1- senescence. *Cell* 73: 347-360.

Luo, K.; Vega-Palas, M. A. & Grunstein, M. 2002. Rap1-Sir4 binding independent of other Sir, yKu, or histone interactions initiates the assembly of telomeric heterochromatin in yeast. *Genes Dev* 16: 1528-1539.

Mankouri, H. W. & Hickson, I. D. 2007. The RecQ helicase-topoisomerase III-Rmi1 complex: a DNA structure-specific 'dissolvasome'? *Trends Biochem Sci* 32: 538-546.

Marahrens, Y. & Stillman, B. 1992. A yeast chromosomal origin of DNA replication defined by multiple functional elements. *Science* 255: 817-823.

Marcello, L. & Barry, J. D. 2007. Analysis of the *VSG* gene silent archive in *Trypanosoma brucei* reveals that mosaic gene expression is prominent in antigenic variation and is favored by archive substructure. *Genome Res* 17: 1344-1352.

Martin, S. G.; Laroche, T.; Suka, N.; Grunstein, M. & Gasser, S. M. 1999. Relocalization of telomeric Ku and SIR proteins in response to DNA strand breaks in yeast. *Cell* 97: 621-633.

Martinez, P.; Thanasoula, M.; Carlos, A. R.; Gomez-Lopez, G.; Tejera, A. M. et al. 2010. Mammalian Rap1 controls telomere function and gene expression through binding to telomeric and extratelomeric sites. *Nat Cell Biol*

Martino, F.; Kueng, S.; Robinson, P.; Tsai-Pflugfelder, M.; van Leeuwen, F. et al. 2009. Reconstitution of yeast silent chromatin: multiple contact sites and O-AADPR binding load SIR complexes onto nucleosomes in vitro. *Mol Cell* 33: 323-334.

Mason, J. M.; Konev, A. Y.; Golubovsky, M. D. & Biessmann, H. 2003. Cis- and trans-acting influences on telomeric position effect in Drosophila melanogaster detected with a subterminal transgene. *Genetics* 163: 917-930.

Matthews, K. R. 2005. The developmental cell biology of Trypanosoma brucei. *J Cell Sci* 118: 283-290.

McCulloch, R. & Barry, J. D. 1999. A role for RAD51 and homologous recombination in *Trypanosoma brucei* antigenic variation. *Genes & Development* 13: 2875-2888.

McEachern, M. J. & Blackburn, E. H. 1996. Cap-prevented recombination between terminal telomeric repeat arrays (telomere CPR) maintains telomeres in Kluyveromyces lactis lacking telomerase. *Genes Dev* 10: 1822-1834.

McEachern, M. J. & J. E. Haber. 2006. Telomerase-independent Telomere Maintenance in Yeast. *In* Telomeres. *Edited by* de lange, T.; V. Lundblad & E. H. Blackburn. Cold Spring Harbor Laboratory Press, Cold Spring Harbor, New York, pp 199-224.

Mefford, H. C. & Trask, B. J. 2002. The complex structure and dynamic evolution of human subtelomeres. *Nat Rev Genet* 3: 91-102.

Mehlert, A.; Zitzmann, N.; Richardson, J. M.; Treumann, A. & Ferguson, M. A. J. 1998. The glycosylation of the variant surface glycoproteins and procyclic acidic repetitive proteins of *Trypanosoma brucei*. *Molecular & Biochemical Parasitology* 91: 145-152.

Melville, S. E.; Leech, V.; Navarro, M. & Cross, G. A. M. 2000. The molecular karyotype of the megabase chromosomes of *Trypanosoma brucei* stock 427. *Mol. Biochem. Parasitol.* 111: 261-273.

Merrick, C. J. & Duraisingh, M. T. 2007. Plasmodium falciparum Sir2: an unusual sirtuin with dual histone deacetylase and ADP-ribosyltransferase activity. *Eukaryot Cell* 6: 2081-2091.

Micklem, G.; Rowley, A.; Harwood, J.; Nasmyth, K. & Diffley, J. F. 1993. Yeast origin recognition complex is involved in DNA replication and transcriptional silencing. *Nature* 366: 87-89.

Miyake, Y.; Nakamura, M.; Nabetani, A.; Shimamura, S.; Tamura, M. et al. 2009. RPA-like mammalian Ctc1-Stn1-Ten1 complex binds to single-stranded DNA and protects telomeres independently of the Pot1 pathway. *Mol Cell* 36: 193-206.

Moazed, D.; Kistler, A.; Axelrod, A.; Rine, J. & Johnson, A. D. 1997. Silent information regulator protein complexes in *Saccharomyces cerevisiae* - a sir2/sir4 complex and evidence for a regulatory domain in sir4 that inhibits its interaction with sir3. *Proceedings of the National Academy of Sciences of the United States of America* 94: 2186-2191.

Mok, B. W.; Ribacke, U.; Rasti, N.; Kironde, F.; Chen, Q. et al. 2008. Default Pathway of var2csa switching and translational repression in Plasmodium falciparum. *PLoS One* 3: e1982.

Moretti, P.; Freeman, K.; Coodly, L. & Shore, D. 1994. Evidence that a complex of SIR proteins interacts with the silencer and telomere-binding protein RAP1. *Genes Dev* 8: 2257-2269.

Moretti, P. & Shore, D. 2001. Multiple interactions in sir protein recruitment by Rap1p at silencers and telomeres in yeast. *Molecular and Cellular Biology* 21: 8082-8094.

Mottram, J. C.; Murphy, W. J. & Agabian, N. 1989. A transcriptional analysis of the Trypanosoma brucei hsp83 gene cluster. *MBP* 37: 115-127.

Munoz-Jordan, J. L. & Cross, G. A. M. 2001. Telomere shortening and cell cycle arrest in *Trypanosoma brucei* expressing human telomeric repeat factor TRF1. *Mol. Biochem. Parasitol.* 114: 169-181.

Munoz-Jordan, J. L.; Cross, G. A. M.; de Lange, T. & Griffith, J. D. 2001. t-loops at trypanosome telomeres. *EMBO J* 20: 579-588.

Murnane, J. P.; Sabatier, L.; Marder, B. A. & Morgan, W. F. 1994. Telomere dynamics in an immortal human cell line. *Embo J* 13: 4953-4962.

Murray, A. W. & J. W. Szostak. 1983. Construction of artificial chromosomes in yeast. *In* 305 189-305 193.

Murti, K. G. & Prescott, D. M. 1999. Telomeres of polytene chromosomes in a ciliated protozoan terminate in duplex DNA loops. *Proc Natl Acad Sci U S A* 96: 14436-14439.

Myler, P. J.; Aline, R. F. J.; Scholler, J. K. & Stuart, K. D. 1988. Changes in telomere length associated with antigenic variation in *Trypanosoma brucei*. *MBP* 29: 243-250.

Nabetani, A. & Ishikawa, F. 2011. Alternative lengthening of telomeres pathway: recombination-mediated telomere maintenance mechanism in human cells. *J Biochem* 149: 5-14.

Nagy, P. L.; Griesenbeck, J.; Kornberg, R. D. & Cleary, M. L. 2002. A trithorax-group complex purified from Saccharomyces cerevisiae is required for methylation of histone H3. *Proc Natl Acad Sci U S A* 99: 90-94.

Nakayama, J.; Rice, J. C.; Strahl, B. D.; Allis, C. D. & Grewal, S. I. 2001. Role of histone H3 lysine 9 methylation in epigenetic control of heterochromatin assembly. *Science* 292: 110-113.

Naumov, G. I.; Naumova, E. S.; Turakainen, H. & Korhola, M. 1992. A new family of polymorphic metallothionein-encoding genes MTH1 (CUP1) and MTH2 in Saccharomyces cerevisiae. *Gene* 119: 65-74.

Navarro, M. & Gull, K. 2001. A pol I transcriptional body associated with *VSG* mono-allelic expression in *Trypanosoma brucei*. *Nature* 414: 759-763.

Ness, F. & Aigle, M. 1995. RTM1: a member of a new family of telomeric repeated genes in yeast. *Genetics* 140: 945-956.

Ng, H. H.; Feng, Q.; Wang, H.; Erdjument-Bromage, H.; Tempst, P. et al. 2002. Lysine methylation within the globular domain of histone H3 by Dot1 is important for telomeric silencing and Sir protein association. *Genes Dev* 16: 1518-1527.

Niida, H.; Shinkai, Y.; Hande, M. P.; Matsumoto, T.; Takehara, S. et al. 2000. Telomere maintenance in telomerase-deficient mouse embryonic stem cells: characterization of an amplified telomeric DNA. *Mol Cell Biol* 20: 4115-4127.

Nikitina, T. & Woodcock, C. L. 2004. Closed chromatin loops at the ends of chromosomes. *J Cell Biol* 166: 161-165.

Noma, K.; Sugiyama, T.; Cam, H.; Verdel, A.; Zofall, M. et al. 2004. RITS acts in cis to promote RNA interference-mediated transcriptional and post-transcriptional silencing. *Nat Genet* 36: 1174-1180.

Norris, S. J. 2006. Antigenic variation with a twist--the Borrelia story. *Mol Microbiol* 60: 1319-1322.

Nugent, C. I.; Hughes, T. R.; Lue, N. F. & Lundblad, V. 1996. Cdc13p: a single-strand telomeric DNA-binding protein with a dual role in yeast telomere maintenance. *Science* 274: 249-252.

O'Connor, M. S.; Safari, A.; Liu, D.; Qin, J. & Songyang, Z. 2004. The human Rap1 protein complex and modulation of telomere length. *J Biol Chem* 279: 28585-28591.

Opitz, O. G.; Suliman, Y.; Hahn, W. C.; Harada, H.; Blum, H. E. et al. 2001. Cyclin D1 overexpression and p53 inactivation immortalize primary oral keratinocytes by a telomerase-independent mechanism. *J Clin Invest* 108: 725-732.

Palm, W. & de Lange, T. 2008. How shelterin protects mammalian telomeres. *Annu Rev Genet* 42: 301-334.

Pardue, M. L. & DeBaryshe, P. G. 2008. Drosophila telomeres: A variation on the telomerase theme. *Fly (Austin)* 2: 101-110.

Park, M. J.; Jang, Y. K.; Choi, E. S.; Kim, H. S. & Park, S. D. 2002. Fission yeast Rap1 homolog is a telomere-specific silencing factor and interacts with Taz1p. *Mol Cells* 13: 327-333.

Pays, E.; Laurent, M.; Delinte, K.; Van Meirvenne, N. & Steinert, M. 1983a. Differential size variations between transcriptionally active and inactive telomeres of Trypanosoma brucei. *Nucleic Acids Res* 11: 8137-8147.

Pays, E.; van Assel, S.; Laurent, M.; Dero, B.; Michiels, F. et al. 1983b. At least two transposed sequences are associated in the expression site of a surface antigen gene in different trypanosome clones. *Cell* 34: 359-369.

Pedram, M.; Sprung, C. N.; Gao, Q.; Lo, A. W.; Reynolds, G. E. et al. 2006. Telomere position effect and silencing of transgenes near telomeres in the mouse. *Mol Cell Biol* 26: 1865-1878.

Pedram, M. & Donelson, J. E. 1999. The anatomy and transcription of a monocistronic expression site for a metacyclic variant surface glycoprotein gene in *Trypanosoma brucei*. *J Biol Chem* 274: 16876-16883.

Petrie, V. J.; Wuitschick, J. D.; Givens, C. D.; Kosinski, A. M. & Partridge, J. F. 2005. RNA interference (RNAi)-dependent and RNAi-independent association of the Chp1 chromodomain protein with distinct heterochromatic loci in fission yeast. *Mol Cell Biol* 25: 2331-2346.

Pham, V. P.; Qi, C. C. & Gottesdiener, K. M. 1996. A detailed mutational analysis of the VSG gene expression site promoter. *Mol Biochem Parasitol* 75: 241-254.

Pizzi, E. & Frontali, C. 2001. Fine structure of Plasmodium falciparum subtelomeric sequences. *Mol. Biochem. Parasitol.* 118: 253-258.

Pologe, L. G. & Ravetch, J. V. 1988. Large deletions result from breakage and healing of P. falciparum chromosomes. *Cell* 55: 869-874.

Proudfoot, C. & McCulloch, R. 2005. Distinct roles for two RAD51-related genes in *Trypanosoma brucei* antigenic variation. *Nucleic Acids Res* 33: 6906-6919.

Pryde, F. E. & Louis, E. J. 1999. Limitations of silencing at native yeast telomeres. *EMBO J.* 18: 2538-2550.

Purser, J. E. & Norris, S. J. 2000. Correlation between plasmid content and infectivity in Borrelia burgdorferi. *Proc Natl Acad Sci U S A* 97: 13865-13870.

Ralph, S. A.; Scheidig-Benatar, C. & Scherf, A. 2005. Antigenic variation in Plasmodium falciparum is associated with movement of var loci between subnuclear locations. *Proc Natl Acad Sci U S A* 102: 5414-5419.

Ralph, S. A. & Scherf, A. 2005. The epigenetic control of antigenic variation in Plasmodium falciparum. *Curr Opin Microbiol* 8: 434-440.

Rao, H.; Marahrens, Y. & Stillman, B. 1994. Functional conservation of multiple elements in yeast chromosomal replicators. *Mol Cell Biol* 14: 7643-7651.

Reddel, R. R.; Bryan, T. M. & Murnane, J. P. 1997. Immortalized cells with no detectable telomerase activity. A review. *Biochemistry (Mosc)* 62: 1254-1262.

Reifsnyder, C.; Lowell, J.; Clarke, A. & Pillus, L. 1996. Yeast SAS silencing genes and human genes associated with AML and HIV-1 Tat interactions are homologous with acetyltransferases. *Nat Genet* 14: 42-49.

Renauld, H.; Aparicio, O. M.; Zierath, P. D.; Billington, B. L.; Chhablani, S. K. et al. 1993. Silent domains are assembled continuously from the telomere and are defined by promoter distance and strength, and by SIR3 dosage. *Genes Dev* 7: 1133-1145.

Reynolds, T. B. & Fink, G. R. 2001. Bakers' yeast, a model for fungal biofilm formation. *Science* 291: 878-881.

Riha, K.; Heacock, M. L. & Shippen, D. E. 2006. The role of the nonhomologous end-joining DNA double-strand break repair pathway in telomere biology. *Annu Rev Genet* 40: 237-277.

Roberts, D. J.; Craig, A. G.; Berendt, A. R.; Pinches, R.; Nash, G. et al. 1992. Rapid switching to multiple antigenic and adhesive phenotypes in malaria. *Nature* 357: 689-692.

Robinson, N. P.; Burman, N.; Melville, S. E. & Barry, J. D. 1999. Predominance of duplicative VSG gene conversion in antigenic variation in African trypanosomes. *Mol Cell Biol* 19: 5839-5846.

Roguev, A.; Schaft, D.; Shevchenko, A.; Pijnappel, W. W.; Wilm, M. et al. 2001. The Saccharomyces cerevisiae Set1 complex includes an Ash2 homologue and methylates histone 3 lysine 4. *EMBO J* 20: 7137-7148.

Rubio, J. P.; Thompson, J. K. & Cowman, A. F. 1996. The *var* genes of *Plasmodium falciparum* are located in the subtelomeric region of most chromosomes. *EMBO Journal* 15: 4069-4077.

Rudenko, G. & Van der Ploeg, L. H. 1989. Transcription of telomere repeats in protozoa. *Embo J* 8: 2633-2638.

Rudenko, G.; McCulloch, R.; Dirksmulder, A. & Borst, P. 1996. Telomere exchange can be an important mechanism of variant surface glycoprotein gene switching in *Trypanosoma brucei*. *Molecular & Biochemical Parasitology* 80: 65-75.

Rusche, L. N.; Kirchmaier, A. L. & Rine, J. 2002. Ordered nucleation and spreading of silenced chromatin in *Saccharomyces cerevisiae*. *Mol Biol Cell* 13: 2207-2222.

Sadaie, M.; Iida, T.; Urano, T. & Nakayama, J. 2004. A chromodomain protein, Chp1, is required for the establishment of heterochromatin in fission yeast. *EMBO J* 23: 3825-3835.

Salanti, A.; Staalsoe, T.; Lavstsen, T.; Jensen, A. T.; Sowa, M. P. et al. 2003. Selective upregulation of a single distinctly structured var gene in chondroitin sulphate A-adhering Plasmodium falciparum involved in pregnancy-associated malaria. *Mol Microbiol* 49: 179-191.

Scherf, A.; Figueiredo, L. M. & Freitas-Junior, L. H. 2001. Plasmodium telomeres: a pathogen's perspective. *Current Opinion in Microbiology* 4: 409-414.

Schwan, T. G.; Karstens, R. H.; Schrumpf, M. E. & Simpson, W. J. 1991. Changes in antigenic reactivity of Borrelia burgdorferi, the Lyme disease spirochete, during persistent infection in mice. *Can J Microbiol* 37: 450-454.

Serizawa, S.; Miyamichi, K. & Sakano, H. 2004. One neuron-one receptor rule in the mouse olfactory system. *Trends Genet* 20: 648-653.

Sfeir, A.; Kabir, S.; van Overbeek, M.; Celli, G. B. & de Lange, T. 2010. Loss of Rap1 induces telomere recombination in the absence of NHEJ or a DNA damage signal. *Science* 327: 1657-1661.

Shi, H. F.; Djikeng, A.; Mark, T.; Wirtz, E.; Tschudi, C. et al. 2000. Genetic interference in *Trypanosoma brucei* by heritable and inducible double-stranded RNA. *RNA-A Publication of the RNA Society* 6: 1069-1076.

Shykind, B. M. 2005. Regulation of odorant receptors: one allele at a time. *Hum Mol Genet* 14 Spec No 1: R33-9.

Singer, M. S. & Gottschling, D. E. 1994. TLC1: template RNA component of Saccharomyces cerevisiae telomerase [see comments]. *Science* 266: 404-409.

Smith, J. D.; Chitnis, C. E.; Craig, A. G.; Roberts, D. J.; Hudson-Taylor, D. E. et al. 1995. Switches in expression of *Plasmodium falciparum var* genes correlate with changes in antigenic and cytoadherent phenotypes of infected erythrocytes. *Cell* 82: 101-110.

Smith, J. S.; Brachmann, C. B.; Celic, I.; Kenna, M. A.; Muhammad, S. et al. 2000. A phylogenetically conserved NAD+-dependent protein deacetylase activity in the Sir2 protein family. *Proc Natl Acad Sci U S A* 97: 6658-6663.

Smith, S.; Banerjee, S.; Rilo, R. & Myung, K. 2008. Dynamic regulation of single-stranded telomeres in Saccharomyces cerevisiae. *Genetics* 178: 693-701.

Stanne, T. M. & Rudenko, G. 2010. Active VSG expression sites in *Trypanosoma brucei* are depleted of nucleosomes. *Eukaryot Cell* 9: 136-147.

Stanne, T. M.; Kushwaha, M.; Wand, M.; Taylor, J. E. & Rudenko, G. 2011. TbISWI regulates multiple polymerase I (Pol I)-transcribed loci and is present at Pol II transcription boundaries in Trypanosoma brucei. *Eukaryot Cell* 10: 964-976.

Steere, A. C.; Coburn, J. & Glickstein, L. 2004. The emergence of Lyme disease. *J Clin Invest* 113: 1093-1101.

Stewart, J. A.; Chaiken, M. F.; Wang, F. & Price, C. M. 2011. Maintaining the end: Roles of telomere proteins in end-protection, telomere replication and length regulation. *Mutat Res*

Strahl-Bolsinger, S.; Hecht, A.; Luo, K. & Grunstein, M. 1997. SIR2 and SIR4 interactions differ in core and extended telomeric heterochromatin in yeast. *Genes Dev* 11: 83-93.

Strahl, B. D.; Grant, P. A.; Briggs, S. D.; Sun, Z. W.; Bone, J. R. et al. 2002. Set2 is a nucleosomal histone H3-selective methyltransferase that mediates transcriptional repression. *Mol Cell Biol* 22: 1298-1306.

Stringer, J. R. 2005. Surface antigens. *In Pneumocystis Pneumonia. Edited by* Walzer, P. D. & M. T. Cushion. New York: Marcel Dekker, New York, pp 95-126.

Su, X.; Heatwole, V. M.; Wertheimer, S. P.; Guinet, F.; Herrfeldt, J. A. et al. 1995. The large diverse gene family var encodes proteins involved in cytoadherence and antigenic variation of Plasmodium falciparum-infected erythrocytes. *Cell* 82: 89-100.

Su, Y.; Barton, A. B. & Kaback, D. B. 2000. Decreased meiotic reciprocal recombination in subtelomeric regions in Saccharomyces cerevisiae. *Chromosoma* 109: 467-475.

Sugioka-Sugiyama, R. & Sugiyama, T. 2011. Sde2: a novel nuclear protein essential for telomeric silencing and genomic stability in Schizosaccharomyces pombe. *Biochem Biophys Res Commun* 406: 444-448.

Sugiyama, T.; Cam, H. P.; Sugiyama, R.; Noma, K.; Zofall, M. et al. 2007. SHREC, an effector complex for heterochromatic transcriptional silencing. *Cell* 128: 491-504.

Suka, N.; Luo, K. & Grunstein, M. 2002. Sir2p and Sas2p opposingly regulate acetylation of yeast histone H4 lysine16 and spreading of heterochromatin. *Nat Genet* 32: 378-383.

Sunkin, S. M. & Stringer, J. R. 1997. Residence at the expression site is necessary and sufficient for the transcription of surface antigen genes of Pneumocystis carinii. *Mol Microbiol* 25: 147-160.

Sunkin, S. M.; Linke, M. J.; McCormack, F. X.; Walzer, P. D. & Stringer, J. R. 1998. Identification of a putative precursor to the major surface glycoprotein of Pneumocystis carinii. *Infect Immun* 66: 741-746.

Taddei, A. & Gasser, S. M. 2004. Multiple pathways for telomere tethering: functional implications of subnuclear position for heterochromatin formation. *Biochim Biophys Acta* 1677: 120-128.

Tanny, J. C.; Dowd, G. J.; Huang, J.; Hilz, H. & Moazed, D. 1999. An enzymatic activity in the yeast Sir2 protein that is essential for gene silencing. *Cell* 99: 735-745.

Teng, S. C. & Zakian, V. A. 1999. Telomere-telomere recombination is an efficient bypass pathway for telomere maintenance in Saccharomyces cerevisiae. *Molecular & Cellular Biology* 19: 8083-8093.

Teng, S. C.; Chang, J.; McCowan, B. & Zakian, V. A. 2000. Telomerase-independent lengthening of yeast telomeres occurs by an abrupt Rad50p-dependent, Rif-inhibited recombinational process. *Mol Cell* 6: 947-952.

Teytelman, L.; Eisen, M. B. & Rine, J. 2008. Silent but not static: accelerated base-pair substitution in silenced chromatin of budding yeasts. *PLoS Genet* 4: e1000247.

Thompson, J. K.; Rubio, J. P.; Caruana, S.; Brockman, A.; Wickham, M. E. et al. 1997. The chromosomal organization of the Plasmodium falciparum var gene family is conserved. *Mol Biochem Parasitol* 87: 49-60.

Tompa, R. & Madhani, H. D. 2007. Histone H3 lysine 36 methylation antagonizes silencing in Saccharomyces cerevisiae independently of the Rpd3S histone deacetylase complex. *Genetics* 175: 585-593.

Tonkin, C. J.; Carret, C. K.; Duraisingh, M. T.; Voss, T. S.; Ralph, S. A. et al. 2009. Sir2 paralogues cooperate to regulate virulence genes and antigenic variation in *Plasmodium falciparum*. *PLoS Biol* 7: e84.

Trask, B. J.; Friedman, C.; Martin-Gallardo, A.; Rowen, L.; Akinbami, C. et al. 1998. Members of the olfactory receptor gene family are contained in large blocks of DNA duplicated polymorphically near the ends of human chromosomes. *Hum Mol Genet* 7: 13-26.

Triolo, T. & Sternglanz, R. 1996. Role of interactions between the origin recognition complex and SIR1 in transcriptional silencing. *Nature* 381: 251-253.

Tsukamoto, Y.; Kato, J. & Ikeda, H. 1997. Silencing factors participate in DNA repair and recombination in *Saccharomyces cerevisiae*. *Nature* 388: 900-903.

Turakainen, H.; Naumov, G.; Naumova, E. & Korhola, M. 1993. Physical mapping of the MEL gene family in Saccharomyces cerevisiae. *Curr Genet* 24: 461-464.

Turner, C. M. R.; Barry, J. D.; Maudlin, I. & Vickerman, K. 1988. An estimate of the size of the metacyclic variable antigen repertoire of Trypanosoma brucei rhodensiense. *Parasitology* 97: 269-276.

van der Ploeg, L. H. T.; Liu, A. Y. C. & Borst, P. 1984. Structure of the growing telomeres of trypanosomes. *Cell* 36: 459-468.

van Leeuwen, F.; Gafken, P. R. & Gottschling, D. E. 2002. Dot1p modulates silencing in yeast by methylation of the nucleosome core. *Cell* 109: 745-756.

Van Mulders, S. E.; Christianen, E.; Saerens, S. M.; Daenen, L.; Verbelen, P. J. et al. 2009. Phenotypic diversity of Flo protein family-mediated adhesion in Saccharomyces cerevisiae. *FEMS Yeast Res* 9: 178-190.

Vanhamme, L.; Poelvoorde, P.; Pays, A.; Tebabi, P.; Van Xong, H. et al. 2000. Differential RNA elongation controls the variant surface glycoprotein gene expression sites of *Trypanosoma brucei*. *Mol. Microbiol.* 36: 328-340.

Venkatasubrahmanyam, S.; Hwang, W. W.; Meneghini, M. D.; Tong, A. H. & Madhani, H. D. 2007. Genome-wide, as opposed to local, antisilencing is mediated redundantly by the euchromatic factors Set1 and H2A.Z. *Proc Natl Acad Sci U S A* 104: 16609-16614.

Viswanathan, M.; Muthukumar, G.; Cong, Y. S. & Lenard, J. 1994. Seripauperins of Saccharomyces cerevisiae: a new multigene family encoding serine-poor relatives of serine-rich proteins. *Gene* 148: 149-153.

Volpe, T. A.; Kidner, C.; Hall, I. M.; Teng, G.; Grewal, S. I. et al. 2002. Regulation of heterochromatic silencing and histone H3 lysine-9 methylation by RNAi. *Science* 297: 1833-1837.

Voss, T. S.; Thompson, J. K.; Waterkeyn, J.; Felger, I.; Weiss, N. et al. 2000. Genomic distribution and functional characterisation of two distinct and conserved Plasmodium falciparum var gene 5' flanking sequences. *Mol Biochem Parasitol* 107: 103-115.

Voss, T. S.; Healer, J.; Marty, A. J.; Duffy, M. F.; Thompson, J. K. et al. 2006. A var gene promoter controls allelic exclusion of virulence genes in Plasmodium falciparum malaria. *Nature* 439: 1004-1008.

Wada, M.; Sunkin, S. M.; Stringer, J. R. & Nakamura, Y. 1995. Antigenic variation by positional control of major surface glycoprotein gene expression in Pneumocystis carinii. *J Infect Dis* 171: 1563-1568.

Wada, M. & Nakamura, Y. 1996. Unique telomeric expression site of major-surface-glycoprotein genes of Pneumocystis carinii. *DNA Res* 3: 55-64.

Wallrath, L. L. & Elgin, S. C. R. 1995. Position effect variegation in Drosophila is associated with an altered chromatin structure. *Genes Dev* 9: 1263-1277.

Walter, M. F.; Jang, C.; Kasravi, B.; Donath, J.; Mechler, B. M. et al. 1995. DNA organization and polymorphism of a wild-type Drosophila telomere region. *Chromosoma* 104: 229-241.

Wan, M.; Qin, J.; Songyang, Z. & Liu, D. 2009. OB fold-containing protein 1 (OBFC1), a human homolog of yeast Stn1, associates with TPP1 and is implicated in telomere length regulation. *J Biol Chem* 284: 26725-26731.

Wang, Q. P.; Kawahara, T. & Horn, D. 2010. Histone deacetylases play distinct roles in telomeric VSG expression site silencing in African trypanosomes. *Mol Microbiol* 77: 1237-1245.

Wang, R. C.; Smogorzewska, A. & de Lange, T. 2004. Homologous recombination generates T-loop-sized deletions at human telomeres. *Cell* 119: 355-368.

Weaver, D.; Boubnov, N.; Wills, Z.; Hall, K. & Staunton, J. 1995. V(D)J recombination: double-strand break repair gene products used in the joining mechanism. *Ann N Y Acad Sci* 764: 99-111.

Wilkie, A. O.; Higgs, D. R.; Rack, K. A.; Buckle, V. J.; Spurr, N. K. et al. 1991. Stable length polymorphism of up to 260 kb at the tip of the short arm of human chromosome 16. *Cell* 64: 595-606.

Wyrick, J. J.; Holstege, F. C.; Jennings, E. G.; Causton, H. C.; Shore, D. et al. 1999. Chromosomal landscape of nucleosome-dependent gene expression and silencing in yeast. *Nature* 402: 418-421.

Wyrick, J. J.; Aparicio, J. G.; Chen, T.; Barnett, J. D.; Jennings, E. G. et al. 2001. Genome-wide distribution of ORC and MCM proteins in S. cerevisiae: high-resolution mapping of replication origins. *Science* 294: 2357-2360.

Yang, X.; Figueiredo, L. M.; Espinal, A.; Okubo, E. & Li, B. 2009. RAP1 is essential for silencing telomeric variant surface glycoprotein genes in *Trypanosoma brucei*. *Cell* 137: 99-109.

Ye, J. Z.; Hockemeyer, D.; Krutchinsky, A. N.; Loayza, D.; Hooper, S. M. et al. 2004. POT1-interacting protein PIP1: a telomere length regulator that recruits POT1 to the TIN2/TRF1 complex. *Genes Dev* 18: 1649-1654.

Zakian, V. A. & Blanton, H. M. 1988. Distribution of telomere-associated sequences on natural chromosomes in Saccharomyces cerevisiae. *Mol Cell Biol* 8: 2257-2260.

Zhang, J. R.; Hardham, J. M.; Barbour, A. G. & Norris, S. J. 1997. Antigenic variation in Lyme disease borreliae by promiscuous recombination of VMP-like sequence cassettes. *Cell* 89: 275-285.

Zhang, J. R. & Norris, S. J. 1998a. Kinetics and in vivo induction of genetic variation of vlsE in Borrelia burgdorferi. *Infect Immun* 66: 3689-3697.

———. 1998b. Genetic variation of the Borrelia burgdorferi gene vlsE involves cassette-specific, segmental gene conversion. *Infect Immun* 66: 3698-3704.

Zomerdijk, J. C. B. M.; Ouellete, M.; ten Asbroek, A. L. M. A.; Kieft, R.; Bommer, A. M. M. et al. 1990. The promoter for a variant surface glycoprotein gene expression site in *Trypanosoma brucei*. *EMBO J.* 9: 2791-2801.

Zomerdijk, J. C. B. M.; Kieft, R.; Duyndam, M.; Shiels, P. G. & Borst, P. 1991. Antigenic variation in *Trypanosoma brucei*: a telomeric expression site for variant-specific surface glycoprotein genes with novel features. *Nucl Acids Res.* 19: 1359-1368.

Zvereva, M. I.; Shcherbakova, D. M. & Dontsova, O. A. 2010. Telomerase: structure, functions, and activity regulation. *Biochemistry (Mosc)* 75: 1563-1583.

Section 3

Noncanonical Functions of the Telomere

9

Extra-Telomeric Roles of Telomeric Proteins

Arkasubhra Ghosh* and Vinay Tergaonkar
Laboratory of NFkB signalling, Institute of Molecular and Cell Biology
Singapore

1. Introduction

Telomeres are tandem repeats of (TTAGGG)n sequence at the ends of chromosomes bound by a complex of proteins which are known to protect these ends from degradation and DNA repair activities. "Shelterin" is a dynamic multi-protein complex (Refer to previous chapters) (de Lange 2005) with DNA remodeling activity that acts together with several associated DNA repair factors to modify the structure of the telomeric DNA, thereby protecting chromosome ends (Bianchi et al. 1999; Griffith et al. 1999; Karlseder et al. 2002; Kim et al. 2003; Wang et al. 2011). While the main function of shelterin proteins is to bind and protect the telomeric repeats, telomere length per se is maintained and replenished by the ribonucleoprotein enzyme called "telomerase" which has a very specific TTAGGG repeat dependent reverse transcriptase activity (Blackburn 2000). Telomeres progressively shorten with each cell division in cultured primary human cells until a critically shortened length is reached, upon which the cells enter replicative senescence. Although the relevance of replicative senescence to aging in vivo remains poorly understood, numerous reports suggest that telomere shortening may be associated with organismal aging (Epel et al. 2009; Monaghan 2010), with concomitant metabolic decline and increased risk for disease and death (Jaskelioff et al. 2011; Jeon et al. 2011). Likewise, shorter telomere length has been shown to be associated with age-related diseases including coronary heart disease (Calvert et al. 2011; Krauss et al. 2011), hypertension (Dimitroulis et al. 2011), and dementia (Rolyan et al. 2011; Takata et al. 2011), as well as with a general risk for diseases such as insulin resistance and obesity (Al-Attas et al. 2010; Al-Attas et al. 2010; Makino et al. 2010; Njajou et al. 2011). However, the moleluar basis, if any, of these correlations and associations are not yet clear. Increasing amount of evidence suggests that telomeric proteins may also be involved in non-canonical activities at extra-telomeric sites or organelles within the cell. These novel, non-canonical functions may partially explain the mechanistic link between the telomere phenotypes found to be associated with physiological mechanisms, disease and organismal homeostasis (Teo et al. 2010; Gizard et al. 2011; Indran et al. 2011; Li et al. 2011; Martinez and Blasco 2011).

Since the discovery of telomeres, telomere-associated proteins have been thought to primarily function in telomere maintenance and homeostasis. Given that visualizing telomeric proteins by immunofluorescence techniques indicated that these proteins are exclusively present only at the telomeres gave rise to the notion that their function too is restricted at the telomeres. These conclusions gained further ground since the effect of loss of function of the telomeric proteins on organismal viability was also attributed entirely to the telomere dysfunction. Yet the actual underlying mechanistic basis of the phenotypes exhibited by telomeric proteins have just started to unravel through interesting work by a number of laboratories. In this chapter, we will define some of the novel "extra-telomeric roles" of telomeric proteins since their functional locations and contexts are away from the telomere and/or they are independent of the telomere length or status in the cell. We will discuss the studies that led to these novel roles, the discrepancies amongst the different observations and the evidence that these functions indeed are telomere-independent and finally the possible reason why these non-telomeric functions of telomeric proteins can have an effect on a number of human ailments.

2. Discovery of extra-telomeric roles of telomeric proteins

Although numerous studies have been carried out to elucidate protein-protein interactions and telomere localizations of telomeric proteins, the analysis of their subcellular and extra-telomeric localization and function has gained attention only recently (Takai et al. 2010). The shelterin components TPP1, Rap1 and POT1 were shown to be present in non-chromatin bound fractions of the cell (Takai et al. 2010). This has been driven by the discovery of extra-telomeric roles for members of the telomeric complex like TRF2 at DNA damage foci (Bradshaw et al. 2005; Kaminker et al. 2005) and TIN2 at HP1 marked extra-telomeric sites (Kaminker et al. 2005). Interestingly, several studies proposed recently that mammalian Rap1 is present in many subnuclear locations (Takai et al. 2010; Teo et al. 2010) which also suggested multiple roles of Rap1 away from the telomere. Notably, whereas neither the de Lange nor Blasco group found a significant role for Rap1 in inhibiting telomere fusions in mouse cells, a recent report by Baumann and colleagues suggests that this may be the case in human cells (Bae and Baumann 2007; Sarthy et al. 2009). The difference in these findings may be due to the species under investigation (i.e., mouse versus human) or the experimental approaches taken by each group. Indeed, the de Lange and Blasco groups used a loss of function approach whereas the Baumann group utilized ectopic expression of a fusion protein, which could account for the differences in the studies. Interestingly, while Rap1 was initially suggested to be stabilized in the nucleus by TRF2 in the murine cells, we and others have observed that in human cells Rap1 is stable in the cytosol even in the absence of TRF2 (Teo et al. 2010). We further discovered a novel role of Rap1 in regulation of the NFkB signaling cascade.

Elongation of chromosomal ends by telomerase(Blackburn et al. 1989) during cell division prevents senescence in cells (allowing cells to overcome the Hayflick limit (Hayflick 1965)). Consequently, telomerase activity in cancer cells is thought to assist in overcoming the replicative crisis by addition of telomeric repeats. It has been known for a while that telomerase activity is highly upregulated in a number of human cancers and that aberrant expression of telomerase is a common occurrence in a number of human diseases. It is assumed that elongation of telomeres is the primary function of the reactivated telomerase in human cancers (Counter et al. 1994; Shay and Wright 2005; Blackburn et al. 2006). However, various studies have highlighted novel roles for telomerase, which are independent of its function on the telomeres. Interestingly, a number of these roles are now being suggested to be important for the functional basis for the molecular function of telomerase's role in human cancers as well as diseases like atherosclerosis (Gizard et al. 2011). These functions include roles of telomerase in Wnt signaling (Park et al. 2009), mitochondrial regulation (Gordon and Santos 2010; Indran et al. 2011; Mukherjee et al. 2011) and DNA damage response (Beliveau and Yaswen 2007; Chenette 2009; Tamakawa et al. 2010).

3. The multi-faceted roles of telomerase

Some of these novel, non-canonical functions of telomerase were initially described in murine studies (Gonzalez-Suarez et al. 2001; Artandi et al. 2002). It has been shown that TERT overexpression in mice leads to spontaneous tumorigenesis, although telomere length did not change appreciably (Blasco et al. 1996). However, murine telomeres are very long and pathologies related to telomere shortening and accelerated aging are only observed in fifth or sixth generation telomerase knockout mice (Blasco et al. 1997; Wynford-Thomas and Kipling 1997; Goytisolo et al. 2000; Herrera et al. 2000). Also, there is low-level telomerase activity in most somatic murine tissues including breast epithelia, a primary site of TERT overexpression mediated carcinogenesis (Greenberg et al. 1998; Artandi et al. 2002). Furthermore, recent studies in primary human mammary epithelial cells have identified an apparently telomere-independent function of hTERT that enables human mammary epithelial cells (HMECs) to proliferate in mitogen deficient conditions, a hallmark of cancer (Smith et al. 2003; Mukherjee et al. 2011). Another study demonstrates that overexpressing mTERT in skin epithelia causes proliferation of hair follicle stem cells (Sarin et al. 2005). This function was traced to mTERT's function as a co-factor on β-catenin containing transcriptional regulation of the Wnt signaling pathway (Park et al. 2009). Transgenic mice overexpressing TERT are susceptible to carcinogen induced tumor formation as well as increased wound healing. Ectopic telomerase overexpression protects cells from antiproliferative or apoptotic stimuli (Bodnar et al. 1998; Ren et al. 2001). Conversely, in a wide variety of cell types, telomerase inhibition can enhance sensitivity to cytotoxic drugs (Harley 2008; Joseph et al. 2010; Roth et al. 2010). Additionally, hTERT can function as a RNA dependent RNA polymerase that can bind to non hTR RNAs and mediate independent functions, especially in the mitochondria as well as regulate mitochondrial functions (Maida et al. 2009; Esakova and Krasilnikov 2010; Indran et al. 2011; Mukherjee et al. 2011; Nitta et al. 2011). This multitude of alternative functions of telomerase is suggestive of its broader role in regulating cellular physiology, especially in diseased states.

3.1 Role of telomerase in Wnt transcriptional control

The role of telomerase in cell growth and stem cell function has been well documented (Lansdorp 2008; Flores and Blasco 2010). By using an RNAi screen, Coussens and coworkers discovered HIF1α as a novel regulator of telomerase in murine embryonic stem cells, thereby hinting at a feedback mechanism that is relevant to stem cell survival in cancers (Coussens et al. 2010). Sarin et al. reported that forced overexpression of mTERT in mouse skin triggered hair follicles to enter or remain in the active phase (Sarin et al. 2005). The result was furry mice in which the normal regulation of hair growth was disrupted. Even more striking was the observation that this effect of mTERT overexpression occurred in mice lacking mTR (Sarin et al. 2005) and was supported by a catalytically inactive protein ($mTERT^{ci}$) (Choi et al. 2008), ruling out the possibility that mTERT's enzymatic role in telomere maintenance was responsible.

3.1.1 The Wnt signaling pathway

Wnt proteins are secreted morphogens that are required for basic developmental processes, such as cell-fate specification, progenitor-cell proliferation (Willert et al. 2003) and the control of asymmetric cell division, in many different species and organs(Lyuksyutova et al. 2003; Logan and Nusse 2004). Recently, its importance in embryogenesis and cancer (Lie et al. 2005) has gained attention. There are at least three different Wnt pathways: the canonical pathway, the planar cell polarity (PCP) pathway (Schlessinger et al. 2007) and the Wnt/ Ca2+ pathway (Miller et al. 1999). In the canonical Wnt pathway, the major effect of Wnt ligand binding to its receptor is the stabilization of cytoplasmic ß-catenin through inhibition of the ß-catenin degradation complex. ß-catenin is then free to enter the nucleus and activate Wnt-regulated genes through its interaction with TCF (T-cell factor) family transcription factors and concomitant recruitment of coactivators. Planar cell polarity (PCP) signaling leads to the activation of the small GTPases RHOA (RAS homologue gene-family member A) and RAC1, which activates the stress kinase JNK (Jun N-terminal kinase) and ROCK (RHO-associated coiled-coil-containing protein kinase 1) and this leads to remodeling of the cytoskeleton and changes in cell adhesion and motility (Malliri and Collard 2003; Hall 2005; Angers and Moon 2009; Hoogeboom and Burgering 2009). WNT-Ca2+ signaling is mediated through G proteins and phospholipases and leads to transient increases in cytoplasmic free calcium that subsequently activates the kinase PKC (protein kinase C) and CAMKII (calcium calmodulin mediated kinase II) and the phosphatase calcineurin. Calcineurin induces activation of transcription factor NFAT, which regulates ventral patterning(Komiya and Habas 2008). CamKII activates TAK1 and NLK kinases, which can interfere with TCF/ß-Catenin signaling in the canonical pathway (Miller et al. 1999; Komiya and Habas 2008; Dodge and Lum 2011).

3.1.2 Telomerase regulates Wnt signaling by associating with Brg1 to regulate beta-catenin dependent transcriptional targets

To identify genomic targets that might explain the effect of telomerase function observed previously in hair follicle stem cells (Sarin et al. 2005), gene expression changes following rapid downregulation of mTERT^{ci} in skin were monitored. Affected genes strongly correlated with those regulated by the Myc and Wnt pathways (Choi et al. 2008), and Park et al. demonstrated that telomerase ablation resulted in altered mRNA expression levels of genes involved in signal transduction and development of epithelia and cytoskeleton of mice (Park et al. 2009). They then analyzed, using pattern-matching algorithms, the genome-wide transcriptional response after modulating TERT levels in mice. The results of this analysis revealed that the transcriptional response for TERT was similar to that observed for Wnt and Myc signaling pathways. Similar to telomerase, both Myc (Wolfer and Ramaswamy 2011) and Wnt (Ramachandran et al. 2011) have critical roles in carcinogenesis, metastasis and stem cell biology (Reya and Clevers 2005; Smith et al. 2010). The ability of telomerase is therefore similar to the effect of ß-catenin in activating stem cells. Artandi et al then establish that TERT functions as a transcriptional co-factor for the Wnt/ß-catenin transcriptional complex. TERT achieves this function by specific interactions with BRG-1, an ATP-dependent SWI/SNF chromatin-remodeling factor that is required for ß-catenin transcriptional function. Consistent with this interaction, a T-cell factor (TCF)-binding site reporter construct (TOP-FLASH) was upregulated by overexpression of either mTERT or mTERT^{ci} (where the catalytic subunit does not bind the RNA component TERC) in a BRG1-dependent, but mTERC-independent manner (Park et al. 2009), establishing that the enzymatic activity of telomerase is not required for this function. Although these results have the caveat that overexpression might create gain-of-function phenotypes, the results presented by Park and colleagues build a strong case for TERT mediated regulation of Wnt signaling. The authors provided evidences for specific binding of an epitope-tagged version of mTERT at Wnt-regulated promoters under conditions in which the protein was not overexpressed (Park et al. 2009). Furthermore, to demonstrate a role for TERT in Wnt pathway activation, they examined the consequences of TERT loss in three different contexts. In conditional mTERT knockout ES cells, basal and induced expression of the Wnt target genes like Axin2 was reduced upon mTERT excision. In another model, the impact of Xenopus TERT (xTERT) knockdown was examined in embryonic growth since Wnt signaling is important during Xenopus laevis development (Lyuksyutova et al. 2003). The injection of two different morpholinos directed against xTERT into frog embryos caused striking defects in anterior-posterior axis formation. These defects were rescued by co-injection of morpholino-resistant xTERT or xTERTci mRNAs, thereby suggesting that these effects are specific and due to a noncatalytic role of TERT. Remarkably, first-generation mTERT-deficient mice (which still have long and functional telomeres), while superficially normal, revealed a partially penetrant (~50% of animals) homeotic transformation of the vertebrae, observed as loss of the 13th rib on one or both sides, proving the novel, extratelomeric role for TERT dependent Wnt signaling during development.

3.2 Role of telomerase in DNA damage repair

It has been shown that telomerase, together with other telomere-specific binding proteins, maintains telomere heterochromatin, thereby preventing telomere degradation and the activation of the DNA damage response pathway (Chan and Blackburn 2002). DNA repair proteins (such as ATM, WRN, MRN complex) have been found to play essential roles in the telomere maintenance (Machwe et al. 2004; Blasco 2005; de Lange 2005; Burma et al. 2006; van Overbeek and de Lange 2006). Prior work in both budding yeast (Flint et al. 1994; Myung et al. 2001) and mammalian cells (Sprung et al. 1999; Stellwagen et al. 2003; Gao et al. 2008) indicates that chromosome breaks at locations distinct from telomeres are occasionally repaired by telomere addition; however, this mechanism for chromosome healing occurs much less frequently than other forms of DNA repair. However, it is also possible that telomerase may participate in other forms of DNA repair. This was elegantly shown in a study by Masutomi and coworkers, which implicates hTERT as a regulator of the DNA damage response pathway and in regulating histone dependent chromatin reorganization (Masutomi et al. 2005).

3.2.1 DNA double strand break repair pathways

DNA double-strand breaks (DSBs) pose a serious threat to cell viability and genome stability. Under homeostasis, DSB are generated during replication by blocking lesions resulting from reactive oxygen species (ROS) leading to fork collapse; during genomic rearrangements such as yeast mating-type switching, V(D)J recombination, class-switch recombination, meiosis; and from physical stress when dicentric or catenated chromosomes are pulled to opposite poles during mitosis (Franco et al. 2006; Keeney and Neale 2006;

Chaudhuri et al. 2007). DSBs are also produced when cells are exposed to DNA damaging agents including ionizing radiation (IR), which creates DSBs directly and indirectly via production of ROS; chemical agents and UV light that create replication blocking lesions (alkyl adducts, pyrimidine dimers, and crosslinks) e.g Doxorubicin; and cancer chemotherapeutics that poison topoisomerase I (which produces replication-blocking lesions) e.g. Camptothecin, or topoisomerase II, (which traps the enzyme-DNA complex) after DSB induction and can potentially produce DSBs during any phase of the cell cycle (Limoli et al. 2002; Furuta et al. 2003; Bryant et al. 2010). Failure to repair DSBs, or misrepair, can result in cell death or large-scale chromosome rearrangements including deletions, translocations, and chromosome fusions that enhance genome instability, a hallmark of cancer cells (Rothkamm et al. 2001; Degrassi et al. 2004; Su 2006; Puig et al. 2008; Sliwinska et al. 2009). Cells have evolved groups of proteins that function in signaling networks that sense DSBs or other DNA damage, arrest cell cycle, and activate DNA repair pathways (Franco et al. 2006). The cellular responses can occur at various stages of the cell cycle and are collectively called DNA damage checkpoints, but when cells suffer too much damage overlapping signaling pathways can trigger apoptosis to prevent propagation of cells with unstable genomes (Rothkamm et al. 2001; Franco et al. 2006; Su 2006; Jeggo and Lavin 2009).

Eukaryotic cells repair DSBs primarily by two mechanisms: nonhomologous end-joining (NHEJ) and homologous recombination (HR); also known as "error-prone" and "error-free" repair, respectively (Natarajan and Palitti 2008). Upon induction of a DSB, NHEJ proceeds in a stepwise manner beginning with limited end-processing by the MRE11/RAD50/NBS1 (MRN) complex, end-binding by Ku comprising the Ku70 and Ku80 subunits, and recruitment of the DNA-dependent protein kinase catalytic subunit (DNA-PKcs), forming the trimeric DNA-PK holoenzyme (Burma et al. 2006). Once bound to broken ends, DNA-PK is activated, consequently phosphorylating itself and other targets including RPA, WRN, and Artemis; in cells lacking ATM, DNA-PK can also phosphorylate histone H2AX, termed γ-H2AX (Stiff et al. 2004). In the final step, DNA ligase IV, with its binding partners XRCC4 and XLF, seals the break (Gu et al. 2007). An alternative Ligase III-mediated NHEJ pathway is promoted by PARP-1 and is more error-prone than classical NHEJ (Simsek et al. 2011). HR is considered a more accurate mechanism for DSB repair because broken ends use homologous sequences elsewhere in the genome (sister chromatids, homologous chromosomes, or repeated regions on the same or different chromosomes) to prime repair synthesis (Helleday 2003). With the exception of sister chromatids, repair templates are often not perfectly homologous, and in these cases HR results in loss of heterozygosity, with information transferred non-reciprocally from the unbroken (donor) locus to the broken (recipient) locus, a process termed gene conversion. HR initiates with extensive 5′ to 3′ end-processing at broken ends, which is regulated by MRN (Langerak et al. 2011). The resulting 3′ ssDNA tails are bound by hSSB (single-strand binding protein), which is replaced with Rad51 in a reaction mediated by various related proteins like RAD52, BRCA1 & 2, etc. (Qing et al. 2011). The resulting Rad51 nucleoprotein filament searches for and invades a homologous sequence, which can dissociate and anneal with the processed end of the non-invading strand on the opposite side of the DSB in a RAD54 dependent manner (Mazin et al. 2010), or both ends may invade producing a double-Holliday junction that is resolved to yield crossover or non-crossover recombinants. Thereafter, the remaining ssDNA gaps and nicks are repaired by DNA polymerase and DNA ligase (Lieber 2010).

3.2.2 Extra-telomeric role of telomerase in DNA damage repair

In an attempt to understand novel roles of telomerase, Masutomi et al analyzed the effects of suppressing hTERT function on the cells response to ionizing radiation. They examined previously characterized phosphorylation changes in several proteins of the DNA damage response (DDR) pathway in diploid human fibroblasts, which only transiently express low levels of hTERT in S-phase(Masutomi et al. 2003). Irradiation of human BJ or WI38 fibroblasts led to the phosphorylation of H2AX (γ-H2AX), ATM and BRCA1 proteins and up-regulated the p53 protein with similar results when treated with the chemotherapeutic agents irinotecan or etoposide. However, such treatments of these fibroblasts stably expressing either an hTERT-coding sequence-specific shRNA (hTERT shRNA) or an hTERT 3′ untranslated region-specific shRNA (hTERT 3′ UTR shRNA) to ionizing radiation, irinotecan, or etoposide failed to induce a similar degree of H2AX or ATM phosphorylation or stabilization of p53 protein. These findings indicate that in cells lacking hTERT, the DNA damage response is dampened. Conversely, the expression of WT hTERT, which is resistant to the effects of the hTERT 3′ UTR-specific shRNA in cells expressing this shRNA rescued telomerase activity and the DDR defect. They also found that fibroblasts expressing a catalytically inactive hTERT mutant (DN hTERT) as well as select other mutants that impair the catalytic activity of telomerase(Hahn et al. 1999), also showed an impaired DNA damage response, suggesting that chronic loss of hTERT function either by RNA interference or catalytic inhibition abrogates the cellular response to DNA damage, implicating hTERT as a critical regulator of the DNA damage response pathway. Interestingly, over the short time periods of these experiments (low population doublings), there were no detectable alterations in overall telomere length or changes in the length of the 3′ telomeric single-stranded overhang either before or after irradiation of cells expressing an hTERT-specific shRNA as compared with cells expressing a control shRNA. Furthermore, since they observed only 7% of nuclear foci containing γ-H2AX colocalized with telomeres after treatment with ionizing radiation, it is not possible to attribute the effects to a telomere specific effect. These observations are in line with a previous study, which demonstrates that during senescence in human cell culture or in mice, there is an accumulation of irreparable DNA damage lesions (Sedelnikova et al. 2004). They further show that hTERT ablation reduced ATM autophosphorylation in response to ionizing radiation, as well as to agents such as trichostatin A (TSA). These findings suggest that suppression of hTERT expression modulates overall chromatin architecture. Therefore, they went on to demonstrate that chromatin derived from cells lacking hTERT was slightly more susceptible to MN (micrococcal nuclease) digestion, particularly at earlier time points compared with control cell lines. Remarkably, they found decreased levels of histone H3-lysine (K) 9 dimethylation and increased amounts of H3-K9 acetylation in cells lacking hTERT. The heterochromatic proteins 1 (HP1) associate with di- and tri-methylated but not to acetylated forms of H3-K9 to form heterochromatin (Murr 2010). Supportive of this observation, they also demonstrate by acid extraction of histones, that H2Ax levels in soluble fractions were higher than the chromatin bound insoluble fraction in hTERT ablated cells compared to controls. However, there were no appreciable differences in the amounts of soluble macro H2A.1, H2B, H3, and H4 in cells that expressed or lacked hTERT expression, suggesting that it is the stress dependent chromatin remodeling that is dependent on TERT. This is experimentally proven by altered migration of chromatin in pulsed-field gel electrophoresis.

Telomerase knockout mice lacking the RNA component mTerc also show impaired responses to agents that damage DNA (Wong et al. 2000); although the effects are apparent only in late generation mTerc-null mice that show significant telomere shortening and dysfunction (Goytisolo et al. 2000). Recent studies however report that there are no detectable effects of mTert or mTerc deficiency on chromatin structure and DNA damage responses (Vidal-Cardenas and Greider 2010). Although, regulation of chromatin plays a critical role in mammalian development(Meehan 2003; Kim et al. 2009; Cheng and Blumenthal 2010), developmental compensation in murine genetic models or species differences may account for the differences observed in the studies. Such developmental compensation, as has been observed in mice lacking the retinoblastoma gene (Sage et al. 2003), might similarly mask the effects of germ-line telomerase loss on chromatin structure and DNA damage.

Telomerase is reactivated in 80-90% of all cancers, providing the cancer cells with increased proliferative and survival properties (Harley 2008). Mouse tumors also show evidence of increased telomerase activity (Blasco et al. 1996), despite harboring long telomeres and basal telomerase activity. Because recent work in both transgenic mice and human cells suggests that increased TERT expression contributes to malignant transformation even in cells harboring long telomeres (Blasco and Hahn 2003; Blasco 2005; Jones et al. 2011), the effects of hTERT on chromatin may provide a plausible mechanism for such additional functions of hTERT in maintaining chromosomal stability and may suggest how TERT can contribute to cell transformation independently of its effects on telomere maintenance.

3.3 Role of telomerase in mitochondria

3.3.1 Mechanisms of oxidative-stress

Tissue homeostasis is controlled by the balance between the rates of cell proliferation and cell death, which in turn is tightly regulated by diverse intracellular signaling cascades. It has been shown that the intracellular redox milieu which is driven by a balance between rate of generation of intracellular reactive oxygen species (ROS) and the efficiency of their scavenging play a critical role in controlling cellular signaling, protein turnover, ion transport and ultimately cell survival. Abnormal accumulation of ROS contributes to cellular aging and the senescence process whilst the ability to withstand oxidative stress leads to enhanced longevity in several species (Finkel and Holbrook 2000; Ma 2010). Although telomere length and its attrition contribute to senescence, telomere attrition is not the only stimulus for replicative senescence. A growing body of evidence suggests that oxidative stress can induce or accelerate the onset of replicative senescence, a phenomenon referred to as stress-induced replicative senescence (Toussaint et al. 2000; Duan et al. 2005). Interestingly, depending upon intracellular levels and the nature of the ROS species, the effects could be as diverse as activation of gene transcription and proliferation to DNA damage and cell death induction (Valko et al. 2006; Valko et al. 2007), which is intimately correlative to associated diseases phenotypes. The correlation between a "pro-oxidant" state and cell survival has been further consolidated by findings using oncogene-induced models of cell transformation, such as activated Rac, Bcl-2, and Akt/PKB (Clement et al. 2003; Lim and Clement 2007; Ma 2010).

Along with membrane bound NADPH oxidase complex (Nox family), the mitochondrial electron transport chain (ETC) also serves as a major intracellular source of ROS. The high flux of O_2 through ETC (almost 90% for oxidative phosphorylation) is accompanied by leakage of electrons, resulting in the generation of superoxide anions, predominantly involving complexes I and III of the ETC (Vercesi et al. 2006; Orrenius et al. 2007). The presence of Mn superoxide dismutase (MnSOD; SOD2) in the mitochondrial matrix coordinates with GSH to scavenge these superoxide anions, thereby limiting the excessive accumulation of H_2O_2. The cytosolic Cu/Zn SOD (SOD1) serves a similar function in scavenging ROS generated outside of the mitochondria or directly released from the mitochondria. Therefore, efficient shuttling of electrons across the ETC coupled with mitochondrial O_2 consumption is important for normal mitochondrial physiology including ATP synthesis. In addition to mitochondrial DNA damage, excessive ROS accumulation in the mitochondria could trigger mitochondrial outer membrane permeabilization and facilitate the egress of apoptosis amplification factors such cytochrome C, apoptosis inducing factor (AIF), and Smac/Diablo.

3.3.2 Effects of telomerase on oxidative stress

TERT expression itself is regulated by many transcription factors, including AP1, SP1 and NF-κB, all of which are redox regulated (Poole et al. 2001; Akiyama et al. 2003; Takakura et al. 2005; Cong and Shay 2008). AP1 has been shown to suppress hTERT expression whilst SP1 and NF-κB are strong activators of TERT. Furthermore, prevention of nuclear export of hTERT enhances the anti-apoptotic activity of TERT against ROS-dependent apoptosis (Haendeler et al. 2004; Kurz et al. 2004).

Extra-nuclear hTERT has been shown to translocate to the mitochondria following oxidative stress (Santos et al. 2004; Santos et al. 2006; Kovalenko et al. 2010) however, its mechanistic role in mitochondrial function only emerged recently (Kovalenko et al. 2010; Indran et al. 2011; Mukherjee et al. 2011; Nitta et al. 2011). Dairkee et al. suggested a signature pattern characteristic of tumor cell immortalization (immortalization signature or ImmSig) wherein overexpression of oxidoreductase genes was identified as an important marker (Dairkee et al. 2004). As expected, hTERT ablation reversed ImmSig expression, increased cellular ROS levels, altered mitochondrial membrane potential, and induced apoptotic and proliferative changes in immortalized cells (Dairkee et al. 2004). While certain reports suggested that the localization of hTERT to the mitochondria resulted in increased mitochondrial DNA damage following acute oxidative stress, hTERT expression did not alter the rate of H_2O_2 breakdown, although levels of chelatable metal ions were higher, suggesting that the damaging effects of hTERT could be attributed to the elevated levels of divalent metal ions via Fenton chemistry (Santos et al. 2004). However, other studies demonstrate anti-apoptotic effects of mitochondrial localization of hTERT (Massard et al. 2006; Cong and Shay 2008) suggesting that Bax oligomerisation on mitochondrial membranes could be hTERT regulated. Several recent studies confirmed the protective response against oxidative stress in hTERT expressing cells (Massard et al. 2006; Mondello et al. 2006; Ahmed et al. 2008; Lee et al. 2008; Haendeler et al. 2009) and indicated that the function at the mitochondria is independent of its telomere synthesis activity.

3.3.3 Mitochondria specific functions of telomerase

Ahmed et al report that telomerase expressing MRC-5 lung fibroblasts demonstrated a significant translocation of hTERT to the mitochondria following oxidative stress, which was followed by lower mitochondrial DNA damage, reduced mitochondrial peroxide levels and an increase in mitochondrial membrane potential. In addition, reports have also suggested that hTERT expression positively impacts mitochondrial function by improving its calcium buffering capacity and reducing O_2^- production (Massard et al. 2006). Haelender et al demonstrate that mitochondrial hTERT exerted a novel protective function by binding to mitochondrial DNA, increasing respiratory chain activity, and protecting against oxidative stress-induced damage (Haendeler et al. 2009). Studies also suggest that hTERT expression in cells improves mitochondrial function by maintaining mitochondrial membrane potential, improving calcium storage and reducing mitochondrial formation (Massard et al. 2006; Passos et al. 2007; Ahmed et al. 2008). Microarray profiling of gene expression in cancer cells established that telomerase activity controlled several glycolytic pathway genes, suggesting modulation of the energy state of tumor cells and telomerase ablation decreased glucose consumption, lactate production, cell proliferation and viability while bulk telomere length remained relatively unchanged (Li et al. 2005; Bagheri et al. 2006). In studies done by Haelender et al, mitochondria isolated from $TERT^{-/-}$ mice displayed a significant reduction in complex I dependent respiration as compared to mitochondria from TERT wild type mice. The study also identified two TERT binding regions in mitochondrial DNA containing the coding sequences for NADH:ubiquinone oxidoreductase (complex I) subunit 1 and 2 (ND1, ND2). They therefore hypothesized that mitochondrial TERT may counteract ROS production by complex I via binding to ND1 and ND2, thereby increasing the synthesis of functional complex I subunits, which in turn can reduce the formation of damaged complex I that leaks electrons onto oxygen. Indran et al reported that cells overexpressing hTERT have greater basal COX (cyclooxygenase) activity, suggesting improved mitochondrial efficiency leading to reduced ROS production (Indran et al. 2011). Therefore, hTERT may be regulating COX either by direct interaction, given hTERT's mitochondrial localization, or indirectly by binding to other COX interacting proteins such as Bcl-2. Alternatively, hTERT seems to modulate intracellular redox status by improving cellular antioxidant capacity via modulating glutathione levels in the cells and conferring survival advantages as evidenced by enhanced GSH/GSSG ratio in a variety of cell lines (Indran et al. 2011).

3.3.4 Mutational analysis of telomerase catalytic component hTERT decouples its functions at the telomere vs. mitochondria

Mukherjee et al studied a panel of hTERT mutants (Counter et al. 1998; Armbruster et al. 2001; Banik et al. 2002) and demonstrated that the ability of hTERT to enhance proliferation, which was a result of increased cell division and decreased apoptosis, could be genetically uncoupled from its functions in telomere elongation, lifespan extension, and DNA damage responses. Remarkably, they identified telomere elongation-deficient mutants that were still able to extend cellular lifespan. Loss of this specific ability was seen upon hPOT1 ablation, suggesting that the ability to recruit telomere-capping proteins is critical for the survival advantage of ectopic hTERT expression. They also discovered a novel role for telomerase in regulating mitochondrial RMRP (RNA component of mitochondrial RNA processing endoribonuclease) level (Maida et al. 2009) that was crucial for enhancing proliferation. They further demonstrated that the hTERT–RMRP pathway, which results in generation of siRNAs and feedback suppression of RMRP, is linked to the enhanced cell proliferation phenotype in HMECs (human mammary epithelial cells). RMRP has varied cellular functions, including processing RNAs required to generate primers for mitochondrial DNA replication, pre-rRNA processing during rRNA maturation, mRNA cleavage of cell cycle genes, and potential regulation of gene expression via complexing with hTERT to generate siRNAs (Maida et al. 2009; Esakova and Krasilnikov 2010). These results therefore provide critical genetic support for the idea that hTERT has at least four biological functions—regulation of cell survival/proliferation, telomere elongation, cellular lifespan extension, and regulation of DNA damage responses. Interestingly, these studies concluded that all the diverse biological roles of hTERT require hTERT catalytic activity, even though all but telomere elongation are functionally independent of telomere. This observation differed from that observed by Park et al., in Wnt signaling (previous section) where the TERC was dispensable. One hTERT mutant that was predominantly cytoplasmic localized but retained catalytic activity was unable to enhance proliferation, indicating the requirement for nuclear localisation and decoupling its function in mitochondria. This observation has importance in diseases like CHH (cartilage hair hypoplasia), a pleiotropic disorder characterized by a short stature with other skeletal abnormalities, hypoplastic hair, immune deficiency and neuronal dysplasia of the intestine (Ridanpaa et al. 2001). Patients with CHH show a predisposition to lymphomas and other cancers. Mutations in RMRP, encoding a structural RNA molecule, have been linked to CHH (Ridanpaa et al. 2001). The details of underlying mechanisms by which RMRP might impact the pro-proliferative effect of hTERT require further elucidation. Further investigation of these pathways, as well as of alternative hTERT activities and its other binding partners, would not only improve our understanding of how hTERT exerts its anti-ROS effects at the mitochondria but also suggest novel ways for the development of anti-telomerase cancer therapeutic agents.

4. Diverse roles of shelterin proteins

Shelterin is composed of six core members that include TRF1, TRF2 (Telomeric Repeat binding Factor 1 and 2), TIN2 (TRF1- and TRF2-Interacting Nuclear Factor 2), POT1 (Protection Of Telomeres 1), TPP1 (formerly known as TINT1, PTOP or PIP1) and RAP1 (Repressor/Activator Protein 1) (Broccoli et al. 1997; Smith et al. 1998; Ye and de Lange 2004; de Lange 2005; Xin et al. 2007; Kendellen et al. 2009; Abreu et al. 2010). Three members of this complex, TRF1, TRF2 and POT1, bind directly to telomeric DNA repeats and anchor the rest of the complex along the length of the telomeres. The actual length of the telomeres varies in various species and also within mammals. TRF1 and TRF2 bind the double-stranded (TTAGGG)n repeats of telomeres while POT1 binds to 3' single-stranded G overhangs (Broccoli et al. 1997; Smith et al. 1998; Ye and de Lange 2004; de Lange 2005; Xin et al. 2007; Kendellen et al. 2009; Abreu et al. 2010). Rap1 was discovered as a TRF2 interacting factor and named such due to its sequence homology with the yeast Rap1 (Li et al. 2000). The yeast Rap1 has a multitude of functions both at the telomere and at other sites on the chromatin. These extra telomeric roles of yeast Rap1 include working as a transcription factor, and also participating in chromatin boundary formation and silencing at subtelomeric sites through the recruitment of Sir proteins (Morse 2000). Unlike the yeast Rap1 that can bind directly to DNA at telomeric and non-telomeric sites due to its two Myb domains, the human homolog contains a single Myb domain, which renders it unable to bind to DNA on its own. Hence, the mammalian Rap1 is recruited by its high affinity binding partner TRF2 to the telomeres. Mammalian Rap1 has been suggested to be required for telomere length maintenance (Li and de Lange 2003; O'Connor et al. 2004) and prevention of telomere recombination and fragility (Sfeir et al. 2009; Sfeir et al. 2010). Genetic abrogation of many of the shelterin complex components individually results in early embryonic lethality in mice (Blasco 2005). The recent availability of several transgenic mouse models of shelterin complex components, as well as the generation of tissue-specific conditional mouse models of these components, has revealed a role for these proteins in cancer susceptibility and age related pathologies even in the presence of normal telomerase activity and under conditions when telomere length is normal (Blasco 2005). Recent work from different laboratories has suggested that Rap1 may not be directly involved in telomere protection, but rather in regulation of DNA repair activities at the telomere (Pardo and Marcand 2005; Bae and Baumann 2007; Sarthy et al. 2009; Bombarde et al. 2010; Sfeir et al. 2010; Chen et al. 2011). Sfeir et al have reported that conditional loss of Rap1 alone had little effect on telomere stability (i.e., no overt changes in telomere length, telomere DNA damage foci, or telomeric fusions were noted). However, when combined with loss of Ku, there was a marked increase in telomere sister chromatid exchanges, suggesting that Rap1 participates in inhibiting homology-directed repair (HR or HDR) at the telomere (Sfeir et al. 2010). Whole body or targeted depletion of Rap1 in stratified epithelia (in Rap1Δ/Δ K5-cre mice) does not affect the viability and fertility of the animals (Martinez et al. 2010; Sfeir et al. 2010). While skin specific deletion of Rap1 has been reported to cause both early onset of skin hyperpigmentation during adulthood and an obese phenotype in females (Martinez et al. 2010), there are no specific indications from these mouse models if Rap1 deletion has any role in longevity and cancer.

Clearly, the underlying molecular mechanisms by which telomerase and the shelterin complex proteins regulate processes critical for cancers like cell proliferation, survival upon genotoxic stress and invasion cannot be explained by the function of these proteins only on the telomere. Indeed recent studies have also indicated that telomeric proteins like Rap1 do have functional roles in diverse sub cellular locations (Martinez et al. 2010; Takai et al. 2010; Teo et al. 2010). In line with this, the expression levels of several other components of the shelterin proteins are altered in various human cancers (Blanco et al. 2007; Teo et al. 2010). These novel, non-telomeric roles of telomeric proteins could provide a useful Achilles' heel for developing drugs for a number of human ailments including cancer.

4.1 Rap1 in NFκB signaling

Using an unbiased screen we reported the identification of Rap1, as a novel adaptor of IKK and a critical regulator of NFkB. Our results documented the first, telomere independent, cytoplasmic role for mammalian Rap1 in transcription of NFkB target genes (Teo et al. 2010). We showed that Rap1 is part of the IKK complex and promotes IKK activity towards p65 subunit of NFkB by working as an adaptor (Teo et al. 2010).

4.1.1 The mediator of inflammation – NFκB (Nuclear factor κ-light chain enhancer of activated B cells)

Transcription factor NFkB is activated by a variety of cellular and developmental signals (Ghosh and Hayden 2008). Both activation and inactivation of NFkB signaling are rapid and tightly controlled events under normal physiological settings in most healthy cell types. Deregulated activation of NFkB has been observed and causally linked to development of several human pathologies including cancers (Ben-Neriah and Karin 2011). The NFκB family is composed of, RelA, RelB, c-Rel proteins and also includes the processed forms of p105 and p100 proteins, namely p50 and p52, respectively (Hayden and Ghosh 2008). All the Rel proteins contain a RHD (Rel Homology Domain), within which lies the DNA binding, dimerization and IκB binding domains. The rate-limiting step in the activation of NFkB in response to stimulation is the degradation of the inhibitory IkB proteins that inhibit NFκB function mainly because they prevent the binding of NFκB dimers to DNA. IκBα, IκBβ, IκBε, IκBζ, IκBγ and BCL3 and the precursor p100 and p105 proteins are the identified members of the IkB family. Phosphorylation of IkBs by IkB kinases (IKK), IKK1 and IKK2, is critical for their subsequent ubiquitination and proteolytic degradation in response to stimulation(Hayden and Ghosh 2008; Ben-Neriah and Karin 2011). In particular, recent evidence has highlighted that IKK mediated covalent modification of free p65 subunit is critical for NFkB to function as an efficient transcription factor.

4.1.2 Cytosolic function of telomeric protein Rap1 in NFκB signaling

Gel filtration analysis of macromolecular complexes as well as direct biochemistry identified cytosolic Rap1 to be physically associated with the functional IKK complex, the primary node of NFkB activation. Biochemical experiments demonstrated that Rap1 was crucial for efficient recruitment of IKKs and phosphorylation of p65, an essential step for rendering NF-κB transcriptionally competent. Specifically, Rap1 was required in the IKK complex for it to be proficient in phosphorylating p65 on serine-536 in response to inflammatory stimuli. However, the phosphorylation and degradation of IkB was not significantly influenced in loss-of-function experiments. Rap1 was shown in kinase assays to be required by the IKK kinase complex to define specificity of the substrate; i.e., p65 compared to IkB or c-Rel. Moreover, the authors found that NF-κB signalling could in turn regulate Rap1 expression through NF-κB binding sites in the Rap1 promoter region. When NF-κB pathway activation was abrogated, total Rap1 expression was diminished; however, when the p65 subunit was overexpressed, more Rap1 was found in total cellular extracts, suggesting the existence of a feedback loop for Rap1 self-activation. In case of NFkB signaling, both the human and murine model are in agreement; Rap1 functions as an adapter that determines the substrate specificity of the IKK complex, thereby regulating inflammatory gene expression patterns (Teo et al. 2010). These findings also suggest the interesting possibility that Rap1 has additional partners, which stabilize it in various subcellular locations and that Rap1 functions, both in the nucleus (at the telomere and on chromatin) and in the cytoplasm. We further established the importance of this NFkB regulation in homeostasis by uncovering the effect of its dysregulation in cancer. Significantly, in human breast cancer tissue microarrays, we observed higher levels of cytosolic Rap1 corresponding with higher levels of activated NFkB, but also higher grades of tumor (Teo et al. 2010). These findings suggest that Rap1 and NFkB function in concert to enhance tumor survival and metastasis by upregulating NFkB dependent anti-apoptotic mechanisms.

4.2 Extratelomeric role of shelterin complex proteins Rap1, TRF1 and TRF2 in transcriptional control

Telomeric factors have long been known to play a role in binding at internal chromosomal locations. The first example of this kind was yeast Rap1, which specifically binds to telomeric DNA and was identified, at first, as a general regulatory factor. Interestingly, in yeast, telomere alterations can lead to the delocalization from telomeres of Rap1-associated heterochromatin factors that are able to operate at extratelomeric or interstitial genomic sites (Maillet et al. 1996; Marcand et al. 1996). Based on these yeast results, it is tempting to propose that telomeric factors are released from the telomeres after telomere shortening or alteration and subsequently relocalize to extra-telomeric sites, where they modify the cellular transcriptional program.

In another evidence of a prominent non-telomeric transcriptional role of a telomeric protein, Martinez et al. performed chromatin immunoprecipitation sequencing (ChIP–seq) using RAP1 antibodies and discovered that it not only binds to telomeres but also to other non-telomeric sites throughout the murine genome, via recognition of the $(TTAGGG)_2$ consensus motif (Martinez et al. 2010). Extratelomeric RAP1 was shown to bind to non-coding regions in chromosomes 2, 11 and 17, which are enriched in TTAGGG tandem repeats, raising the possibility that RAP1 might prevent fragility and recombination at these genomic sites. Similar to its yeast counterpart, murine RAP1 binding sites were enriched at subtelomeric regions, leading to derepression of subtelomeric genes in Rap1-deficient cells, thereby indicating an evolutionarily conserved role for RAP1 in subtelomeric silencing. Although mammalian RAP1 was initially thought to have diverged from yeast Rap1 due to loss of its DNA-binding domain, these observations suggest that Rap1 may still be functionally conserved. The observation that RAP1 also binds to genomic sites lacking TTAGGG repeats and the fact that many of these sites were also associated with genes that are deregulated on Rap1 deletion suggests that RAP1 may interact with factors other than TRF2 to help gene transcriptional regulation. Gene set enrichment analysis (GseA) on genes downregulated in Rap1-null MEFs revealed significant downregulation of imprinted genes, as well as downregulation of genes involved in cancer, cell adhesion and metabolism (like peroxisome proliferator-activated receptor signaling, growth hormone and insulin secretion pathways) in Rap1-null cells. In turn, Rap1-null cells showed significant upregulation of ABC transporters and genes involved in type II diabetes, suggesting a negative effect of Rap1 deletion on metabolism. In agreement with a role of RAP1 in transcriptional regulation, RAP1-binding sites were shown to have RAP1-dependent enhancer activity. It should be noted that this Rap1 localization to various sites was not in response to any cellular stress. However, these data are slightly divergent from two subsequent reports also analyzed binding of telomeric proteins to extra-telomeric chromosomal sites by ChIP-seq (Simonet et al. 2011; Yang et al. 2011).

In the first study by Yang et al, analysis of genome-wide chromatin-binding patterns of two telomeric proteins RAP1 and TRF2 revealed that these proteins can associate with interstitial sites, too. In agreement with the study by Martinez et al, they demonstrate that TRF2 and Rap1 could bind distinct and overlapping extratelomeric chromatin binding sites (also called interstitial binding sites or ITS) that not only contained the TTAGGG repeat, but also non-telomeric repeat motifs. The binding overlap between Rap1 and TRF2 is expected given that these two proteins form stable protein heterodimers. In addition, they also identified unique bindings for RAP1 and TRF2, respectively, indicating TRF2-independent function of RAP1. The data suggest that while the binding of RAP1 to TTAGGG repeats could be TRF2 dependent, the mechanism by which RAP1 associates with non-telomere-repeat sequences could be dependent on its interaction with other chromatin-associated factors. Using stringent criteria, they predict ~ 300 potential TRF2 binding sites that contain telomeric repeats which was confirmed by TRF2 overexpression. They also observed that overexpression of TRF2 did not lead to an increase in the binding of endogenous RAP1 lending credence to the notion that extratelomeric binding of these telomeric proteins is not dependent on their interactions with each other.

A novel finding of the second study of TRF1 and TRF2 genome-wide binding by Simonet et al was the identification of non-ITS binding sites centered on (ATTCC)n satellite 2/3 repeats or alphoid DNA satellite sequences, which form part of the most prominent autosomal heterochromatin blocks (Simonet et al. 2011). Given the reported role of TRF1 and TRF2 in the control of replication fork progression through telomeric chromatin(Sfeir et al. 2009; Ye et al. 2010), it is possible that these shelterin components play a similar role in other regions of DNA that are difficult to replicate, such as those packaged as heterochromatin. Gene ontology data (Simonet et al. 2011) suggested that a large subset of TRF binding sites may have functional relevance since they occur more frequently within or in close proximity to genes, which agrees with results from Martinez et al., since TRF sites are frequently located in intronic regions or distant from promoters(Simonet et al. 2011). Thus, TRF1 and TRF2 possibly regulate gene expression through looping mechanisms or by modifying the chromatin landscape. It is possible that cellular levels of TRF proteins influence their binding to the ITSs, and thus the expression of neighboring genes. Interestingly, they also observe from sequence alignments of bound and unbound extratelomeric sites that TRF1 and TRF2 discriminate between different sites on the basis of their length and sequence (Simonet et al. 2011). This observation suggests that other features such as accessibility and/or the chromatin structure of the surrounding DNA region may influence TRF binding. Thus, additional sites might be bound if the TRF protein concentration and/or chromatin context is altered.

However, in both studies in human cells (Simonet et al. 2011; Yang et al. 2011), the authors identified only a limited number of interstitial binding sites for RAP1, TRF2 and TRF1. Along those lines, it is possible that the number of RAP1 and TRF binding sites may have been underestimated, due to potential antibody-epitope sensitivity differences or due to species differences. Furthermore the general technical difficulty in identifying and calling peaks in repeat elements could be an additional reason for under-representation of binding sites. The data from Yang et al suggests that the cellular concentration of TRF2 may play a role in selective binding of TRF2 to its target sites. Since mouse telomeres are much longer than humans, it is plausible that differences in telomeric protein concentration may, at least in part account for the different binding site numbers observed between human and mouse.

4.3 Role of TRF2 in DNA damage repair pathway

Various laboratories have reported TRF2 association with proteins involved in DSB repair at the telomeres, including the MRE11/Rad50/NBS1 (MRN) complex, Ku70, WRN and BLM (Song et al. 2000; Zhu et al. 2000; Opresko et al. 2002; Dimitrova and de Lange 2009). Interestingly, Bradshaw et al demonstrate that TRF2 localizes to DSB (DNA double strand break; see description in previous section) sites at the early stages of cellular response to DSBs, appearing in the first few seconds after DSB induction and leaving as DSBs are being processed (Bradshaw et al. 2005). They created DSBs in defined nuclear regions of SV40-transformed human fibroblasts using pulsed laser microbeam irradiation followed by immunofluorescence monitoring of TRF2, ATM and H2AX. These data indicated involvement of TRF2 in an ATM-independent DNA-damage response at extra-telomeric sites. This data also demonstrated that the N-terminal basic domain is essential for TRF2 to associate with nontelomeric DSBs in vivo in contrast to the requirement of both Myb and basic domains of TRF2 for telomere localization. Given earlier reports that TRF2 preferentially localizes to double-strand–single-strand junctions of artificial telomeres as opposed to related, blunt-ended DNA (Stansel et al. 2001), the data suggested that the TRF2 DSB response may be DNA structure dependent rather than sequence based. However, these data were questioned by another study that could not find TRF2 localization to DSB (Williams et al. 2007). Yet, the differences in the studies could be attributed to differences in the method of inducing DSB and the cellular context, indicating that the TRF2 response may be limited to specific kind and level of the damage.

A subsequent report also demonstrated that TRF2 is involved in DSB repair of non-telomeric DNA (Mao et al. 2007). Their results corroborated earlier findings that TRF2 represses NHEJ (non-homologous end joining) but show that it is required for HR (homologous recombination). TRF2 stimulated HR at nontelomeric DSB as demonstrated by ectopic expression of the full-length TRF2 and C-terminally truncated TRF2 ($TRF2^{\Delta M}$). The N-terminal domain of TRF2 has DNA binding activity independent of the TTAGGG sequence (Fouche et al. 2006). They also show that the TRF2 mutant ($TRF2^{\Delta M}$) that contains this unspecific DNA-binding domain and lacks the C-terminal domain stimulates HR when overexpressed (Mao et al. 2007). Thus, it is likely that the N-terminal domain of TRF2 is involved in strand invasion during HR repair of DSBs, and the C-terminal domain plays a regulatory role by limiting the HR activity of TRF2. Conversely, depletion of TRF2 strongly inhibited HR evidenced by delayed Rad51 foci formation after irradiation without affecting NHEJ. These results suggest that TRF2 plays a functional role in HR and may inhibit NHEJ by directing DSB repair toward HR pathway. Although TRF2 inhibits HR at telomeres, the observation that it mediates formation of T-loop formation at telomeres (Stansel et al. 2001), which resemble the structure of Holliday junctions is indicative of a role in HR. The basic domain of TRF2 binds to Holliday junctions in a sequence-unspecific manner (Fouche et al. 2006) suggesting that TRF2 may participate in HR of nontelomeric DNA.

Interestingly, since depletion of TRF2 delays Rad51 foci formation after irradiation by ≈4 h, it is speculated that TRF2 is required to directly recruit Rad51 or its paralogs such as Rad52 and BRCA2. TRF2 may interact with these proteins and facilitate further recruitment of Rad51. Collectively these findings suggest that, based on the configuration of DNA ends or other factors, certain breaks are preferentially processed by NHEJ, and others are preferentially processed by HR. Since TRF2 is recruited to the site of DSB very early, within 2 sec of irradiation (Bradshaw et al. 2005), a possible scenario could be that TRF2 arrives early, marks certain DSBs for repair by HR, and facilitates strand invasion by Rad51. These data exemplify another distinct extra-telomeric role for TRF2 in regulation of the DNA damage repair pathways.

5. Conclusion

The discovery of varied novel extra telomeric functions of telomeric proteins may have critical implications not only for tumorigenesis and telomerase-targeted anticancer therapeutics but also for tissue regeneration, genetic disorders associated with defects in telomeric proteins, apart from normal biological processes such as tissue homeostasis and organismal aging. A key to realizing this potential lies in determining whether these extratelomeric functions are mediated by the same or different biochemical or molecular activities of these proteins and who their cellular partners are in such specific functions. This would not only help us understand how telomeric proteins perform these diverse roles, but also determine whether these different pathways could be selectively targeted to provide multiple independent therapeutic targets for distinct human ailments.

6. References

Abreu, E., E. Aritonovska, et al. (2010). "TIN2-tethered TPP1 recruits human telomerase to telomeres in vivo." *Molecular and cellular biology* 30(12): 2971-2982.

Ahmed, S., J. F. Passos, et al. (2008). "Telomerase does not counteract telomere shortening but protects mitochondrial function under oxidative stress." *Journal of cell science* 121(Pt 7): 1046-1053.

Akiyama, M., T. Hideshima, et al. (2003). "Nuclear factor-kappaB p65 mediates tumor necrosis factor alpha-induced nuclear translocation of telomerase reverse transcriptase protein." *Cancer research* 63(1): 18-21.

Al-Attas, O. S., N. Al-Daghri, et al. (2010). "Telomere length in relation to insulin resistance, inflammation and obesity among Arab youth." *Acta paediatrica* 99(6): 896-899.

Al-Attas, O. S., N. M. Al-Daghri, et al. (2010). "Adiposity and insulin resistance correlate with telomere length in middle-aged Arabs: the influence of circulating adiponectin." *European journal of endocrinology / European Federation of Endocrine Societies* 163(4): 601-607.

Angers, S. and R. T. Moon (2009). "Proximal events in Wnt signal transduction." *Nature reviews. Molecular cell biology* 10(7): 468-477.

Armbruster, B. N., S. S. Banik, et al. (2001). "N-terminal domains of the human telomerase catalytic subunit required for enzyme activity in vivo." *Molecular and cellular biology* 21(22): 7775-7786.

Artandi, S. E., S. Alson, et al. (2002). "Constitutive telomerase expression promotes mammary carcinomas in aging mice." *Proceedings of the National Academy of Sciences of the United States of America* 99(12): 8191-8196.

Bae, N. S. and P. Baumann (2007). "A RAP1/TRF2 complex inhibits nonhomologous end-joining at human telomeric DNA ends." *Molecular cell* 26(3): 323-334.

Bagheri, S., M. Nosrati, et al. (2006). "Genes and pathways downstream of telomerase in melanoma metastasis." *Proceedings of the National Academy of Sciences of the United States of America* 103(30): 11306-11311.

Banik, S. S., C. Guo, et al. (2002). "C-terminal regions of the human telomerase catalytic subunit essential for in vivo enzyme activity." *Molecular and cellular biology* 22(17): 6234-6246.

Beliveau, A. and P. Yaswen (2007). "Soothing the watchman: telomerase reduces the p53-dependent cellular stress response." *Cell cycle* 6(11): 1284-1287.

Ben-Neriah, Y. and M. Karin (2011). "Inflammation meets cancer, with NF-kappaB as the matchmaker." *Nature immunology* 12(8): 715-723.

Bianchi, A., R. M. Stansel, et al. (1999). "TRF1 binds a bipartite telomeric site with extreme spatial flexibility." *The EMBO journal* 18(20): 5735-5744.

Blackburn, E. H. (2000). "The end of the (DNA) line." *Nature structural biology* 7(10): 847-850.

Blackburn, E. H., C. W. Greider, et al. (1989). "Recognition and elongation of telomeres by telomerase." *Genome / National Research Council Canada = Genome / Conseil national de recherches Canada* 31(2): 553-560.

Blackburn, E. H., C. W. Greider, et al. (2006). "Telomeres and telomerase: the path from maize, Tetrahymena and yeast to human cancer and aging." *Nature medicine* 12(10): 1133-1138.

Blanco, R., P. Munoz, et al. (2007). "Telomerase abrogation dramatically accelerates TRF2-induced epithelial carcinogenesis." *Genes & development* 21(2): 206-220.

Blasco, M. A. (2005). "Telomeres and human disease: ageing, cancer and beyond." *Nature reviews. Genetics* 6(8): 611-622.

Blasco, M. A. and W. C. Hahn (2003). "Evolving views of telomerase and cancer." *Trends in cell biology* 13(6): 289-294.

Blasco, M. A., H. W. Lee, et al. (1997). "Telomere shortening and tumor formation by mouse cells lacking telomerase RNA." *Cell* 91(1): 25-34.

Blasco, M. A., M. Rizen, et al. (1996). "Differential regulation of telomerase activity and telomerase RNA during multi-stage tumorigenesis." *Nature genetics* 12(2): 200-204.

Bodnar, A. G., M. Ouellette, et al. (1998). "Extension of life-span by introduction of telomerase into normal human cells." *Science* 279(5349): 349-352.

Bombarde, O., C. Boby, et al. (2010). "TRF2/RAP1 and DNA-PK mediate a double protection against joining at telomeric ends." *The EMBO journal* 29(9): 1573-1584.

Bradshaw, P. S., D. J. Stavropoulos, et al. (2005). "Human telomeric protein TRF2 associates with genomic double-strand breaks as an early response to DNA damage." *Nature genetics* 37(2): 193-197.

Broccoli, D., A. Smogorzewska, et al. (1997). "Human telomeres contain two distinct Myb-related proteins, TRF1 and TRF2." *Nature genetics* 17(2): 231-235.

Bryant, P. E., A. C. Riches, et al. (2010). "Mechanisms of the formation of radiation-induced chromosomal aberrations." *Mutation research* 701(1): 23-26.

Burma, S., B. P. Chen, et al. (2006). "Role of non-homologous end joining (NHEJ) in maintaining genomic integrity." *DNA repair* 5(9-10): 1042-1048.

Calvert, P. A., T. V. Liew, et al. (2011). "Leukocyte telomere length is associated with high-risk plaques on virtual histology intravascular ultrasound and increased proinflammatory activity." *Arteriosclerosis, thrombosis, and vascular biology* 31(9): 2157-2164.

Chan, S. W. and E. H. Blackburn (2002). "New ways not to make ends meet: telomerase, DNA damage proteins and heterochromatin." *Oncogene* 21(4): 553-563.

Chaudhuri, J., U. Basu, et al. (2007). "Evolution of the immunoglobulin heavy chain class switch recombination mechanism." *Advances in immunology* 94: 157-214.

Chen, Y., R. Rai, et al. (2011). "A conserved motif within RAP1 has diversified roles in telomere protection and regulation in different organisms." *Nature structural & molecular biology* 18(2): 213-221.

Chenette, E. J. (2009). "DNA damage response: Keeping telomerase at bay." *Nature reviews. Molecular cell biology* 10(12): 813.

Cheng, X. and R. M. Blumenthal (2010). "Coordinated chromatin control: structural and functional linkage of DNA and histone methylation." *Biochemistry* 49(14): 2999-3008.

Choi, J., L. K. Southworth, et al. (2008). "TERT promotes epithelial proliferation through transcriptional control of a Myc- and Wnt-related developmental program." *PLoS genetics* 4(1): e10.

Clement, M. V., J. L. Hirpara, et al. (2003). "Decrease in intracellular superoxide sensitizes Bcl-2-overexpressing tumor cells to receptor and drug-induced apoptosis independent of the mitochondria." *Cell death and differentiation* 10(11): 1273-1285.

Cong, Y. and J. W. Shay (2008). "Actions of human telomerase beyond telomeres." *Cell research* 18(7): 725-732.

Counter, C. M., W. C. Hahn, et al. (1998). "Dissociation among in vitro telomerase activity, telomere maintenance, and cellular immortalization." *Proceedings of the National Academy of Sciences of the United States of America* 95(25): 14723-14728.

Counter, C. M., H. W. Hirte, et al. (1994). "Telomerase activity in human ovarian carcinoma." *Proceedings of the National Academy of Sciences of the United States of America* 91(8): 2900-2904.

Coussens, M., P. Davy, et al. (2010). "RNAi screen for telomerase reverse transcriptase transcriptional regulators identifies HIF1alpha as critical for telomerase function in murine embryonic stem cells." *Proceedings of the National Academy of Sciences of the United States of America* 107(31): 13842-13847.

Dairkee, S. H., Y. Ji, et al. (2004). "A molecular 'signature' of primary breast cancer cultures; patterns resembling tumor tissue." *BMC genomics* 5(1): 47.

de Lange, T. (2005). "Shelterin: the protein complex that shapes and safeguards human telomeres." *Genes & development* 19(18): 2100-2110.

Degrassi, F., M. Fiore, et al. (2004). "Chromosomal aberrations and genomic instability induced by topoisomerase-targeted antitumour drugs." *Current medicinal chemistry. Anti-cancer agents* 4(4): 317-325.

Dimitroulis, D., A. Katsargyris, et al. (2011). "Telomerase expression on aortic wall endothelial cells is attenuated in abdominal aortic aneurysms compared to healthy nonaneurysmal aortas." *Journal of vascular surgery : official publication, the Society for Vascular Surgery [and] International Society for Cardiovascular Surgery, North American Chapter.*

Dimitrova, N. and T. de Lange (2009). "Cell cycle-dependent role of MRN at dysfunctional telomeres: ATM signaling-dependent induction of nonhomologous end joining (NHEJ) in G1 and resection-mediated inhibition of NHEJ in G2." *Molecular and cellular biology* 29(20): 5552-5563.

Dodge, M. E. and L. Lum (2011). "Drugging the cancer stem cell compartment: lessons learned from the hedgehog and Wnt signal transduction pathways." *Annual review of pharmacology and toxicology* 51: 289-310.

Duan, J., Z. Zhang, et al. (2005). "Irreversible cellular senescence induced by prolonged exposure to H2O2 involves DNA-damage-and-repair genes and telomere shortening." *The international journal of biochemistry & cell biology* 37(7): 1407-1420.

Epel, E. S., S. S. Merkin, et al. (2009). "The rate of leukocyte telomere shortening predicts mortality from cardiovascular disease in elderly men." *Aging* 1(1): 81-88.

Esakova, O. and A. S. Krasilnikov (2010). "Of proteins and RNA: the RNase P/MRP family." *RNA* 16(9): 1725-1747.

Finkel, T. and N. J. Holbrook (2000). "Oxidants, oxidative stress and the biology of ageing." *Nature* 408(6809): 239-247.

Flint, J., C. F. Craddock, et al. (1994). "Healing of broken human chromosomes by the addition of telomeric repeats." *American journal of human genetics* 55(3): 505-512.

Flores, I. and M. A. Blasco (2010). "The role of telomeres and telomerase in stem cell aging." *FEBS letters* 584(17): 3826-3830.

Fouche, N., A. J. Cesare, et al. (2006). "The basic domain of TRF2 directs binding to DNA junctions irrespective of the presence of TTAGGG repeats." *The Journal of biological chemistry* 281(49): 37486-37495.

Franco, S., F. W. Alt, et al. (2006). "Pathways that suppress programmed DNA breaks from progressing to chromosomal breaks and translocations." *DNA repair* 5(9-10): 1030-1041.

Furuta, T., H. Takemura, et al. (2003). "Phosphorylation of histone H2AX and activation of Mre11, Rad50, and Nbs1 in response to replication-dependent DNA double-strand breaks induced by mammalian DNA topoisomerase I cleavage complexes." *The Journal of biological chemistry* 278(22): 20303-20312.

Gao, Q., G. E. Reynolds, et al. (2008). "Telomerase-dependent and -independent chromosome healing in mouse embryonic stem cells." *DNA repair* 7(8): 1233-1249.

Ghosh, S. and M. S. Hayden (2008). "New regulators of NF-kappaB in inflammation." *Nature reviews. Immunology* 8(11): 837-848.

Gizard, F., E. B. Heywood, et al. (2011). "Telomerase activation in atherosclerosis and induction of telomerase reverse transcriptase expression by inflammatory stimuli in macrophages." *Arteriosclerosis, thrombosis, and vascular biology* 31(2): 245-252.

Gonzalez-Suarez, E., E. Samper, et al. (2001). "Increased epidermal tumors and increased skin wound healing in transgenic mice overexpressing the catalytic subunit of telomerase, mTERT, in basal keratinocytes." *The EMBO journal* 20(11): 2619-2630.

Gordon, D. M. and J. H. Santos (2010). "The emerging role of telomerase reverse transcriptase in mitochondrial DNA metabolism." *Journal of nucleic acids* 2010.

Goytisolo, F. A., E. Samper, et al. (2000). "Short telomeres result in organismal hypersensitivity to ionizing radiation in mammals." *The Journal of experimental medicine* 192(11): 1625-1636.

Greenberg, R. A., R. C. Allsopp, et al. (1998). "Expression of mouse telomerase reverse transcriptase during development, differentiation and proliferation." *Oncogene* 16(13): 1723-1730.

Griffith, J. D., L. Comeau, et al. (1999). "Mammalian telomeres end in a large duplex loop." *Cell* 97(4): 503-514.

Gu, J., H. Lu, et al. (2007). "Single-stranded DNA ligation and XLF-stimulated incompatible DNA end ligation by the XRCC4-DNA ligase IV complex: influence of terminal DNA sequence." *Nucleic acids research* 35(17): 5755-5762.

Haendeler, J., S. Drose, et al. (2009). "Mitochondrial telomerase reverse transcriptase binds to and protects mitochondrial DNA and function from damage." *Arteriosclerosis, thrombosis, and vascular biology* 29(6): 929-935.

Haendeler, J., J. Hoffmann, et al. (2004). "Antioxidants inhibit nuclear export of telomerase reverse transcriptase and delay replicative senescence of endothelial cells." *Circulation research* 94(6): 768-775.

Hahn, W. C., S. A. Stewart, et al. (1999). "Inhibition of telomerase limits the growth of human cancer cells." *Nature medicine* 5(10): 1164-1170.

Hall, A. (2005). "Rho GTPases and the control of cell behaviour." *Biochemical Society transactions* 33(Pt 5): 891-895.

Harley, C. B. (2008). "Telomerase and cancer therapeutics." *Nature reviews. Cancer* 8(3): 167-179.

Hayden, M. S. and S. Ghosh (2008). "Shared principles in NF-kappaB signaling." *Cell* 132(3): 344-362.

Hayflick, L. (1965). "The Limited in Vitro Lifetime of Human Diploid Cell Strains." *Experimental cell research* 37: 614-636.

Helleday, T. (2003). "Pathways for mitotic homologous recombination in mammalian cells." *Mutation research* 532(1-2): 103-115.

Herrera, E., A. C. Martinez, et al. (2000). "Impaired germinal center reaction in mice with short telomeres." *The EMBO journal* 19(3): 472-481.

Hoogeboom, D. and B. M. Burgering (2009). "Should I stay or should I go: beta-catenin decides under stress." *Biochimica et biophysica acta* 1796(2): 63-74.

Indran, I. R., M. P. Hande, et al. (2011). "hTERT overexpression alleviates intracellular ROS production, improves mitochondrial function, and inhibits ROS-mediated apoptosis in cancer cells." *Cancer research* 71(1): 266-276.

Jaskelioff, M., F. L. Muller, et al. (2011). "Telomerase reactivation reverses tissue degeneration in aged telomerase-deficient mice." *Nature* 469(7328): 102-106.

Jeggo, P. and M. F. Lavin (2009). "Cellular radiosensitivity: how much better do we understand it?" *International journal of radiation biology* 85(12): 1061-1081.

Jeon, B. G., E. J. Kang, et al. (2011). "Comparative Analysis of Telomere Length, Telomerase and Reverse Transcriptase Activity in Human Dental Stem Cells." *Cell transplantation*.

Jones, A. M., A. D. Beggs, et al. (2011). "TERC polymorphisms are associated both with susceptibility to colorectal cancer and with longer telomeres." *Gut*.

Joseph, I., R. Tressler, et al. (2010). "The telomerase inhibitor imetelstat depletes cancer stem cells in breast and pancreatic cancer cell lines." *Cancer research* 70(22): 9494-9504.

Kaminker, P., C. Plachot, et al. (2005). "Higher-order nuclear organization in growth arrest of human mammary epithelial cells: a novel role for telomere-associated protein TIN2." *Journal of cell science* 118(Pt 6): 1321-1330.

Karlseder, J., A. Smogorzewska, et al. (2002). "Senescence induced by altered telomere state, not telomere loss." *Science* 295(5564): 2446-2449.

Keeney, S. and M. J. Neale (2006). "Initiation of meiotic recombination by formation of DNA double-strand breaks: mechanism and regulation." *Biochemical Society transactions* 34(Pt 4): 523-525.

Kendellen, M. F., K. S. Barrientos, et al. (2009). "POT1 association with TRF2 regulates telomere length." *Molecular and cellular biology* 29(20): 5611-5619.

Kim, J. K., M. Samaranayake, et al. (2009). "Epigenetic mechanisms in mammals." *Cellular and molecular life sciences : CMLS* 66(4): 596-612.

Kim, S. H., S. Han, et al. (2003). "The human telomere-associated protein TIN2 stimulates interactions between telomeric DNA tracts in vitro." *EMBO reports* 4(7): 685-691.

Komiya, Y. and R. Habas (2008). "Wnt signal transduction pathways." *Organogenesis* 4(2): 68-75.

Kovalenko, O. A., M. J. Caron, et al. (2010). "A mutant telomerase defective in nuclear-cytoplasmic shuttling fails to immortalize cells and is associated with mitochondrial dysfunction." *Aging cell* 9(2): 203-219.

Krauss, J., R. Farzaneh-Far, et al. (2011). "Physical fitness and telomere length in patients with coronary heart disease: findings from the heart and soul study." *PloS one* 6(11): e26983.

Kurz, D. J., S. Decary, et al. (2004). "Chronic oxidative stress compromises telomere integrity and accelerates the onset of senescence in human endothelial cells." *Journal of cell science* 117(Pt 11): 2417-2426.

Langerak, P., E. Mejia-Ramirez, et al. (2011). "Release of Ku and MRN from DNA ends by Mre11 nuclease activity and Ctp1 is required for homologous recombination repair of double-strand breaks." *PLoS genetics* 7(9): e1002271.

Lansdorp, P. M. (2008). "Telomeres, stem cells, and hematology." *Blood* 111(4): 1759-1766.

Lee, J., Y. H. Sung, et al. (2008). "TERT promotes cellular and organismal survival independently of telomerase activity." *Oncogene* 27(26): 3754-3760.

Li, B. and T. de Lange (2003). "Rap1 affects the length and heterogeneity of human telomeres." *Molecular biology of the cell* 14(12): 5060-5068.

Li, B., S. Oestreich, et al. (2000). "Identification of human Rap1: implications for telomere evolution." *Cell* 101(5): 471-483.

Li, C. T., Y. M. Hsiao, et al. (2011). "Vorinostat represses telomerase activity via epigenetic regulation of telomerase reverse transcriptase in non-small cell lung cancer cells." *Journal of cellular biochemistry*.

Li, S., J. Crothers, et al. (2005). "Cellular and gene expression responses involved in the rapid growth inhibition of human cancer cells by RNA interference-mediated depletion of telomerase RNA." *The Journal of biological chemistry* 280(25): 23709-23717.

Lie, D. C., S. A. Colamarino, et al. (2005). "Wnt signalling regulates adult hippocampal neurogenesis." *Nature* 437(7063): 1370-1375.

Lieber, M. R. (2010). "The mechanism of double-strand DNA break repair by the nonhomologous DNA end-joining pathway." *Annual review of biochemistry* 79: 181-211.

Lim, S. and M. V. Clement (2007). "Phosphorylation of the survival kinase Akt by superoxide is dependent on an ascorbate-reversible oxidation of PTEN." *Free radical biology & medicine* 42(8): 1178-1192.

Limoli, C. L., E. Giedzinski, et al. (2002). "UV-induced replication arrest in the xeroderma pigmentosum variant leads to DNA double-strand breaks, gamma -H2AX formation, and Mre11 relocalization." *Proceedings of the National Academy of Sciences of the United States of America* 99(1): 233-238.

Logan, C. Y. and R. Nusse (2004). "The Wnt signaling pathway in development and disease." *Annual review of cell and developmental biology* 20: 781-810.

Lyuksyutova, A. I., C. C. Lu, et al. (2003). "Anterior-posterior guidance of commissural axons by Wnt-frizzled signaling." *Science* 302(5652): 1984-1988.

Ma, Q. (2010). "Transcriptional responses to oxidative stress: pathological and toxicological implications." *Pharmacology & therapeutics* 125(3): 376-393.

Machwe, A., L. Xiao, et al. (2004). "TRF2 recruits the Werner syndrome (WRN) exonuclease for processing of telomeric DNA." *Oncogene* 23(1): 149-156.

Maida, Y., M. Yasukawa, et al. (2009). "An RNA-dependent RNA polymerase formed by TERT and the RMRP RNA." *Nature* 461(7261): 230-235.

Maillet, L., C. Boscheron, et al. (1996). "Evidence for silencing compartments within the yeast nucleus: a role for telomere proximity and Sir protein concentration in silencer-mediated repression." *Genes & development* 10(14): 1796-1811.

Makino, N., M. Sasaki, et al. (2010). "Telomere biology in cardiovascular disease - role of insulin sensitivity in diabetic hearts." *Experimental and clinical cardiology* 15(4): e128-133.

Malliri, A. and J. G. Collard (2003). "Role of Rho-family proteins in cell adhesion and cancer." *Current opinion in cell biology* 15(5): 583-589.

Mao, Z., A. Seluanov, et al. (2007). "TRF2 is required for repair of nontelomeric DNA double-strand breaks by homologous recombination." *Proceedings of the National Academy of Sciences of the United States of America* 104(32): 13068-13073.

Marcand, S., S. W. Buck, et al. (1996). "Silencing of genes at nontelomeric sites in yeast is controlled by sequestration of silencing factors at telomeres by Rap 1 protein." *Genes & development* 10(11): 1297-1309.

Martinez, P. and M. A. Blasco (2011). "Telomeric and extra-telomeric roles for telomerase and the telomere-binding proteins." *Nature reviews. Cancer* 11(3): 161-176.

Martinez, P., M. Thanasoula, et al. (2010). "Mammalian Rap1 controls telomere function and gene expression through binding to telomeric and extratelomeric sites." *Nature cell biology* 12(8): 768-780.

Massard, C., Y. Zermati, et al. (2006). "hTERT: a novel endogenous inhibitor of the mitochondrial cell death pathway." *Oncogene* 25(33): 4505-4514.

Masutomi, K., R. Possemato, et al. (2005). "The telomerase reverse transcriptase regulates chromatin state and DNA damage responses." *Proceedings of the National Academy of Sciences of the United States of America* 102(23): 8222-8227.

Masutomi, K., E. Y. Yu, et al. (2003). "Telomerase maintains telomere structure in normal human cells." *Cell* 114(2): 241-253.

Mazin, A. V., O. M. Mazina, et al. (2010). "Rad54, the motor of homologous recombination." *DNA repair* 9(3): 286-302.

Meehan, R. R. (2003). "DNA methylation in animal development." *Seminars in cell & developmental biology* 14(1): 53-65.

Miller, J. R., A. M. Hocking, et al. (1999). "Mechanism and function of signal transduction by the Wnt/beta-catenin and Wnt/Ca2+ pathways." *Oncogene* 18(55): 7860-7872.

Monaghan, P. (2010). "Telomeres and life histories: the long and the short of it." *Annals of the New York Academy of Sciences* 1206: 130-142.

Mondello, C., M. G. Bottone, et al. (2006). "Oxidative stress response in telomerase-immortalized fibroblasts from a centenarian." *Annals of the New York Academy of Sciences* 1091: 94-101.

Morse, R. H. (2000). "RAP, RAP, open up! New wrinkles for RAP1 in yeast." *Trends in genetics : TIG* 16(2): 51-53.

Mukherjee, S., E. J. Firpo, et al. (2011). "Separation of telomerase functions by reverse genetics." *Proceedings of the National Academy of Sciences of the United States of America*.

Murr, R. (2010). "Interplay between different epigenetic modifications and mechanisms." *Advances in genetics* 70: 101-141.

Myung, K., A. Datta, et al. (2001). "Suppression of spontaneous chromosomal rearrangements by S phase checkpoint functions in Saccharomyces cerevisiae." *Cell* 104(3): 397-408.

Natarajan, A. T. and F. Palitti (2008). "DNA repair and chromosomal alterations." *Mutation research* 657(1): 3-7.

Nitta, E., M. Yamashita, et al. (2011). "Telomerase reverse transcriptase protects ATM-deficient hematopoietic stem cells from ROS-induced apoptosis through a telomere-independent mechanism." *Blood* 117(16): 4169-4180.

Njajou, O. T., R. M. Cawthon, et al. (2011). "Shorter telomeres are associated with obesity and weight gain in the elderly." *International journal of obesity*.

O'Connor, M. S., A. Safari, et al. (2004). "The human Rap1 protein complex and modulation of telomere length." *The Journal of biological chemistry* 279(27): 28585-28591.

Opresko, P. L., C. von Kobbe, et al. (2002). "Telomere-binding protein TRF2 binds to and stimulates the Werner and Bloom syndrome helicases." *The Journal of biological chemistry* 277(43): 41110-41119.

Orrenius, S., V. Gogvadze, et al. (2007). "Mitochondrial oxidative stress: implications for cell death." *Annual review of pharmacology and toxicology* 47: 143-183.

Pardo, B. and S. Marcand (2005). "Rap1 prevents telomere fusions by nonhomologous end joining." *The EMBO journal* 24(17): 3117-3127.

Park, J. I., A. S. Venteicher, et al. (2009). "Telomerase modulates Wnt signalling by association with target gene chromatin." *Nature* 460(7251): 66-72.

Passos, J. F., G. Saretzki, et al. (2007). "DNA damage in telomeres and mitochondria during cellular senescence: is there a connection?" *Nucleic acids research* 35(22): 7505-7513.

Poole, J. C., L. G. Andrews, et al. (2001). "Activity, function, and gene regulation of the catalytic subunit of telomerase (hTERT)." *Gene* 269(1-2): 1-12.

Puig, P. E., M. N. Guilly, et al. (2008). "Tumor cells can escape DNA-damaging cisplatin through DNA endoreduplication and reversible polyploidy." *Cell biology international* 32(9): 1031-1043.

Qing, Y., M. Yamazoe, et al. (2011). "The epistatic relationship between BRCA2 and the other RAD51 mediators in homologous recombination." *PLoS genetics* 7(7): e1002148.

Ramachandran, I., E. Thavathiru, et al. (2011). "Wnt inhibitory factor 1 induces apoptosis and inhibits cervical cancer growth, invasion and angiogenesis in vivo." *Oncogene*.

Ren, J. G., H. L. Xia, et al. (2001). "Expression of telomerase inhibits hydroxyl radical-induced apoptosis in normal telomerase negative human lung fibroblasts." *FEBS letters* 488(3): 133-138.

Reya, T. and H. Clevers (2005). "Wnt signalling in stem cells and cancer." *Nature* 434(7035): 843-850.

Ridanpaa, M., H. van Eenennaam, et al. (2001). "Mutations in the RNA component of RNase MRP cause a pleiotropic human disease, cartilage-hair hypoplasia." *Cell* 104(2): 195-203.

Rolyan, H., A. Scheffold, et al. (2011). "Telomere shortening reduces Alzheimer's disease amyloid pathology in mice." *Brain : a journal of neurology* 134(Pt 7): 2044-2056.

Roth, A., C. B. Harley, et al. (2010). "Imetelstat (GRN163L)--telomerase-based cancer therapy." *Recent results in cancer research. Fortschritte der Krebsforschung. Progres dans les recherches sur le cancer* 184: 221-234.

Rothkamm, K., M. Kuhne, et al. (2001). "Radiation-induced genomic rearrangements formed by nonhomologous end-joining of DNA double-strand breaks." *Cancer research* 61(10): 3886-3893.

Sage, J., A. L. Miller, et al. (2003). "Acute mutation of retinoblastoma gene function is sufficient for cell cycle re-entry." *Nature* 424(6945): 223-228.

Santos, J. H., J. N. Meyer, et al. (2004). "Mitochondrial hTERT exacerbates free-radical-mediated mtDNA damage." *Aging cell* 3(6): 399-411.

Santos, J. H., J. N. Meyer, et al. (2006). "Mitochondrial localization of telomerase as a determinant for hydrogen peroxide-induced mitochondrial DNA damage and apoptosis." *Human molecular genetics* 15(11): 1757-1768.

Sarin, K. Y., P. Cheung, et al. (2005). "Conditional telomerase induction causes proliferation of hair follicle stem cells." *Nature* 436(7053): 1048-1052.

Sarthy, J., N. S. Bae, et al. (2009). "Human RAP1 inhibits non-homologous end joining at telomeres." *The EMBO journal* 28(21): 3390-3399.

Schlessinger, K., E. J. McManus, et al. (2007). "Cdc42 and noncanonical Wnt signal transduction pathways cooperate to promote cell polarity." *The Journal of cell biology* 178(3): 355-361.

Sedelnikova, O. A., I. Horikawa, et al. (2004). "Senescing human cells and ageing mice accumulate DNA lesions with unrepairable double-strand breaks." *Nature cell biology* 6(2): 168-170.

Sfeir, A., S. Kabir, et al. (2010). "Loss of Rap1 induces telomere recombination in the absence of NHEJ or a DNA damage signal." *Science* 327(5973): 1657-1661.

Sfeir, A., S. T. Kosiyatrakul, et al. (2009). "Mammalian telomeres resemble fragile sites and require TRF1 for efficient replication." *Cell* 138(1): 90-103.

Shay, J. W. and W. E. Wright (2005). "Senescence and immortalization: role of telomeres and telomerase." *Carcinogenesis* 26(5): 867-874.

Simonet, T., L. E. Zaragosi, et al. (2011). "The human TTAGGG repeat factors 1 and 2 bind to a subset of interstitial telomeric sequences and satellite repeats." *Cell research* 21(7): 1028-1038.

Simsek, D., E. Brunet, et al. (2011). "DNA ligase III promotes alternative nonhomologous end-joining during chromosomal translocation formation." *PLoS genetics* 7(6): e1002080.

Sliwinska, M. A., G. Mosieniak, et al. (2009). "Induction of senescence with doxorubicin leads to increased genomic instability of HCT116 cells." *Mechanisms of ageing and development* 130(1-2): 24-32.

Smith, K. N., A. M. Singh, et al. (2010). "Myc represses primitive endoderm differentiation in pluripotent stem cells." *Cell stem cell* 7(3): 343-354.

Smith, L. L., H. A. Coller, et al. (2003). "Telomerase modulates expression of growth-controlling genes and enhances cell proliferation." *Nature cell biology* 5(5): 474-479.

Smith, S., I. Giriat, et al. (1998). "Tankyrase, a poly(ADP-ribose) polymerase at human telomeres." *Science* 282(5393): 1484-1487.

Song, K., D. Jung, et al. (2000). "Interaction of human Ku70 with TRF2." *FEBS letters* 481(1): 81-85.

Sprung, C. N., G. E. Reynolds, et al. (1999). "Chromosome healing in mouse embryonic stem cells." *Proceedings of the National Academy of Sciences of the United States of America* 96(12): 6781-6786.

Stansel, R. M., T. de Lange, et al. (2001). "T-loop assembly in vitro involves binding of TRF2 near the 3' telomeric overhang." *The EMBO journal* 20(19): 5532-5540.

Stellwagen, A. E., Z. W. Haimberger, et al. (2003). "Ku interacts with telomerase RNA to promote telomere addition at native and broken chromosome ends." *Genes & development* 17(19): 2384-2395.

Stiff, T., M. O'Driscoll, et al. (2004). "ATM and DNA-PK function redundantly to phosphorylate H2AX after exposure to ionizing radiation." *Cancer research* 64(7): 2390-2396.

Su, T. T. (2006). "Cellular responses to DNA damage: one signal, multiple choices." *Annual review of genetics* 40: 187-208.

Takai, K. K., S. Hooper, et al. (2010). "In vivo stoichiometry of shelterin components." *The Journal of biological chemistry* 285(2): 1457-1467.

Takakura, M., S. Kyo, et al. (2005). "Function of AP-1 in transcription of the telomerase reverse transcriptase gene (TERT) in human and mouse cells." *Molecular and cellular biology* 25(18): 8037-8043.

Takata, Y., M. Kikukawa, et al. (2011). "Association Between ApoE Phenotypes and Telomere Erosion in Alzheimer's Disease." *The journals of gerontology. Series A, Biological sciences and medical sciences.*

Tamakawa, R. A., H. B. Fleisig, et al. (2010). "Telomerase inhibition potentiates the effects of genotoxic agents in breast and colorectal cancer cells in a cell cycle-specific manner." *Cancer research* 70(21): 8684-8694.

Teo, H., S. Ghosh, et al. (2010). "Telomere-independent Rap1 is an IKK adaptor and regulates NF-kappaB-dependent gene expression." *Nature cell biology* 12(8): 758-767.

Toussaint, O., E. E. Medrano, et al. (2000). "Cellular and molecular mechanisms of stress-induced premature senescence (SIPS) of human diploid fibroblasts and melanocytes." *Experimental gerontology* 35(8): 927-945.

Valko, M., D. Leibfritz, et al. (2007). "Free radicals and antioxidants in normal physiological functions and human disease." *The international journal of biochemistry & cell biology* 39(1): 44-84.

Valko, M., C. J. Rhodes, et al. (2006). "Free radicals, metals and antioxidants in oxidative stress-induced cancer." *Chemico-biological interactions* 160(1): 1-40.

van Overbeek, M. and T. de Lange (2006). "Apollo, an Artemis-related nuclease, interacts with TRF2 and protects human telomeres in S phase." *Current biology : CB* 16(13): 1295-1302.

Vercesi, A. E., A. J. Kowaltowski, et al. (2006). "Mitochondrial Ca2+ transport, permeability transition and oxidative stress in cell death: implications in cardiotoxicity, neurodegeneration and dyslipidemias." *Frontiers in bioscience : a journal and virtual library* 11: 2554-2564.

Vidal-Cardenas, S. L. and C. W. Greider (2010). "Comparing effects of mTR and mTERT deletion on gene expression and DNA damage response: a critical examination of telomere length maintenance-independent roles of telomerase." *Nucleic acids research* 38(1): 60-71.

Wang, H., G. J. Nora, et al. (2011). "Single molecule studies of physiologically relevant telomeric tails reveal POT1 mechanism for promoting G-quadruplex unfolding." *The Journal of biological chemistry* 286(9): 7479-7489.

Willert, K., J. D. Brown, et al. (2003). "Wnt proteins are lipid-modified and can act as stem cell growth factors." *Nature* 423(6938): 448-452.

Williams, E. S., J. Stap, et al. (2007). "DNA double-strand breaks are not sufficient to initiate recruitment of TRF2." *Nature genetics* 39(6): 696-698; author reply 698-699.

Wolfer, A. and S. Ramaswamy (2011). "MYC and metastasis." *Cancer research* 71(6): 2034-2037.

Wong, K. K., S. Chang, et al. (2000). "Telomere dysfunction impairs DNA repair and enhances sensitivity to ionizing radiation." *Nature genetics* 26(1): 85-88.

Wynford-Thomas, D. and D. Kipling (1997). "Telomerase. Cancer and the knockout mouse." *Nature* 389(6651): 551-552.

Xin, H., D. Liu, et al. (2007). "TPP1 is a homologue of ciliate TEBP-beta and interacts with POT1 to recruit telomerase." *Nature* 445(7127): 559-562.

Yang, D., Y. Xiong, et al. (2011). "Human telomeric proteins occupy selective interstitial sites." *Cell research* 21(7): 1013-1027.

Ye, J., C. Lenain, et al. (2010). "TRF2 and apollo cooperate with topoisomerase 2alpha to protect human telomeres from replicative damage." *Cell* 142(2): 230-242.

Ye, J. Z. and T. de Lange (2004). "TIN2 is a tankyrase 1 PARP modulator in the TRF1 telomere length control complex." *Nature genetics* 36(6): 618-623.

Zhu, X. D., B. Kuster, et al. (2000). "Cell-cycle-regulated association of RAD50/MRE11/NBS1 with TRF2 and human telomeres." *Nature genetics* 25(3): 347-352.

Section 4

Telomere DNA and Its Evolution

10

Genomic Distribution of Telomeric DNA Sequences – What Do We Learn from Fish About Telomere Evolution?

Konrad Ocalewicz
University of Warmia and Mazury in Olsztyn
Poland

1. Introduction

Ends of the eukaryotic chromosomes are capped with nucleoprotein complexes named telomeres. The DNA component of the telomeres usually is consisted of tandemly repeated G-rich DNA short sequences like TTTAGGG in plants (Cox et al., 1993; Fuchs et al., 1995), G_{2-8}TTAC(A) in the fission yeast (*Schizosaccharomyces pombe*) (Murray et al., 1986) and $T(G)_{2-3}(TG)_{1-6}$ in baker's yeast (*Saccharomyces cerevisiae*) (Shampay et al., 1984), TTGGGG in *Tetrahymena thermophila* (Blackburn et al., 1978), TTAGGC in *Ceanerhabditis elegans* (Cangiano and La Volpe, 1993) or TTAGG in the insects (Okazaki et al. 1993), among others (for more telomeric DNA sequences see Telomerase Database, http://telomerase.asu.edu/). In all vertebrates studied to date, telomeres contains tandemly repeated G-rich hexanucleotide sequence (TTAGGG/CCCTAA)n and the associated proteins comprising six subunits: TRF1, TRF2, POT1, TIN2, TPP1 and RAP1 (Bolzán and Bianchi, 2006). The telomeric DNA length shows huge interspecies variation and ranged from less than 100 bp (base pairs) in the ciliate *Oxytricha* (Klobutcher et al., 1981), hundreds of base pairs in the baker's yeast to 50 - 150 kb (kilo base) in the laboratory mouse (*Mus musculus*) (Kipling and Cooke, 1990) or even more (up to 2 Mb in chicken *Galus galus domesticus*) (Delany et al. 2003). The human normal cells show telomeric DNA of 5-20 kb length (Moyzis et al., 1988). Variation in the length of the telomeric arrays have been observed between non-homologous and even homologous chromosomes within individual cells in human and mice, among others (Landsorp et al., 1996; Zijlmans et al., 1997). Moreover, p-arm telomeres have been shown to be shorter that their q-arm counterparts in the mouse and Chinese hamster chromosomes (Slijepcevic et al., 1997). Mammalian telomeres replicate throughout S phase: some of the telomeres replicate early while other telomeres replicate later (Zou et al., 2004). Moreover, asynchronous replication of the mammalian p- and q-arm telomeres of the same chromosome has been observed (Zou et al., 2004).

Telomeres prevent chromosomes from end-to-end fusions, allowing DNA repair machinery distinguish natural chromosomal ends from the ends that appear in the course of breakage events (de Lange, 2002; Bolzán and Bianchi 2006). Telomeres ensure proper chromosome topology in the nucleus and may silence genes located in the vicinity of the telomeric region, and this phenomenon is called a "telomere position effect" (Luderus et al., 1996;

Copenhaver and Pikaard, 1996). As the linear DNA cannot be entirely replicated by the DNA polymerases because of the "end replication problem" (Watsan, 1972; Olovnikov, 1973), telomeres ensure complete replication of the chromosomal DNA and protect chromosomes from degradation (de Lange, 2002). Thus, telomeres shorten after each round of the cell division. In the cultured human cells, the loss of the telomeric repeats during each S phase has been estimated for 50-200 bp (Huffman et al., 2000). This loss may be compensated by telomerase, an enzyme whose catalytic protein subunit (TERT, telomerase reverse transcriptase) adds telomeric DNA repeats to the end of telomeres using as a template an integral RNA component (TR, telomerase RNA). Moreover, different cellular mechanisms may be used for the telomere length maintenance/elongation such as reciprocal recombination and transposition of the chromosomal terminal elements when telomerase is not active or inactivated (Biessmann and Mason, 1997).

Although telomeres, by definition, are terminal elements of the chromosomes, telomeric DNA repeats are also observed at internal chromosomal sites and are called Interstitial (or Interchromosomal) Telomeric Sequences (ITSs), Interstitial Telomeric Repeat sequences (ITRs) or Interstitial Telomeric Bands (ITBs). ITSs may be located close to the centromeres or between centromere and the real telomeres. The first and the most well-known description of the existence of unusual locations of telomeric DNA sequences far from their natural occurrence at the ends of the chromosomes was brought to light in 1990 by Meyne and collaborators. These authors identified telomeric repeats at non-telomeric locations in 55 out of 100 vertebrate species studied. ITSs have been observed in the exponents of four classes of vertebrates: Mammalia, Aves, Reptilia and Amphibia. The majority of the intrachromosomally located $(TTAGGG)_n$ sequences were observed at the pericentromeric areas of the bi-armed chromosomes within or at the margin of the constitutive heterochromatin (Meyne et al., 1990). This observation led to a conclusion that ITSs might have been left by the ancient centric fusions of ancestral chromosome. Since then, more sensitive FISH techniques enabling identification of telomeric repeats such as PNA-FISH using peptide telomeric probe and PRINS using $(TTAGGG)_7$/ $(CCCTAA)_7$ primers for amplification of telomeric DNA have been developed (Koch et al., 1989; Terkelsen et al., 1993). Application of such approaches together with chromosome banding techniques, molecular cloning, and genome sequencing led to identification of ITSs in species that were not studied previously to this regard as well as re-examination of the species that did not show any ITSs formerly.

Below, patterns of the chromosomal distribution of telomeric DNA sequences in several chosen vertebrates have been reviewed in the context of the chromosomal rearrangements and other mechanisms that may lead to the internal insertion of the telomeric repeats. Special attention has been paid to the distribution of the telomeric DNA sequences in the fish genome. Fishes with more than 30 000 species are the most numerous and diverse group of vertebrates (Nelson, 1994). This group of vertebrates comprises jawless fishes (hagfishes, lampreys), cartilaginous fishes (sharks and rays), and bony fishes (lobe-finned fish and ray-finned fish) (Nelson, 1994). Ray-finned fishes species represent more than 95% of all the extant fishes. More than 99.8% of ray-finned fishes belong to Teleostei (Volf, 2004). Although ancestral teleostean karyotype comprising 48-50 of one-armed chromosomes is still the most frequently observed pattern within teleosts, species with more derived karyotypes composed of both - one- and bi-armed chromosomes - have been also observed. Diversification of teleostean karyotypes is attributed to whole genome duplication event in the Teleost ancestor and chromosomal rearrangements (Zhou et al., 2002). Moreover, some of the Teleost fish families like Salmonidae are thought to have a tetraploid origin. Tetraploidization event in the Salmonid ancestor has been followed by the rediploidization process leading to the recovery of disomic segregation and performed by the various chromosomal rearrangements like fusions and inversions (Phillips and Rab, 2001). On top of that, androgenetic fish developing in the gamma/X radiation-enucleated eggs seem to be promising models for studying the role of telomerase in the fish DNA Double Strand Breaks repair machinery (Ocalewicz et al., 2004a, 2009).

2. Classification of interstitial telomeric DNA sequences

Based on the chromosomal location, length, DNA composition and the origin, several kinds of the ITSs have been described (Nergadze et al., 2004; Bolzán and Bianchi, 2006; Lin and Yan, 2008; Ruiz-Herrera et al., 2008). In the human genome, three classes of ITSs have been proposed based on the sequence organization, localization, and flanking sequences by Azzalin et al. (2001): (Class 1) so-called short ITSs, composed of a few exact telomeric repeats up to 20 hexamers; (Class 2) subtelomeric ITSs consisted of several hundred base pairs of tandem repeats, many of which differ from the TTAGGG repeat sequence by one or more base substitutions and (Class 3) ITS sites formed by the ancestral chromosome fusions and composed of head-to-head arrays of repeats. Short ITSs may be further divided into five subclasses based upon their flanking sequences (Lin and Yan, 2008). Subtelomeric ITSs are observed at all human chromosomes, and short ITSs have been identified at 50 loci in human chromosomes, while only one ITSs derived from the fusion event have been described in the human genome (Azzalin et al., 1997; Azzalin et al., 2001; Ijdo et al., 1991). ITSs that represent class 1 and 2 may appear in the course of repair of double-strand breaks (DSBs) by the mechanism employing action of telomerase and/or recombination involving chromosome ends in the germ lines during evolution (Nergadze et al., 2004). Further rearrangements like amplifications, deletions, or transpositions of ITSs may cause its uneven distribution in the genome, for example (Lin and Yan, 2008).

One of the recent proposition based on the purely cytogenetic characteristic of non-telomeric distribution of $(TTAGGG)_n$ repeats in mammalian species is to differentiate two kinds of ITSs: short stretches (from a few to a few hundred base pairs) of internally located telomeric repeats (s-ITSs) and long stretches (up to hundreds of kilo base) of the heterochromatic ITSs (het-ITSs) mainly assigned to the centromeric chromosomal regions (Ruiz-Herrera et al., 2008). Short ITSs composed of head-to-tail tandem arrays are widely distributed in human, chimpanzee, mouse, or rat (Azzalin et al., 2001; Nergadze et al., 2007). Analysis of DNA sequences adjacent to the s-ITSs suggested that telomeric sequences were internally inserted by transposition or synthesized by telomerase to repair DNA double-strand breaks (DSB) (Ruiz-Herrera et al., 2008). Heterochromatic ITSs on the other hand, seem to originate in the course of the ancestral chromosomal rearrangements, mostly fusions, accompanying evolution of mammalian karyotypes. Such ITSs are usually co-localized with heterochromatic regions. Although such classification of ITSs has been attributed to mammalian genome, ITSs of various origin have been also observed in the non-mammalian species.

3. Chromosome rearrangements and distribution of telomeric DNA sequences in the vertebrates

3.1 Internally located telomeric repeat sequences as relicts of the chromosome fusions

Telomeric DNA observed at the non-telomeric locations might be associated with known chromosome rearrangements, like centric fusions (Robertsonian translocations) and tandem fusions. Fusion of two one-armed chromosomes leading to the formation of one metacentric or submetacentric chromosome may leave telomeric DNA sequences at the fusion site at the pericentromeric location. This region is usually heterochromatic. Interstitial non-centromeric sites of $(TTAGGG)_n$ sequences may be relicts of the tandem fusions. In such cases, coincidence between ITSs and heterochromatin is rarely observed (Nanda et al. 2002). Irrespective of the origin, such ITSs might be organized in very long arrays that are much longer than those observed at the chromosomal ends. In the Chinese hamster, large pericentromeric interstitial telomeric DNA sites are observed (Bertoni et al., 1996), and telomeric DNA sequences have been discovered to be the main component of the satellite DNA with its abundance reaching up to 5% of the Chinese hamster genome (Bertoni et al., 1996; Slijepcevic et al., 1996; Faravelli et al., 1998; 2002). Moreover, ITSs might be interspersed with other repetitive DNA sequences (Salvadori et al., 1995). Sometimes, chromosome breakage occurs within the ITS region (Alvarez et al., 1993; Slijepcevic et al., 1996).

Internally located telomeric DNA sequences have been observed in many mammalian and non-mammalian species showing more degenerative karyotypes when compared to their plesiomorphic (ancestral) complements. A 2n = 22 karyotype, is thought to be an ancestral for the marsupial family Macropodidae (kangaroos and wallabies) (Metcalfe et al. 2007). In the swamp wallaby (*Wallabia bicolor*) (2n= 10 in female, 2n= 11 in male) telomeric DNA sequences were retained at the fusion sites in four chromosomes formed in the course of centric fusions (Metcalfe et al., 1998). The lowest chromosome number exhibited in the mammalian species equals 6/7 (female/male) and is observed in the Indian muntjac deer (*Muntiacus muntjak vaginalis* MMV). The common ancestor of the muntjacs lived about 1.7-3.7 million years ago and its karyotype was presumably composed of 70 chromosomes. (Hartman and Scherthan, 2004). Cytogenetic survey of the muntjacs revealed that chromosome reduction observed in the genus occurred linearly from the putative ancestral complement 2n= 70 through a Chinese muntjac-like (2n= 46) to a Fea's muntjac-like (2n= 13/14) karyotypes. Further chromosome reduction to 2n= 8/9 observed in the Black and Gongsham muntjac and to 6/7 chromosomes in the Indian muntjac were rather independent events (Wang and Lan, 2000). Such drastic chromosome reduction and karyotype diversification that happened in such a short stretch of time has been supposed to be caused by the multiple tandem fusions and relatively few centric fusions (Hsu et al., 1975). This assumption has been later proved by the comparative and molecular cytogenetic analysis of the muntjac genome (Lee et al., 1993; Schertchan, 1995; Yang et al., 1997; Zou et al., 2002). Several sites of internally located telomeric repeat sequences in the Indian muntjac chromosome were observed to be co-localized with satellite DNA repeats (Lee et al., 1993; Scherthan, 1995; Hartman and Scherthan, 2004). Such interstitial satellite DNA sequences were assumed to be the "footprints" of the breakage of chromosomal syntenies in the Indian muntjac and thus may be treated as relicts of the ancestral fusion points (Fronicke and

Scherthan, 1997). In the Hartman's zebra (*Equus zebra hartmannae*) showing karyotype composed of relatively low chromosome number (2n= 32) when compared to other equids (2n= 44- 66), several sites of internally located telomeric repeats have been described (Santani et al., 2002) Comparison of the chromosomal distribution of ITSs and comparative chromosome painting of human and Hartman's zebra showed that all ITSs are located at the junctions of evolutionary conserved human- Hartman's zebra chromosomal segments, suggesting that ITSs are relicts of the putative fusions of ancestral chromosomes (Santani et al., 2002). Telomeric sequences at the fusion sites have been also observed in other mammalian species like okapi (*Okapia johnstoni*) (Vermeesch et al., 1996), Eulemur species (Garagna et al. 1997), akodont rodents (*Akodon cursor* and *Bolomys lasiurus*) (Fagundes and Yonenaga-Yassuda, 1998), lemurs (Go et al. 2000), rock wallabies (Petrogale) (Metcalfe et al., 2002), among others.

Chromosome fusions seem to play an important role during the avian karyotype evolution. The avian karyotype has a characteristic structure. It comprises several pairs of relatively gene-poor macrochromosomes and numerous microchromosomes enriched with genes, and even distant species show similar karyotypes (Nanda et al., 2002). It has been discover that chicken telomeric DNA sequences range from 0.5 kb to about 2 Mb (Delany et al., 2000, 2003). Telomeric DNA sequences cover up to 4 % of the chicken diploid genome, which is contrasted with a rather low amount of the telomeric DNA in the human diploid cell (about 0, 3%) (Delany et al., 2003). Based on the size and genome location three classes of telomeric DNA arrays were distinguished in the chicken. It has been suggested that telomeric DNA arrays ranging from 0.5 to 10 kb in length (Class I arrays) represent the interstitial telomeric DNA sequences, while the larger tracts arrays ranging from 10 to 40 kb (Class II) and from 200 kb to 2 Mb (Class III) represent telomeric DNA from the chromosome terminus (Dealny et al. 2003). Many of the cytogenetically studied bird species have exhibited telomeric DNA sequences in non-telomeric positions on the macrochromosomes. However, patterns of their distribution are different in the primitive (Palaeognathae) and modern (Neognathae) birds (Meyne et al., 1990; Nanda et al., 2002). The primitive birds like ostrich *(Struthio camelus)*, emu (*Dromaius novaehollandiae)* and the American rhea *(Rhea americana)* show numerous interstitially located telomeric DNA sites along the entire length of most of the macrochromosome arms. Rather few of the macrochromosomes show ITSs at the (peri)centromeric positions. In the rhea and emu most of the interstitially located telomeric sequences did not coincide with the C-banded heterochromatin. Such distribution pattern of the telomeric DNA sequences in these birds has been proposed to be due to the tandem fusions of macro and microchromosomes in their common ancestor. On the other hand, there are only few if any internally located telomeric DNA sequences in the modern birds like duck (*Cairina moschata*), greylag goose (*Anser anser*), the ring-necked pheasant (*Phasianus colchicus*), Japanese quail (*Coturnix coturnix*) and parrots (Nanda et al,. 2002). Centromerically located telomeric DNA sequences that coincide with the heterochromatin observed on the bi-armed macrochromosomes in two owl species are likely relicts of the chromosome centric fusions. (Meyne et al., 1990; Nanda and Schmid, 1994; Delany et al., 2003).

Reduction of the chromosome number from the ancestral 2n= 32 to 2n= 16 in the lizard *Gonatodes taniae* probably occurred through the centric fusions. Telomeric DNA sequences observed at the pericentromeric regions of all *G. taniae* bi-armed chromosomes were presumably the remnants of the above-mentioned rearrangements. On the other hand, interstitially located telomeric repeats could be also a major component of the repetitive DNA in the pericentromeric C band-positive heterochromatin (Schmid et al. 1994) (see chapter 3.3). Similar location of the telomeric repeats in one and three meta-submetacentric chromosomes in the Brazilian lizards, *Leposoma guianense* and *L. oswaldoi*, respectively indicated Roberstonian translocations were involved in the evolution of these lizards' karyotypes (Pellegrino et al., 1999). Centric fusion in the Brazilian gecko, *Gymnodactylus amarali* also left telomeric repeat DNA sequences at the fusion sites of two chromosomes (Pellegrino et al., 2009).

As pericentromeric ITSs quite frequently coincide with the heterochromatin, it has been proposed to describe such ITS sites as heterochromatic ITSs (het-ITSs) by Ruiz-Herrera et al. (2008), who suggested a four-step mechanism to explain the presence of such sites in the fused chromosomes. The first step is the initial fusion event without loss of the telomeric sequences from the fusion site (1). The next step is formation of the (peri)centromeric heterochromatin by expansion of the internally located telomeric arrays including amplification of the telomeric sequences and other repeats (2). Subsequently the heterochromatic ITSs were reorganized via chromosomal rearrangements that may lead to the redistribution of the telomeric DNA, degeneration of the original ITS array, gradual shortening of the array, and even the loss of the ITS. Finally, breakage within the heterochromatic ITS site may result in chromosome fissions (step 4).

3.2 Chromosome fusions and loss of the interstitial telomeric sequences

Not all chromosome fusions occur with retention of the telomeric DNA repeats at the fusion sites. Telomeric DNA sequences from the ancestral chromosomes may be lost during or after the chromosomes fusion process. Chromosome breakage within centromeric satellite DNA followed by Roberstonian fusions leaves no telomeric repeats at the fusion sites (Garagna et al., 1995; Nanda et al., 1995). On the other hand, telomeric DNA sequences that retain at the fusion sites may undergo gradual loss leading to the shortening of the non-functional telomeric repeats and are therefore undetectable by the cytogenetic approaches (Slijepcevic, 1998). Lack of the internally located telomeric DNA sequences at the fusion points was described in the mouse (*Mus musculus*) (Garagna et al., 1995), neotropical water rat (*Nectomys*) (Silva and Yonenaga-Yassuda, 1998) and short-tailed shrew (*Blarina carolinensis*) (Qumsiyeh et al., 1997), among others.

Chicken chromosomes 1 - 4 presumably appeared in the course of the ancestral chromosome fusion events. However, only chromosome 1-3 exhibited ITSs at the fusion sites (Nanda et al., 2002). In comparison to the primitive bird species like ostrich and emu that display voluminous number of ITS sites in their chromosomes, species showing high number of the bi-armed chromosomes and listed as highly evolved such as parrots lack TTAGGG sequences at non-telomeric sites (Nanda et al., 2002). This may suggest that in the Neognathae birds ITS sites were lost after the divergence of the primitive and modern birds (Nanda et al., 2002). The lack of ITSs in the more derived karyotypes when compared to the ancestral models is in opposite to the suggestion made by Meyne et al. (1990) that ITS sites appear in the course of chromosome rearrangements accompanying karyotype evolution and thus can be observed in the evolutionary advanced species.

3.3 Non-telomeric TTAGGG sequences as components of the satellite DNA

Although many ITS sites observed within or at the margin of the constitutive heterochromatin are remnants of chromosome fusion events (Meyne et al., 1990), such coincidence is not a general rule. Australian and American marsupials (Marsupialia) presumed ancestral karyotype (2n= 14) is observed in the exponents of six of the seven extant marsupial orders (Metcalf et al., 2004). Such karyotype includes bi-armed chromosomes showing centromerically located telomeric sequences that overlap with the large amounts of heterochromatin (Pagnozzi et al., 2000, Metcalf et al. 2004). Comparison of the distribution of the telomeric DNA sequences in the ancestral and more evolved karyotypes with known chromosomal rearrangements suggested that pericentromeric and heterochromatic ITSs in the marsupial 2n= 14 complements might be a component of the native satellite DNA rather than relicts of the recent chromosome rearrangements (Pagnozzi et al., 2000; Metcalfe et al. 2004).

Most of the cytogenetically studied amphibians show telomeric DNA sequences exclusively located at the chromosomal ends (Meyne et al., 1990; Schmid et al., 2003, Schmid et al., 2009). Unexpectedly, interstitial location of the telomeric DNA sequences has been described in the quite conserved karyotypes of the American hylid frogs (Wiley et al., 1992), *Xenopus laevis* (Meyne et al., 1990, Nanda et al., 2008) and *Xenopus clivii* (Nanda et al., 2008). Homogeneity of the karyotypes among related species excluded chromosome fusions as the potential source of ITSs. Moreover, the interstitial telomeric sites in these species coincided with the constitutive heterochromatin identified in the course of C-banding. The clear correspondence between ITSs and the constitutive heterochromatin suggest that $(TTAGGG)_n$ sequences might be a component of a repetitive DNA. Although it is still unknown how the telomeric DNA sequences were inserted into the interstitial positions and amplified, the repair of the DNA Double Strand Breaks with the telomerase should be taken into consideration (Nergadze et al., 2004, 2007). Previously, several authors suggested that telomeric or telomeric like DNA sequences were components of the satellite DNA in some vertebrates (Garrido-Ramos et al., 1998). In other species, telomeric DNA sequences are scattered along the NORs (Nucleolus Organizer Region) DNA sequences (see chapter 4.4).

4. Distribution of telomeric DNA sequences in fish

4.1 Telomerase and the length of the fish telomeres

So far, the telomerase gene in fish has been shown to be expressed in most cells throughout the entire fish life (Elmore et al., 2008; Hartman et al., 2009; Lund et al., 2009). This is in contrast to humans where telomerase activity is absent in most somatic cells but present in embryonic stem cells and tumors (Hiyama and Hiyama, 2007). Although some authors presume that high expression of fish telomerase may be related to the longevity, comparative analysis of telomerase activity in the short- and long-lived fish species showed no positive relationship between telomerase activity and the fish longevity (Elmore et al., 2008). Instead, another hypothesis was suggested: retention of the telomerase in adult fish might be crucial to maintain their regenerative capacity. To test this hypothesis, short fragments of the caudal fish tissue have been removed in medaka (*Oryzias latipes*), zebrafish

(*Danio rerio*), and mummichog (*Fundulus heteroclitus*) specimens, and telomerase activities were assayed before and during the regeneration period. Telomerase was shown to be upregulated during the tissue regeneration, which suggested that telomerase is involved in the fish tissue regeneration after injury (Elmore et al., 2008).

The length of the telomeric DNA in fish studied to date varies from 2 kb to 15 kb (Chew et al., 2002, Elmore et al. 2008) and is similar to that observed in normal human cells (Elmore et al., 2008). Furthermore, retention of the telomere length throughout the entire life has been demonstrated in zebrafish, but not in the medaka (Hatekeyama et al., 2008; Lund et al., 2009). Telomere shortening with age has been also observed in the long-lived strain of *Nothobranchius furzeri* while such attrition has not been detected in the short-lived strain of the same species (Hartmann et al. 2009). Thus, age dependent telomere shortening in fish may be species-specific or even strain specific (Lund et al., 2009; Hartman et al., 2009).

Application of PRINS using $(CCTAAA)_7$ primer and PNA-FISH using telomeric probes revealed different intensity of the hybridization foci on fish chromosomes (Ocalewicz and Dobosz, 2008; Pomianowski et al., 2012). As the fluorescence intensity of the telomere hybridization focus reflects the length of the telomeric repeat sequence (Zijlmans et al., 1997), the differences in the telomere hybridization signal intensity observed on different chromosomes are likely related to variations in their respective telomere lengths. Chromosome rearrangements may lead to such variation. In the albino rainbow trout (*Oncorhynchus mykiss*), one of the X chromosome isoforms has shorter p-arm with weak telomeric hybridization signals. Partial deletion or translocation including telomeric region has been suggested to contribute to the p-arm length difference between two morphological variants of the X chromosome (Figure 1a-b) (Ocalewicz and Dobosz, 2009).

4.2 Fish karyotype evolution and distribution of telomeric repeats: Major rearrangements

As mentioned above, internally located telomeric DNA repeat sequences may be the relicts of the chromosomal rearrangements such as fusions that accompanied the karyotype evolution of many vertebrate species. This may be also true for the fish species. Teleostean fish, the major clade of the ray-finned fish (Actinopterygii) is the largest and the most diverse group of vertebrates. More than half of the cytogenetically surveyed actinopterygians have karyotypes composed of 48-50 chromosomes (Mank and Avise, 2006) and the complement of 48 one-armed chromosomes (NF= 48) is supposed to be ancestral in the Teleostei. Such teleostean ancestral like karyotype (2n= 48) may be the plesiomorphic condition in Scorpeanidae fish (Caputo et al., 1998). However, in *Scorpaena notata*, only 34 uni-armed chromosomes (NF= 34) are observed (Caputo et al., 1998). As the karyotype of *S. notata* comprises of only subtelo-acrocentric chromosomes, the reduction of both chromosome and chromosome arm numbers from 48 to 34 likely occurred in the course of the tandem fusions. Nevertheless, only one pair of chromosomes showed interstitial telomeric DNA sequences in the putative fusion sites in this species. Presumably other ITS sites have been lost or exist in very short arrays that may not be detected by fluorescence in situ hybridization (Caputo et al., 1998).

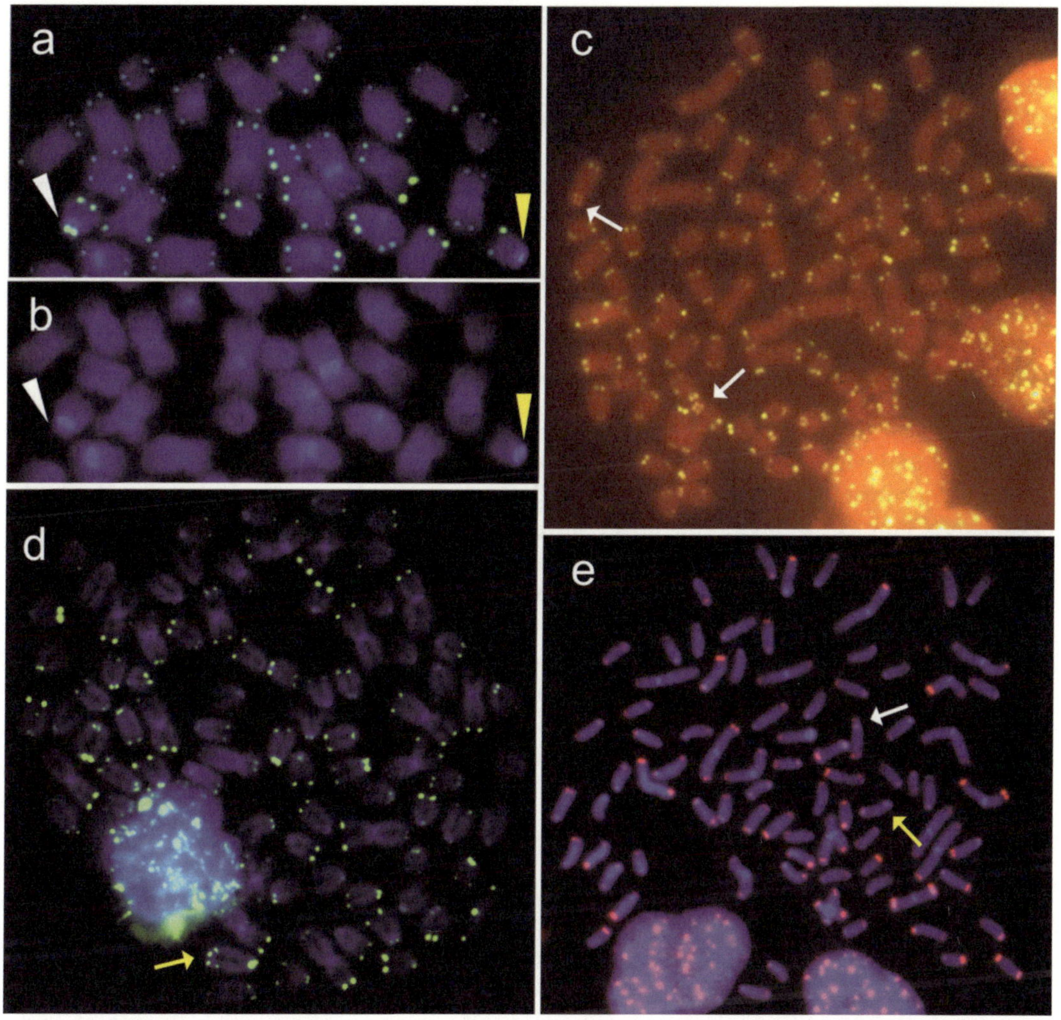

Fig. 1. a-b. Albino rainbow trout (*Oncorhynchus mykiss*) partial metaphase with two morphs of the X chromosome after hybridization with the telomeric probe (PNA-FISH) (a) and staining with DAPI fluorochrome (b). Arrowheads show two morphs of the rainbow trout X chromosomes. White arrowhead - long morph (X^L) with distinct p-arm and bright telomeric signals, yellow arrowhead - short morph (X^L) with reduced p-arm and weak telomeric signals. Fig. 1 c-e. Chromosomes of brook trout (*Salvelinus fontinalis*) (c), Arctic charr (*Salvelinus alpinus*) (d) and their hybrid (e) after PRINS (c, e) and PNA-FISH (d) enabling localization of the telomeric DNA sequences. White arrows indicate brook trout chromosomes with interstitial telomeric sites (ITSs), yellow arrows point the Arctic charr chromosomes with ITSs.

Huge variation in the diploid chromosome number and the karyotype composition are observed in the bitterlings (Acheilognathinae). Diploid chromosome number and the number of chromosome arms vary from 42 to 48 and 50-78, respectively, which was attributed to both Roberstonian and tandem fusions, chromosomal inversions, and some minor rearrangements involving heterochromatic regions (Ueda, 2007). In two bitterling species, The Japanese rosy bitterling (*Rhodeus ocellatus kurumeus*) and the oily bitterling (*Tanakia limbata*), both with similar karyotypes that comprise 8 metacentric, 20 submetacentric and 20 subtelocentric chromosomes (2n= 48, FN= 76) FISH with telomeric probe was applied and showed different distribution patterns of the hybridization signals. In the Japanese bitterling interstitial telomeric sites were observed in the pericentromeric regions of 14-16 chromosomes, which is the highest number of ITSs detected in any of the fish chromosomes studied to date, whereas in the oily bitterling no such location of ITS was exhibited (Sola et al., 2003). Similar phenomenon was observed in the mammalian species that experienced several Roberstonian fusions. ITSs were not described in *Mus musculus domesticus* (Garagna et al., 1995; Nanda et al., 1995) whereas in *M. minutoides* telomeric sequences at the putative fusions sites were retained and observed near the centromeres (Castiglia et al., 2002; Castiglia et al., 2006).

Two interstitial telomeric sites have been detected in the Nile tilapia (*Oreochromis niloticus*) (2n= 44) chromosome 1 that is significantly larger than all the other chromosomes in this organism (Chew et al. 2002). This observation supported hypothesis that chromosome 1 in the Nile tilapia appeared in the course of the fusion of three chromosomes and explained the reduction of chromosome number from the ancestral teleost karyotype of 2n= 48 to 2n= 44 in the Nile tilapia (Chew et al. 2002). In *Oreochromis karongae*, diploid chromosome number is reduced to 38. The *O. karongae* karyotype comprises one large subtelocentric pair of chromosomes, four medium sized pairs (three subtelocentric, one submetacentric) and fourteen small pairs. Three of the medium sized chromosome pairs seem to derive in the course of fusions. Distribution of the telomeric repeats show two interstitial telomeric sites on the chromosome 1 similar to these observed in the Nile tilapia chromosome 1 and one ITS in each of the six fusion chromosomes. Comparison of the position of the current and relic centromeres performed with FISH and the tilapia centromere specific probe and ITS sites in *O. karongae* suggests that the three fusions all occurred in different orientations: the ends of the two q arms to produce pair 2, a p-q fusion in the case of pair 3 and a p-p fusion for pair 4 (Mota-Velasco et al., 2009). In the non-teleostean Elasmobranch fishes (sharks and rays) that are considered as the ancient vertebrates only four species have been studied with FISH and telomeric probe, so far (Rocco 2006). In two of them (*Taeniura lymma* and *Torpedo ocellata*), pericentromeric location of telomeric DNA sequences was detected in four bi-armed chromosomes (Stingo and Rocco, 2001; Rocco et al., 2001; Rocco et al., 2002). This is in agreements with the hypothesis that in cartilaginous fish, karyotype evolution involved a progressive decrease of chromosome number due to the centric fusions (Rocco, 2007).

4.2.1 Salmonid fish species: Chromosome fusions and lack of ITSs

Chromosomal rearrangements like centric and tandem fusions have played important role in the salmonid karyotype evolution during rediploidization process following the whole genome duplication experienced by the salmonid ancestor 100-25 mya (Allendorf and Thorgaard, 1984). The polyploid origin of the Salmonidae has been considerably substantiated (Leong et al., 2010). Both the genome size and the chromosome arms number are approximately twice that of the Salmonid closest relatives, the Esociformes (Phillips and Ráb, 2001). Most of the salmonid species have karyotypes composed of both bi-armed and one-armed chromosomes and have the chromosome arm number (FN) that ranged from 94 to 104, while the related Esocidae fish have the ancestral teleostean karyotype with about 50 one-armed chromosomes. Different chromosome number and the constant chromosome arm number resulted from the centric fusions known as Roberstonian polymorphisms are observed in the salmonid fish from the genera *Hucho, Salmo, Oncorhynchus* and *Salvelinus* (Phillips and Ráb, 2001). Moreover, large acrocentric chromosomes in the Atlantic salmon (*Salmo salar*) karyotype are thought to be the result of tandem fusions (Phillips and Ráb, 2000). Robertsonian fusions, paracentric and pericentric inversions were suggested to be involved in changes leading to the establishment of the present karyotypes of three *Coregonus* species: European whitefish (*Coregonus lavaraetus*), vendace (*Coregonus lavaretus*) and peled (*Coregonus peled*) (Jankun et al., 2007). Unexpectedly, none of the cytogenetically studied salmonid fish species with fused meta- and submetacentric chromosomes showed pericentromeric locations of the telomeric repeats (Abuin et al., 1996; Jankun et al., 2007; Ocalewicz et al., 2008). The lack of ITS at the putative fusion sites in the bi-armed salmonid chromosomes may suggest p-arm telomeres were lost in the course of the chromosome breakage that preceded chromosome fusions. On the other hand, telomeric repeats retained at the fusion sites might have experienced successive loss and degeneration leading to gradual shortening of the non-functional telomeric arrays (Slijepcevic, 1998). Consequently, too short internally located telomeric repeats may be below the resolution of the techniques enabling chromosomal location of DNA sequences. On the other hand, interstitial telomeric DNA sequences located far from the centromeric region have been detected in the Atlantic salmon large subtelocentric chromosomes, which supported hypothesis concerning tandem fusions as the mechanism leading to the formation of some of the chromosomes in this species (Abuin et al., 1996).

4.3 ITSs and minor rearrangements – A *Salvelinus* fish case

Other mechanisms leading to the ITS formation have been suggested in three *Salvelinus* species: lake trout (*Salvelinus namaycush*), brook trout (*Salvelinus fontinalis*) and the Arctic charr (*Salvelinus alpinus*) showing subterminal position of the interstitial telomeric sequences (Figure 1c-d) assigned to the vicinity of the CMA_3 positive GC-rich heterochromatin (Reed and Phillips, 1995; Ocalewicz et al., 2004b; Pomianowski et al., 2012). Guanine-rich chromosomal regions are involved in several rearrangements like transpositions, duplications and (or) translocations resulted in multichromosomal location and variation in size of CMA_3 positively stained chromatin in *Salvelinus* species (Phillips et al., 1988; Phillips and Ráb, 2001). Dispersion of CMA_3 positive chromatin segments among homologous and non-homologous chromosomes could be followed by the insertion of the telomeric repeats linked to the translocated chromosome fragment into the interstitial position. Similar location of ITS in these three species may indicate similar mechanism leading to the insertion of $(TTAGGG)_n$ sequences in the non-telomere position in the *Salvelinus* fish. In the case of the Arctic char metaphase spreads showing extended chromatin, the non-telomeric fluorescent hybridization signal covered a longer stretch of the chromosome than the signal from the telomere position, however the interstitial signal was less intense. This observation suggested that telomeric regions and ITS might have different structures (Pomianowski et al., 2012). It is possible that telomeric DNA sequences were not the only component of the ITS region. Internally inserted short telomeric repeats are frequently flanked by the repetitive or transposable elements and undergo amplification process leading to elongation/expansion of the chromatic region built with different DNA sequences including telomeric repeats (Garrido-Ramos et al., 1998).

It has been also observed that ITSs might be considered as sites fragile for recombination and thus may potentially increase rates of chromosome breaks and rearrangements (Lin and Yan, 2008). This could partially explain the high level of size and location polymorphisms of the heterochromatic regions in *Salvelinus* species (Phillips et al., 1988; Phillips and Ráb, 2001; Pomianowski et al., 2012). Moreover, chromosomes with unusual distribution of telomeric DNA sequences may be useful cytogenetic markers enabling identification of parental chromosomes in hybrid organisms. Recently, Arctic charr and brook trout chromosomes with internally located telomeric repeats have been identified in the karyotype of Arctic charr x brook trout hybrids (Figure 1e) (Ocalewicz, unpublished).

4.4 Other uncommon locations of the telomeric sequences in fish

In addition to the interstitial location of the telomeric DNA, $(TTAGGG)_n$ repeats may also coincide with the nucleolar organizer regions (NORs). Telomeric DNA sequences are observed to scatter along the heterochromatic NORs in the Atlantic eels (*Anguilla anguilla*) (Salvadori et al. 1995), rainbow trout (Abuin et al., 1996), straight-nosed pipefish (*Nerophis ophidion*) (Libertini et al., 2006) and three mullet species (Mugilidae) (Sola et al., 2007). Such unusual distribution of TTAGGG repeats suggests telomeric sequences are interspersed with rDNA sequences. Similar location of telomeric repeats has been previously described in mammalian species including American mole (*Scalopus aquaticus*), Seba's fruit bat (*Carollia perspicillata*) (Meyne et al., 1990), wood lemming (*Myopus schisticolor*) (Liu and Fredga, 1999), and amphibians *Xenopus borealis* and *Xenopus muelleri* (Nanda et al., 2008). The origin of the telomeric sequences interspersed with NORs is unclear. It was suggested that the presence of telomeric repeats within NORs may cause unequal crossing-over and thus give rise to the chromosomal length polymorphism (Salvadori et al., 1996). Moreover, the presence of the telomere sequences may epigenetically inactivate NORs (Guillén et al., 2004; Copenhaver and Pikaard, 1996).

In the sturgeon *Acipenser gueldenstaedti*, two entire chromosomes were light up with the fluorescent signals derived from the telomeric probe in FISH analysis (Fontana et al., 1998). Similar observation has been made in some of the bird microchromosomes. The ability of interstitial telomeric repeats to promote recombination (Ashley and Ward, 1993) may explain enormously high recombination rate in the bird microchromosomes (Nanda et al., 2002).

4.5 Distribution of telomeric DNA sequences in the androgenetic fish

Androgenesis is a reproductive process in which diploid offspring inherit only paternal nuclear DNA. Although natural (spontaneous) androgenesis is observed in limited number of plant and animal species (McKone and Halpern, 2003), paternal chromosome inheritance can be induced intentionally in fish (Komen and Thorgaard, 2007). Artificial androgenesis includes three steps: inactivation of the nuclear DNA in eggs by UV or ionizing (gamma and X) irradiation, insemination of enucleated eggs with untreated or cryopreserved sperm, and diploidization of the paternal chromosomes by exposition of the haploid zygotes to temperature or high pressure shock to suppress the first mitotic division (Komen and Thorgaard, 2007). UV radiation damages chromosomes by inducing thymidine dimers that inhibit process of replication what results in DNA fragmentation, and gamma and X radiations act by inducing chromosome breaks like double strand breaks (DSB). Insufficient dose of radiation results in incomplete inactivation of maternal nuclear genome. Undamaged pieces of the irradiated genome in the forms of chromosome fragments were observed in the androgenetic alevins and adult fish (Parsons and Thorgaard, 1985; Ocalewicz et al. 2004a). In the course of partial inactivation of maternal chromosomes, different chromosome fragments may be provided; acentric terminal fragments with telomeric region at only one end or without any telomeres and centric incomplete chromosomes without telomeres, or telomere at only one arm. Additionally, dicentric chromosome can be formed when the broken end of one centric incomplete chromosome join with a broken end of another incomplete chromosome (Disney et al., 1988). Acentric fragments may be removed from the zygote during the cell divisions or may associate with or even incorporate into paternal intact chromosomes. ITSs observed on the androgenetic rainbow trout chromosomes could be the remnants of the incorporation process (Figure 2a) (Ocalewicz et al., 2004). The centric chromosome fragments with chromosome breaks on both sides of the centromere form ring chromosomes presumably in the course of non-homologous end joining (NHEJ) repair (*e.g.* Pfeifer et al., 2004). On the other hand, the broken ends of the chromosomes could have been repaired with the telomeric DNA repeats synthesized *de novo* by telomerase or another mechanism capable of *de novo* telomere addition (Biessmann et al., 1990). Some of the ionizing radiation induced fish chromosome fragments retained linear construction with telomeric DNA sequences newly added to their broken ends (Figure 2b) (Ocalewicz et al., 2009). Chromosome fragment with two interstitially located telomeric signals observed in the androgenetic brook trout (Figure 2c) might have been also ring chromosome formed in the course of fusion of a radiation-broken chromosome arm with the opposite unbroken arm or arm broken within telomeric region (Henegariu et al., 1997). However we do not exclude that this fragment might have originated from one of the brook trout chromosomes with interstitially located telomeric DNA sequences (Ocalewicz et al., 2004b). Chromosome fragments showing two, always terminally located telomeres detected in the androgenetic brook trout represented another chromatin arrangements (Figure 2d). Such shape and distribution of the hybridization spots suggested formation in the course of the telomere loss in only one chromosome arm and fusion between sister chromatids. On the other hand, both chromosomal ends might have been broken and repaired in the course of two mechanisms - action of the telomerase may heal broken ends of the p-arm while broken ends of the q-arm may undergo fusion. Although telomerase is capable of healing the broken ends of the irradiated fish chromosomes, most of the fragments show spherical shape. It is possible that fish telomerase is not always able to heal the broken chromosome ends with newly synthesized telomeric DNA due to the limited access to DNA breaks (Latre et al., 2004). However, telomerase in fish seems to be involved in the ionizing radiation induced DSB repair, which is in agreement with the observations made in human, chimpanzee, mouse and rats genomes, where analysis of flanking sequences suggested that some of the ITSs were inserted during the repair of DSB (Ruiz-Herrera et al., 2008).

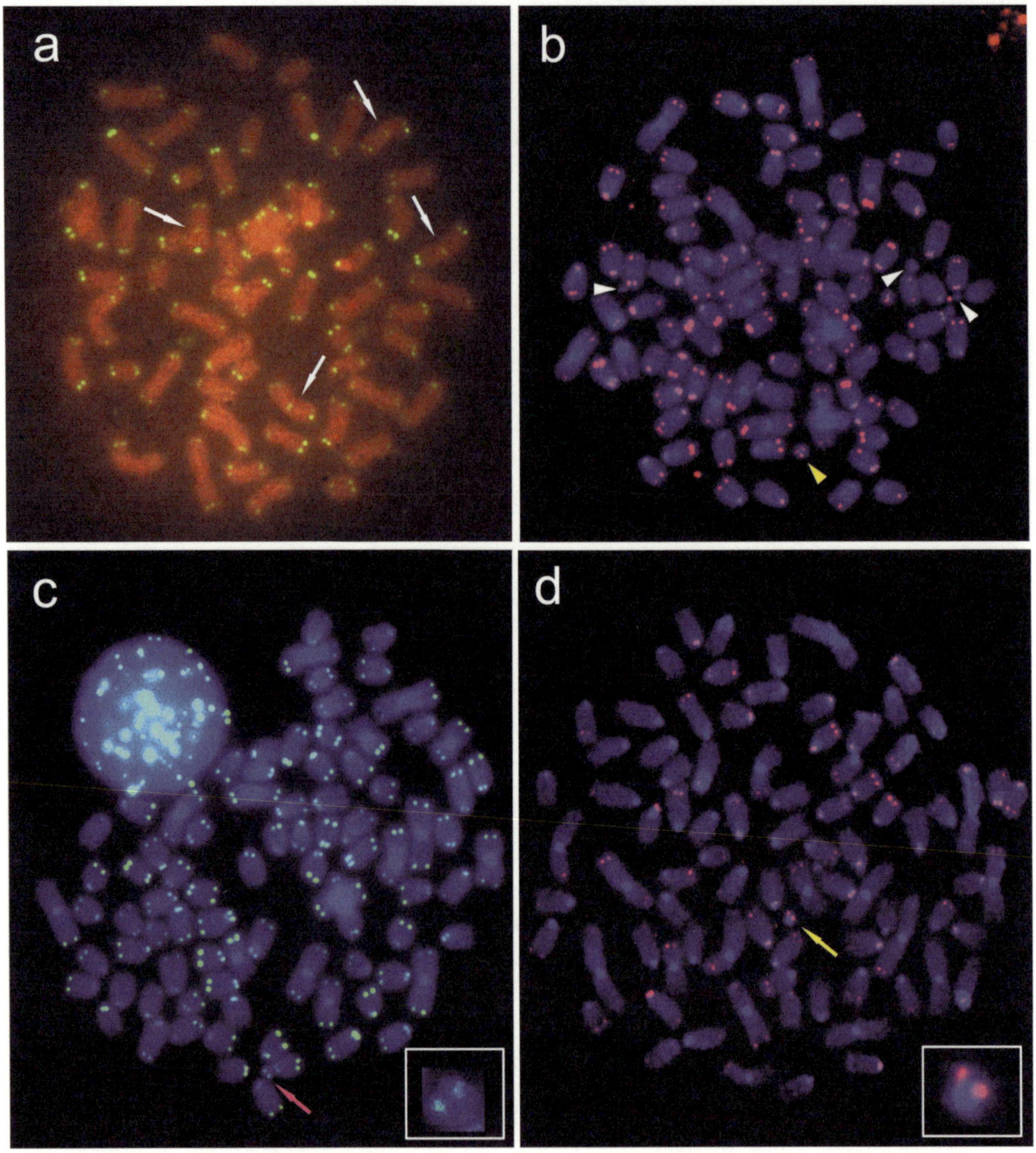

Fig. 2. Chromosomes of androgenetic progenies of rainbow trout (*Oncorhynchus mykiss*) (a), brook trout (*Salvelinus fontinalis*) X Arctic charr (*Salvelinus alpinus*) hybrid (b) and brook trout (c-d) after Primed IN Situ (PRINS) technique with telomeric $(CCCTAA)_7$. White arrows indicate chromosomes with interstitial telomeric DNA sequences (a), yellow arrowhead shows linear chromosome fragment with telomeres (b), white arrowheads point to the telomerless ring chromosome fragments (b), pink arrow indicates chromosome fragment with interstitially located telomeric signals (c) while yellow arrow indicates chromosome fragment with telomeric signals situated terminally (d). Both type of chromosome fragments with telomeric signals are enlarged and framed (c, d).

5. Conclusions

Chromosome fusions are the source of the interstitial telomeric DNA sequences (ITSs) in the vertebrates. On the other hand, quite frequently such rearrangements involve loss of the telomeric repeats at the fusion sites. ITSs can also appear in the course of DNA DSB repair. Internally located telomeric DNA sequences may undergo amplification, degeneration and/or further redistribution. TTAGGG repeats may be part of the centromeric and subterminal satellite DNA or rDNA forming nucleolus organizer regions (NORs). Fish seem to be good models to study the distribution and genomic organization of the ITSs. First, most of the ITSs observed in the fish chromosomes appeared in the course of the similar mechanisms responsible for the ITS formation in the higher vertebrates. Second, apart from the well-known fusion scenario of the ITS origin, other genomic rearrangements such as transposition-mediated translocations of the chromosomal regions including telomeric DNA sequences may result in the interstitial inclusion of the telomeric repeats in fish chromosomes. ITSs observed in the androgenetic fish derive from the incorporation of the ionizing radiation induced terminal acentric chromosome fragments into the intact chromosomes. Moreover, fish telomerase, which is active during the entire ontogenetic development, may be involved in the DSBs repair mechanism in these organisms.

6. Acknowledgments

Results concerning chromosomes of androgenetic brook trout (*Salvelinus fontinalis*) and androgenetic brook trout X Arctic charr (*Salvelinus alpinus*) hybrids described in the chapter 4.5 had been obtained in the course of the research supported by the Polish Ministry of Science and Higher Education, Project No. N311 525240.

7. References

Abuin, M.; Martinez, P. & Sanchez, L. (1996). Localization of the repetitive telomeric sequence $(TTAGGG)_n$ in four salmonid species. *Genome*, Vol. 39, No.5, pp. 1035-1039

Allendorf, F.W. & Thorgaard, G.H. (1984). Tetraploidy and the Evolution of Salmonid Fishes. Evolutionary Genetics of Fishes. (ed. B. J. Turner), pp. 1-53. Plenum Press, New York

Alvarez, L.; Evans, J.W.; Wilks, R.; Lucas, J.N.; Brown, J.M. & Giaccia, A.J. (1993). Chromosomal radiosensitivity at intrachromosomal telomeric sites. Genes Chromosomes Cancer, Vol. 8, No. 1, pp. 8-14

Ashley, T. & Ward, D.C. 1993. A "hot spot" of recombination coincides with an interstitial telomeric sequences in Armenian hamster. *Cytogenetic and Cell Genetics*, Vol. 62, No. 2-3, pp. 169-171

Azzalin, C.M.; Mucciolo, E.; Bertoni, L. & Giulotto, E. (1997). Fluorescence in situ hybridization with a synthetic (T2AG3)n polynucleotide detects several intrachromosomal telomere-like repeats on human chromosomes. Cytogenetics and Cell Genetics, Vol. 78, No. 2, pp. 112–115

Azzalin, C.M.; Nergadze, S.G. & Giulotto, E. (2001). Human intrachromosomal telomeric-like repeats: sequence organization and mechanisms of origin. *Chromosoma*, Vol.110, No.2, pp. 75-82

Bertoni, L.; Attolini, C.; Faravelli, M.; Simi, S. & Giulotto, E. (1996). Intrachromosomal telomere-like DNA sequences in Chinese hamster. *Mammalian Genome*, Vol. 7, No. 11,pp. 853-855

Biessmann, H. & Mason, J.M. (1997). Telomere maintenance without telomerase. *Chromosoma*, Vol.106, No.2, pp. 63-69

Biessmann, H.; Mason, J.; M., Ferry, K.; d'Hulst, M.; Balgeirsdottir, K.; Traverse, K.; L.& Pardue, M-L. (1990). Addition of telomere-associated HeT DNA sequences "heals" broken chromosome ends in Drosophila. *Cell* , Vol.61, No.4, ,No. pp. 663-673

Blackburn, E.H. & Gall, J.G. (1978). A tandemly repeated sequences at the termini of the extrachromosomal ribosomal RNA genes in Tetrahymena. Journal of Molecular Biology, Vol. 120, No. 1, pp. 35-53.

Bolzán, A.D. & Bianchi, M.S. (2006). Telomeres, interstitial telomeric repeat sequences, and chromosomal aberrations. *Mutation Research*, Vol. 612, No3. pp. 189-214

Cangiano, G. & La Volpe, A. (1993). Repetitive DNA sequences located in the terminal portion of the Caenorhabditis elegans chromosomes. Nucleic Acid Research, Vol. 21, No. 5, pp. 1133-1139

Caputo, V.; Sorice, M.; Vitturi, R.; Magistrelli, R. & Olmo, E. (1998). Cytogenetic studies in some species of Scorpaeniformes (Telesotei: Percomorpha). *Chromosome Research*, Vol.6, No.4, pp. 255-262

Castiglia, R.; Gornung, E. & Corti, M. (2002). Cytogenetic analyses of chromosomal rearrangements in *Mus minutoides/musculoides* from North-West Zambia through mapping of the telomeric sequence (TTAGGG)n and banding techniques. *Chromosome Research*, Vol.10, No.5, pp. 399-406

Castiglia, R.; Garagna, S.; Merico, V.; Oguge, N. & Corti, M. (2006). Cytogenetics of a new cytotype of African Mus (subgenus Nanomys) minutoides (Rodentia, Muridae) from Kenya: C- and G- banding and distribution of $(TTAGGG)_n$ telomeric sequences. *Chromosome Research*, Vol. 14, No. ,pp. 587-594

Chew, J.S.K.; Oliveira, C.; Wright, J.M. & Dobson, M.J. (2002). Molecular and cytogenetic analysis of the telomeric $(TTAGGG)_n$ repetitive sequences in the Nile Tilapia, *Oreochromis nilotics* (Teleostei: Cichlidae). *Chromosoma*, Vol.111, No.1, pp. 45-52

Copenhaver, G.P. & Pikaard, C.S. (1996). RFLP and physical mapping with an rDNA-specific endonuclease reveals that nucleolus organizer regions of *Arabidopsis thaliana* adjoin the telomeres on chromosomes 2 and 4. *The Plant Journal* , Vol.9, No.2, pp. 259-272

Cox, A.V.; Bennett, S.T.; Parokonny, A.S.; Kenton, A.; Callimassia, M.A. & Bennett, M.D. (1993). Comparison of plant telomere locations using a PCR-generated synthetic probe. Annals of Boatny, Vol. 72, No. 3, pp. 239-247

de Lange, T. (2002). Protection of mammalian telomeres. Oncogene, Vol. 21, No. 4, pp. 532–534

Delany, M. E., A. B. Krupkin, and M. M. Miller, 2000. Organization of telomere sequences in birds: evidence for arrays of extreme length and for *in vivo* shortening. *Cytogenetics and Cell Genetics*, Vol. 90, No. 1-2, pp. 139–145

Delany, M.E.; Daniels, L.M.; Swanberg, S.E. & Taylor, H.A. 2003. Telomeres in the chicken: genome stability and chromosome ends. *Poultry Science*, Vol. 82, No. 6, pp. 917-926

Disney, J.E.: Johnson, K.R.: Banks, D. K. & Thorgaard, G. H. (1988). Maintenance of foreign gene expression and independent chromosome fragments in adult transgenic rainbow trout and their offspring. *Journal of Experimental Zoology*, Vol.248, No.3, pp. 335-344

Elmore,L.W.; Norris, M.W.; Sircab, S.; Bright, T.; McChesney, P.A.; Winn, R.N. & Holt, S.E. (2008). Upregulation of telomerase function during tissue regeneration. *Experimental Biology and Medicine*, Vol.233, No.8, pp. 958-967

Fagundes, V. & Yonenaga-Yassuda, Y. (1998). Evolutionary conservation of whole homeologous chromosome arms in the Akodont rodents *Bolomys* and *Akodon* (Muridae, Sigmodontidae): maintenance of interstitial telomeric segments (ITBs) in recent event of centric fusions. *Chromosome Research*, Vol. 6, No. 8, pp. 643-648

Faravelli, M.; Azzalin, C.M.; Bertoni, L.; Chernova, O.; Attolini, C.; Mondello, C. & Giulotto, E. (2002). Molecular organization of internal telomeric sequences in Chinese hamster chromosomes. *Gene*, Vol. 283, No 1-2. ,pp. 11-16

Faravelli, M.; Moralli, D.; Bertoni, L.; Attolini, C.; Chernova, O.; Raimondi, E. & Giulott, E. (1998). Two extended arrays of a satellite DNA sequences at the centromere and at the short-arm telomere of Chinese hamster chromosome 5. *Cytogenetics and Cell Genetic*, Vol. 83, No. 3-4 ,pp. 281-286

Fontana, F.; Lanfredi, M.; Chicca, M.; Aiello, V. & Rossi R. (1998). Localization of repetitive telomeric sequences $(TTAGGG)_n$ in four sturgeon species. *Chromosome Research*, Vol.6, No.4, pp. 303-306

Frönicke L, Scherthan H (1997) Zoo-fluorescence in situ hybridization analysis of human and Indian muntjac karyotypes (*Muntiacus muntjac vaginalis*) reveals satellite DNA clusters at the margins of conserved syntenic segments. *Chromosome Research*, Vol.5, No.4, pp. 254–261

Fuchs, J.; Branders, A. & Schubert, I. (1995). Telomere sequences localization and karyotype evolution in higher plants. Plants Systematics and Evolution, Vol. 196, No. 3-4, pp. 227-241.

Garagna, S.; Ronchetti, E.; Mascharetti, S.; Crovella, S.; Foermenti, D.; Rumpler, Y. & Romanini, M.G.M. (1997). Non-telomeric chromosome localization of $(TTAGGG)_n$ repeats in the genus Eulemur. Chromosome Research, Vol.5, No.7, pp. 487-491.

Garagna, S.; Broccoli, D.; Redi, C.A.; Searle, J.B.; Cooke, H.J. & Capanna, E. (1995). Robertsonian metacentrics of the mouse lose telomeric sequences but retain some minor satellite DNA in the pericentromeric area. *Chromosoma*, Vol.103, No. pp. 685-692.

Garrido-Ramos, M.A.; de la Herrán, R.; Ruiz Rejón C. & Ruiz Rejón M. (1998). A satellite DNA of Sparidae family (Pisces, Perciformes) associated with telomeric sequences. *Cytogenetic and Cell Genetics*, Vol. 83, No. (1-2), pp. 3-9

Go, Y.; Rakotoarisoa, G.; Kawamoto, Y.; Randrianjafy, A.; Koyama, N. & Hirai H. (2000). PRINS analysis of the telomeric sequences in seven lemurs. Chromosome Research, Vol. 8, No. 1,pp. 57-65

Guillén, A.K.Z.; Hirai, Y.; Tanoue, T. & Hirai H. (2004). Transcriptional repression mechanisms of nucleolus organizer regions (NORs) in human and chimpanzees. Chromosome Research, Vol.12, No.3, pp. 225-237

Hartmann, N. & Scherthan, H. (2004). Characterization of ancestral chromosome fusion points in the Indian muntjac deer. *Chromosoma*, Vol.112, No.5 , pp. 213-220

Hartmann, N.; Reichwald, K.; Lechel, A.; Graf, M.; Kirschner, J.; Dorn, A.; Terzibasi, E.; Wellner, J.; Platzer, M.; Rudolph, K.L.; Cellerino, A. & Englert, C. (2009). Telomeres shorten while Tert expression increase during ageing of the short-lived fish Nothobranchius furzeri. *Mechanisms of Aging and Development*, Vol.130, No.5, pp. 290-296

Hatekeyama, H.; Nakamura, K.; Izumijama-Shimomura, N.; Ishii, A. & Tsuchida, S. (2008). The teleost Oryzias latipes shows telomere shortening with age despite considerable telomerase activity throughout life. *Mechanisms of Ageing and Development*, Vol. 129, No. 9, pp. 550-557

Henegariu, O.; Kernek, S.; Keating, M.A.; Palmer, C.G. & Heerema, N.A. (1997). PCR and FISH analysis of a ring Y chromosome. *America Journal of Medical Genetics*, Vol. 69, No. 2, pp. 171-176

Hiyama, E. & Hiyama, K. (2007). Telomere and telomerase in stem cells. British Journal of Cancer, Vol. 96, No. , pp. 1020-1024 doi:10.1038/sj.bjc.6603671

Hsu, T.C.; Pathak, S. & Chen, T.R. (1975). The possibility of latent centromeres and a proposed nomenclature system for total chromosome and whole arm translocation. *Cytogenetic and Cell Genetics*, Vol.15, No.1, pp. 41–49

Huffman, K.E.; Levee, S.D.; Tesmer, V.M.; Shay, J.W. & Wright, W.E. 2000. Telomere shortening is proportional to the size of the G-rich telomeric 3′-overhang. Journal of Biological Chemistry, Vol. 275, No. 26, pp. 19-22

Ijdo, J.W.; Baldini, A.; Ward, D.C.; Reeders, S.T. & Wells, R.A. (1991). Origin of human chromosome 2: an ancestral telomere–telomere fusion. Proceedings of the National Academy of Sciences of the United States of America, Vol. 88, No. 20, pp. 9051–9055

Jankun, M.; Woznicki, P.; Ocalewicz, K. & Furgala-Selezniow, G. (2007). Chromosomal evolution in the three species of Holarctic fish of the genus Coregonus (Salmoniformes). *Advances in Limnology*, Vol. 60, pp. 25-37

Kipling, D.& Cooke, H.J. (1990). Hypervariable ultra-long telomeres in mice. Nature, Vol. 347, No. 6291, pp. 400–402

Klobutcher, L.A.; Swanton, M.T.; Donini, P. & Prescott, D.M. (1981). All gene sized DNA molecules in four species of hypotrichs have the same terminal sequence and an unusual 3′ terminus. Proceedings of the National Academy of Sciences of the United States of America, Vol. 78, No. 5, pp. 3015–3019

Koch, J.; Kølvraa, S.; Petersen, K.; Gregersen, N. & Bolend, L. (1989). Oligonucleotide-priming methods for chromosome specific labeling of alpha satellite DNA in situ. *Chromosoma,* Vol. 98, No. 4, pp. 259 – 265

Komen, H. & Thorgaard, G.A. (2007). Androgenesis, gynogenesis and the production of clones in fishes: a review. *Aquaculture,* Vol. 269, No.1-4. pp. 150-173

Lansdorp, P P.M.; Verwoerd, N.P.; van den Rijke, F.M.; Dragowska, V.; Little, M.T.; Dirls, R.W.; Raap, A.K. & Tanke, H.J. (1996). Heterogeneity in telomere length of human chromosomes. Human Molecular Genetics, Vol. 5, No. 5, pp. 685–691

Latre, L.; Genesca, A.; Martin, M.; Ribas, M.; Egozcue, J.; Blasco, M. A.& Tussel, L. (2004). Repair of DNA broken ends is similar in embryonic fibroblass with and without telomerase. *Radiation Research* Vol.162, No.2, pp. 136-142

Lee, C.; Sasi, R. & Lin, C.C. (1993). Interstitial localization of telomeric DNA sequences in the Indian muntjac chromosomes; further evidence for tandem chromosome fusions in the karyotypic evolution of the Asian muntjacs. *Cytogenetic and Cell Genetics*, Vol. 63, No3., pp. 156–159

Leong, J.S.; Jantzen, S.G.; von Schalburg, K.R.; Cooper, G.A.; Messmer, A.M.; Liao, N.Y.; Munro, S.; Moore, R,; Holt, R.A.; Jones, S.J.M.; Davidson, W.S. &Koop, B. (2010). *Salmo salar* and *Esox lucius* full-length cDNA sequences reveal changes in evolutionary pressure on a post-tetraploidization genome. BMC Genomics 2010, 11:279

Libertini, A.; Vitturi, R.; Lannino, A.; Maone, M.C.; Franzoi, P.; Riccato. F. & Colomba, S. (2006). Fish mapping of 18s rDNA and (TTAGGG)n sequences in two pipefish species (Gasteroisteiformes: Syngnathidae). *Journal of Genetics*,Vol. 85, No.2, pp. 153-156

Lin K.W, Yan J. 2008. Endings in the middle: Current knowledge of interstitial telomeric sequences. *Mutation Research/Reviews in Mutation Research*, Vol.658, No.1-2, pp. 95-110. doi:10.1016/j.mrrev.2007.08.006

Lin, K.W. & Yan, J. (2008). Endings in the middle: Current knowledge of interstitial telomeric sequences. *Mutation Research*, Vol. 658, No.1-2., pp. 95-110. doi:10.1016/j.mrrev.2007.08.006

Liu, W.S. & Fredga, K. (1999). Telomeric (TTAGGG) n sequences areassociated with nucleolus organizer regions (NORs) in the wood lemming. *Chromosome Research*, Vol. 7, No.3, pp. 235–240

Luderus, M.E.E.; van Steensel, B.; Chong, L.; Sibon, O.C.M.; Cremers, F.F.M. & de Lange, T. (1996). Structure, subnuclear distribution, and nuclear matrix association of the mammalian telomeric complex. Journal of Cell Biology, Vol. 135, No. 4, pp. 867–881.

Lund, T.C.; Glass, T.J.; Tolar, J. &Blazer, B.R. (2009). Expression of telomerase and telomere length are unaffected by either age or limb regeneration in *Danio rerio*. *PLoS One*, Vol. 4, No. 11, pp. 1-4

Mank, J.E. & Avise, J.C. (2006). Phylogenetic conservation of chromosome numbers in Actinopterygiian fishes. Genetica, Vol. 127, No.1-3, pp. 321-327

McKone, M.J. & Halpern, S.L. (2003). The evolution of androgenesis. *The American Naturalist*, Vol. 161, No. 4, pp. 641-656

Mertcalfe, C.J.; Eldridge, M.D.B. &Johnston, P.G. (2004). Mapping the distribution of the telomeric sequence $(T_2AG_3)_n$ in the 2n= 14 ancestral marsupial complement and in the macropodines (Marsupialia: Macropodidae) by fluorescence in situ hybridization. *Chromosome Research*, Vol.12, No.4 , pp. 405-414

Mertcalfe, C.J.; Eldridge, M.D.B. &Johnston, P.G. (2007). Mapping the distribution of the telomeric sequence (T2AG3)n in the Macropodoidea (Marsupialia), by fluorescence in situ hybridization. II. The ancestral 2n= 22 macropodid karyotype. *Cytogenetic and Genome Research*, Vol. 116, No. 3, pp. 212-217

Metcalfe, C. J.; Eldridge, M.D.B.; Toder, R. & Johnston, P.G. (1998). Mapping the distribution of the telomeric sequence (T2AG3)n in the Macropodoidea (Marsupialia), by fluorescence in situ hybridization. I. The swamp wallaby, *Wallabia bicolor*. *Chromosome Research*, Vol. 6, No. 8, pp. 603-610

Meyne, J.; Baker, R. ; Hobart, H.H.; Hsu, T.C.; Ryder, O.A.; Ward, O.G.; Wiley, J.E.; Wurster-Hill, D,H.; Yates, T.L. & Moyzis, R.K. (1990). Distribution of non-telomeric sites of the $(TTAGGG)_n$ telomeric sequence in vertebrate chromosomes. *Chromosoma*, Vol. 99, No.1, pp. 3-10

Mota-Velasco, J. C.; Alves Ferreira, J.; Cioffi, M. B.; Ocalewicz K.; Campos-Ramos, R.; Shirak, A.; Lee, B.-Y.; Martins, C. & Penman, D. J. (2010). Characterization of the chromosome fusions in *Oreochromis karongae. Chromosome Research*, Vol.18, No.5, pp. 575-586. doi: 10.1007/s10577-010-9141-z

Moyzis, R.K.; Buckingham, J.M.; Cram, L.S.; Dani, M.; Deaven, L.L.; Jones, M.D.; Meyne, J., Ratliff, R.L. & Wu J.R. (1988). A highly conserved repetitive DNA sequence, (TTAGGG) n, present at the telomeres of human chromosomes. *Proceedings of the National Academy of Sciences of the United States of America*, Vol.85, No.18, pp. 6622–6626

Murray, A.W.; Schultes, N.P. & Szostak, J.W. (1986). Chromosome length controls mitotic chromosome segregation in yeast. *Cell*, Vol. 45, No. 4, pp. 529-536.

Nanda, I. & Schmid, M. (1994). Localization of the telomeric $(TTAGGG)_n$ sequences in chicken (Gallus domesticus) chromosomes. *Cytoegentics and Cell Genetics*, Vol. 65, No. 3, pp. 190-193

Nanda, I.; Fugate, M.; Steinlein, C. & Schmid, M. (2008). Distribution of $(TTAGGG)_n$ telomeric sequences in karyotypes of the *Xenopus* species complex. *Cytogenetic and Genome Research*, Vol. 122, No.3-4, pp. 396-400

Nanda, I.; Schneider-Rasp, S.; Winking, H. & Schmid, M. (1995). Loss of telomeric sites in the chromosomes of Mus musculus domesticus (Rodentia: Muridae) during Robertsonian rearrangements. *Chromosome Research*, Vol.3, No.7, pp. 399-409

Nanda, I.; Schrama, D.; Feichtinger, W.; Haaf, T.; Schartl, M. & Schmid, M. (2002). Distribution of telomeric $(TTAGGG)_n$ sequences in avian chromosomes. *Chromosoma*, Vol.111, No.4, pp. 215-227

Nelson JS (1994). Fishes of the World, 3rd edn. John Wiley and Sons: New York.

Nergadze, S.G.; Rocchi, M.; Azzalin, C.M.; Mondello, C. & Giulotto, E. (2004). Insertion of telomeric repeats at intrachromosomal break sites during primate evolution. *Genome Research*, Vol.14, No.9, pp. 1704-1710

Nergadze, S.G.; Santagostino, M.A.; Salzano, A.; Mondello, C. & Giulotto, E. (2007). Contribution of telomerase RNA retrotranscription to DNA double-strand break repair during mammalian genome evolution. *Genome Biology*, Vol.8, No.12, R260

Ocalewicz, K. & Dobosz, S. (2009). Karyotype variation in the albino rainbow trout (*Oncorhynchus mykiss* Walbaum). *Genome*, Vol. 52, No4, pp. 347-352. doi:10.1139/G09-009

Ocalewicz, K.; Babiak, I.; Dobosz, S.; Nowaczyk, J. & Goryczko, K. (2004a). The stability of telomereless chromosome fragments in adult androgenetic rainbow trout. *Journal of Experimental Biology*, Vol. 207 pp. 2229-2236

Ocalewicz, K.; Śliwińska, A. & Jankun M. (2004b). Autosomal localization of internal telomeric sites (ITS) in brook trout, *Salvelinus fontinalis* (Pisces, Salmonidae). *Cytogenetic and Genome Research*, Vol.105, No.1, pp. 79-82. doi: 10.1159/000078012

Ocalewicz, K.; Dobosz, S.; Kuzminski, H. & Goryczko, K. (2009). Formation of chromosome aberrations in androgenetic rainbow trout (*Oncorhynchus mykiss*, Walbaum). *Journal of Fish Biology*, Vol.75, No.9, pp. 2373-2379

Ocalewicz, K.; Woznicki, P.& Jankun M. (2008). Mapping of rRNA genes and telomeric sequences in Danube salmon (*Hucho hucho*) chromosomes using primed in situ labeling technique (PRINS). *Genetica* , Vol. 134, No. 2, pp. 199-203

Okazaki, S.; Tsuchida, K.; Maekawa, H.; Ishikawa, H. & Fujiwara, H. (993). Identification of a pentanucleotide telomeric sequences, $(TTAGG)_n$, in the silkworm Bombyx mori and in other insects. *Molecular and Cellular Biology*, Vol. 13, No. 3, pp. 1424-1432

Olovnikov, A.M. (1973). A theory of marginotomy. Journal of Theoretical Biology, Vol. 41, No. 1, pp. 181–190

Pagnozzi, J.M.; de Jesus Silva, M.J. & Yonenaga-Yassuda, Y. (2000). Intraspecific variation in the distribution of the interstitial telomeric $(TAGGG)_n$ sequences in *Micoureus demerarae* (Marsupialia: Didelphidae). Chromsoome Research, Vol. 8, No. 7,pp. 585-591

Parsons, J.E.& Thorgaard, G.H. (1985). Production of androgenetic diploid rainbow trout. *Journal of Heredity* Vol.76, No.3, pp. 177-181

Pellegrino, K.C.; dos Santos, R.M.; Rodrigues, M.T.; Amaro, R.C. & Yonenaga-Yassuda, Y. (2009). Chromosomal evolution in the Brazilian geckos of the genus Gymnodactylus (Squamata, Phyllodactylidae) from the biomes of Cerrado, Caatinga and Atlantic rain forest: evidence of Roberstonian fusion events and supernumerary chromosomes. Cytogenetics and Genome Research, Vol. 127, No. 2-4, pp. 191-203

Pellegrino, K.C.; Rodrigues, M.T. & Yonenaga-Yassuda, Y. (1999). Chromosomal evolution in the Brazilian lizards of genus *Leposoma* (Squamata, Gymnophthalmidae) from Amazon and Atlantic rain forest: banding patterns and FISH of telomeric sequences. *Hereditas*, Vol. 131, No. 1, pp. 15-21

Pfeifer, P.; Goedecke, W.; Kuhfitting-Kulle, S. & Obe, G. (2004). Pathways of DNA double-strand break repair and their impact on the prevention and formation of chromosomal aberrations. *Cytogenetics and Genome Research,* Vol. 104, No. 1-4, pp. 7-13

Phillips, R.B. & Ráb, P. (2001). Chromosome evolution in the salmonidae (Pisces): an update. *Biological Reviews* Vol.76, No.1, pp. 1-25. doi: 10.1111/j.1469-185X.2000.tb00057.x

Phillips, R.B.; Pleyte, K.A. & Hartley S. E. 1988. Stock-specific differences in the number and chromosome positions of the nucleolar organizer regions in arctic charr (*Salvelinus alpinus*). *Cytogenetic and Cell Genetics*, Vol.48, No.1, pp. 9-12

Pomianowski, L.; Jankun, M. & Ocalewicz, K. (2012). Detection of Interstitial Telomeric Sequences in the Arctic Charr (*Salvelinus alpinus*, Linnaeus 1758) (Teleostei, Salmonidae). Genome, Vol, No. 1, pp. 26–32

Qumsiyeh, M. B., J. L. Choate, J. A. Peppers, P. K. Kennedy, and M. L. Kennedy. 1997. Robertsonian chromosomal rearrangements in the short-tailed shrew, *Blarina carolinensis,* in western Tennessee. Cytogenetics and Cell Genetics, Vol. 76, No. 3-4, pp. 153–158

Reed K., Phillips, R. B. 1995. Molecular cytogenetic analysis of the double-CMA3 chromosome of lake trout, *Salvelinus namaycush. Cytogenetic and Cell Genetics,* Vol.70, No.1-2, pp. 104-107

Rocco, L. (2007). Molecular markers in cartilaginous fish cytogenetics. In: *Fish cytogenetics*. E. Pisano, C. Ozouf-Costaz, F. Foresti & B. G. Kapoor (Eds.), 473-490, Science Publisher, Inc. ISBN 978-1-57808-330-5, New Hampshire, USA

Rocco, L.; Costagliola, D. & Stingo, V. (2001). $(TTAGGG)_n$ telomeric sequence in selachian chromosomes. *Heredity,* Vol. 87, No 5, pp. 583-588. doi:10.1046/j.1365-2540.2001.00945.x

Rocco, L.; Morescalchi, M.A.; Costagliola, D. & Stingo, V. (2002). Karyotype and genome characterization in four cartilaginous fishes. Gene, Vol. 295, No.2, pp. 289-298

Ruiz-Herrera, A.; Nergadze, S.G.; Santagostino, M. and Giulotto, E. (2008). Telomeric repeats far from the ends: mechanisms of origin and role in evolution. *Cytogenetics and Genome Research,* Vol.122, No.3-4, pp. 219-228

Salvadori, S.; Deiana, A.; Coluccia, E.; Florida, G.; Rossi, E. & Zuffardi, O. (1995). Colocalization of $(TTAGGG)_n$ telomeric sequences and ribosomal genes in Atlantic eels. *Chromosome Research,* Vol.3, No1, .pp. 54-58. doi: 10.1007/BF00711162

Santani A, Raudsepp T, Chowdhary BP (2002) Interstitial telomeric sites and NORs in Hartmann's zebra (*Equus zebra hartmannae*) chromosomes. Chromosome Research, Vol.10, No.7, pp. 527–534

Scherthan, H. (1995). Chromosome evolution in muntjac revealed by centromere, telomere and whole chromosome paint probes. In: Brandham PE, Bennet MD (eds) Kew Chromosome Conference IV. Royal Botanic Gardens, Kew, pp 267–281

Schmid, M.; Feichtinger, W.; Nanda, I.; Schakowski, R.; Visbal Garcia, R.; Manzanilla Puppo, J & Fernández Badillo, A. (1994) An extraordinarily low diploid chromosome number in the reptile *Gonatodes taniae* (Squamata, Gekkonidae). *Journal of Heredity,* Vol. 85, No.4 ,pp. 255–260

Shampay, J.; Szostak, J.W. & Blackburn, E.H. (1984). DNA sequences of telomeres maintained in yeast. *Nature,* Vol. 310, No. 5973, pp. 154-157.

Silva, M.J.J. & Yonenaga-Yassuda, Y. (1998). Karyotype and chromosomal polymorphism of an undescribed Akodon from Central Brazil, a species with lowest diploid chromosome number in rodents. *Cytogenetics and Cell Genetics,* Vol. 81, No. 1, pp. 46-50

Slijepcevic, P. (1998). Telomeres and mechanisms of Robertsonian fusions. *Chromosoma,* Vol.107, No.2, pp. 136-140

Slijepcevic, P.; Xiao, Y.; Domingez, J.; Natarajan, A.T. (1996). Spontaneous and radiation-induced chromosomal breakage at interstitial telomeric sites. *Chromosoma,* Vol. 104, No. 8, pp. 594-604

Slijepcevic, P.; Xiao, Y.; Natarajan, A.T. & Bryant, P.E. (1997). Instability of CHO chromosomes containing interstitial telomeric sequences originating from Chinese hamster chromosome 10. *Cytogenetic and Cell Genetics,* Vol.76, No.1-2, pp. 58-60

Sola, L.; Gornung, E.; Mannarelli, M.E. & Rossi, A.R. (2007). Chromosomal evolution of Mugilidae, Mugilomorpha: an overview. In: *Fish cytogenetics*. E. Pisano, C. Ozouf-Costaz, F. Foresti & B. G. Kapoor (Eds.), 165-194, Science Publisher, Inc. ISBN 978-1-57808-330-5, New Hampshire, USA

Sola, L.; Gornung, E.; Naoi, H.; Gunji, R.; Sato, C.; Kawamura, K.; Arai, R. & Ueda, T. (2003). FISH-mapping of 18S ribosomal RNA genes and telomeric sequences in the Japanese bitterlings Rhodeus ocellatus kurumeus and Tanakia limbata (Pisces, Cyprinidae) reveals significant cytogenetic differences in morphologically similar karyotypes. *Genetica*, Vol.119, No.1, pp. 99-106

Stingo, V. & Rocco, L. (2001). Selachian cytogenetics: a review. *Genetica*, Vol.111, No.1-3, pp. 329-347.

Terkelsen, C.; Koch, J.; Kølvraa, S.; Hindkjaer, J.; Pedersen, S. & Bolund, L. (1993). Repeated primed in situ labeling: formation and labeling of specific DNA sequences in chromosomes and nuclei. *Cytogenetics and Cell Genetics*, Vol. 63, No. 4, pp. 235 - 237

Ueda, T. (2007). Chromosomal differentiation in bitterlings (Pisces, Cyprinidae). In: *Fish cytogenetics*. E. Pisano, C. Ozouf-Costaz, F. Foresti & B. G. Kapoor (Eds.), 3-16, Science Publisher, Inc. ISBN 978-1-57808-330-5, New Hampshire, USA

Vermeesch, J.R.; De Meurichy, W.; Van Der Berghe, H.; Marynen, P. & Petit, P. (1996). Differences in the distribution and nature of the interstitial telomeric $(TTAGGG)_n$ sequences in the chromosomes of the Giraffidae, okapi (*Okapia johnstoni*), and giraffe (*Giraffa camelopardis*): evidence for ancestral telomeres at the okapi polymorphic rob(5;26) fusion site. *Cytogenetics and Cell Genetics*, Vol. 72, No. 4, pp. 310-315

Volff, J-N. (2004). Genome evolution and biodiversity in teleost fish. *Heredity*, Vol. 94, No. 3, pp. 280-294

Wang, W.b & Lan, H. (2000). Rapid and parallel chromosomal number reductions in muntjac deer inferred from mitochondrial DNA phylogeny. *Molecular Biology and Evolution* , Vol.17, No.9, pp. 1326–1333

Watson, J.D. (1972). Origin of concatameric T4 DNA. Nature - New Biology, Vol. 239, pp. 197–201

Wiley, J.E.; Meyne, J.; Little, M.L. & Stout, J.C. (1992): Interstitial hybridization sites of the (TTAGGG)n telomeric sequence on the chromosomes of some North American hylid frogs. *Cytogenetic and Cell Genetics*, Vol. 61, No.1, pp. 55–57

Yang, F.; O'Brien, P.C.; Wienberg, J. & Ferguson-Smith, M.A. (1997). A reappraisal of the tandem fusion theory of karyotype evolution in Indian muntjac using chromosome painting. *Chromosome Research*, Vol. 5, No.2, pp. 109–117

Zhou, R.; Cheng, H. & Tiersch, T.R. (2002). Differential genome duplication and fish diversity. Reviews in Fish Biology and Fisheries, Vol. 11, No. ,pp. 331-337

Zijlmans, J. M.; Martens, U. M.; Poon, S. S.; Raap, A. K.; Tanke, H. J.; Ward, R. K. & Lansorp, P. M. (1997). Telomeres in the mouse have large inter-chromosomal variations in the number of T_2AG_3 repeats. *Proceedings of the National Academy of Sciences of the United States of America*, Vol.94, No. p. 7423-7428

Zijlmans, J.M.; Martens, U.M.; Poon, S.S.; Raap, A.K.; Tanke, H.J.; Ward, R.K. & Lansdorp, P.M. (1997). Telomeres in the mouse have large inter-chromosomal variations in the number of T2AG3 repeats. Proceedings of the National Academy of Sciences of the United States of America, Vol. 94, No. 14, pp. 7423–7428

Zou, Y.; Gryaznov, S.M.; Shay, J.W.; Wright, E.W. & Cornforth, M.N. (2004). Asynchronous replication of telomeres at opposite arms of mammalian chromosomes. *Proceedings of the National Academy of Sciences of the United States of America*, Vol.101, No.35, pp. 12928-12933

Zou, Y.; Yi, X.; Wright, W.E. & Shay, J.W. (2002). Human telomerase can immortalize Indian muntjac cells. *Experimental Cell Research*, Vol.281, No.1, pp. 63–76